Textbook of Contemporary Psychiatry

Textbook of Contemporary Psychiatry

Edited by

C. GIBSON DUNN, M.D.
Medical Director
Springwood Psychiatric Institute
Leesburg, Virginia

The Collamore Press
D.C. Heath and Company
Lexington, Massachusetts
Toronto

Every effort has been made to ensure that drug dosage schedules and indications are correct at time of publication. Since ongoing medical research can change standards of usage, and also because of human and typographical error, it is recommended that readers check the *PDR* or package insert before prescription or administration of the drugs mentioned in this book.

Copyright © 1984 by D.C. Heath and Company

All rights reserved. No part of this publication may be reproduced or transmitted in any form or by any means, electronic or mechanical, including photocopy, recording, or any information storage or retrieval system, without permission in writing from the publisher.

Published simultaneously in Canada

Printed in the United States of America

International Standard Book Number: 0-669-04039-8

Library of Congress Catalog Card Number: 80-0604

Library of Congress Cataloging in Publication Data
Main entry under title:

Textbook of contemporary psychiatry.

  Bibliography: p.
  Includes index.
  1. Psychiatry. I. Dunn, C. Gibson.
RC454.T47 1984   616.89   80–0604
ISBN 0-669-04039-8

Contents

	Contributing Authors	vii
	Introduction	ix
I. Evaluation	1. The Psychiatric Evaluation CHERYL T. DUNN, M.D.	3
	2. Psychometric Evaluation NORMAN J. KARL, Ph.D.	15
	3. Psychobiologic Evaluation of Psychiatric Disorders STEVEN D. TARGUM, M.D.	27
II. Clinical Disorders	4. Organic Mental Disorders DANIEL J. O'DONNELL, M.D.	45
	5. Substance Use Disorders C. GIBSON DUNN, M.D.	59
	6. Schizophrenic and Other Nonaffective Psychotic Disorders C. GIBSON DUNN, M.D.	87
	7. Affective Disorders I: Bipolar Disorder (Manic-Depressive Illness) C. GIBSON DUNN, M.D.	105
	8. Affective Disorders II: Depressive Disorders C. GIBSON DUNN, M.D.	119
	9. Anxiety Disorders C. GIBSON DUNN, M.D.	133
	10. Somatoform and Dissociative Disorders CHARLES SCHWARZBECK III, Ph.D., Ed.M.	151
	11. Psychosexual Disorders CHERYL T. DUNN, M.D.	161

	12. Psychological Factors Affecting Physical Condition JESSE RUBIN, M.D.	175
	13. Personality Disorders SYD BROWN, M.D.	187
	14. Eating Disorders ELIOT SOREL, M.D.	207
	15. The Psychiatric Disorders of Adolescence JOHN E. MEEKS, M.D.	217
	16. Geriatric Disorders DAVID H. FRAM, M.D.	233
	17. Psychiatric Manifestations of Medical Disorders and Therapies RALPH W. WADESON, Jr., M.D.	245
III. Treatment	18. Assessment and Management of the Suicidal Patient C. TERRENCE CHASTEK, M.D.	253
	19. Assessment and Management of the Violent Patient C. TERRENCE CHASTEK, M.D.	259
	20. The Psychological Therapies JAMES T. QUATTLEBAUM, M.D.	267
	21. Psychopharmacologic Treatment KENNETH A. KESSLER, M.D. STEVEN D. TARGUM, M.D.	281
	22. Electroconvulsive Therapy C. GIBSON DUNN, M.D.	321
	Index	325

Contributing Authors

Syd Brown, Ph.D.
Clinical Affiliate
Department of Psychology
The American University
Washington, D.C.

Professional Associate
The Psychiatric Institute
Washington, D.C.

C. Terrence Chastek, M.D.
Assistant Clinical Professor of Psychology
The George Washington University
Washington, D.C.

C. Gibson Dunn, M.D.
Medical Director
Springwood Psychiatric Institute
Leesburg, Virginia

Cheryl Taubman Dunn, M.D.
Springwood Psychiatric Institute and
Private Psychiatric Practice
Leesburg, Virginia

David H. Fram, M.D.
Assistant Clinical Professor of Psychiatry
and Behavioral Sciences
The George Washington University
School of Medicine
Washington, D.C.

Attending Psychiatrist
Gerontologic Treatment Service
The Psychiatric Institute
Washington, D.C.

Norman J. Karl, Ph.D.
Chief Psychologist
The Psychiatric Institute
Washington, D.C.

Kenneth A. Kessler, M.D.
President
Metropolitan Mental Health Organization
Washington, D.C.

John E. Meeks, M.D.
Associate Clinical Professor of Psychiatry
The George Washington University
School of Medicine
Washington, D.C.

Medical Director
Psychiatric Institute of Montgomery County
Rockville, Maryland

Daniel J. O'Donnell, M.D.
Attending Psychiatrist
Springwood Psychiatric Institute
Leesburg, Virginia

James T. Quattlebaum, M.D.
Associate Clinical Professor of Psychiatry
The George Washington University
School of Medicine
Washington, D.C.

President, Medical Staff
Psychiatric Institute of Montgomery County
Rockville, Maryland

Jesse Rubin, M.D.
Clinical Professor of Psychiatry
and Behavioral Sciences
The George Washington University
School of Medicine
Washington, D.C.

Charles Schwarzbeck III, Ph.D., Ed.M.
Assistant Clinical Professor of Psychiatry
The George Washington University
School of Medicine
Washington, D.C.

Eliot Sorel, M.D.
Assistant Professor of Psychiatry
Howard University School of Medicine
Washington, D.C.

Assistant Professer of Psychiatry
The George Washington University
School of Medicine
Washington, D.C.

Director, Family Studies Center and
Open Adult Unit
The Psychiatric Institute
Washington, D.C.

Steven D. Targum, M.D.
Medical Director
Sarasota Palms Hospital
Sarasota, Florida

Clinical Associate Professor of Psychiatry
University of Southern Florida
Sarasota, Florida

Ralph W. Wadeson, Jr., M.D.
Assistant Clinical Professor of Psychiatry
The George Washington University
School of Medicine
Washington, D.C.

Acting Director
Psychiatric Institute of Southern Maryland
Clinton, Maryland

Introduction
C. GIBSON DUNN, M.D.

The term *psychiatry* refers to the medical specialty that treats disorders of mental function and associated disturbances of behavior. The description and classification of these disorders and disturbances is called *psychopathology*. The most commonly employed treatments for psychopathology are *psychotherapy* (a psychological method) and *psychopharmacology* (the use of specific medications).

Because of the complexity of mental disorders and the unique obstacles to research, there have been only a limited number of definitive findings concerning etiologies and treatments of psychiatric illnesses. The large areas of uncertainty have allowed and even encouraged investigators and clinicians to use many research and therapeutic methods. When positive results have been observed (or at least perceived), strongly held opinions about the methods have developed. Adherents to the various methods have often advocated their specific approach with a zeal more religious than scientific in its intensity. Nevertheless, a number of basic methods or approaches have yielded crucial knowledge not previously appreciated. Contemporary psychiatry at its best draws on many of these earlier, diverse approaches and attempts to integrate the various bodies of knowledge in treating the individual patient. For any given patient, one approach with its concepts and methods may be more useful than another approach. For some patients, several approaches may be needed in sequence or in parallel. All too often in the past, however, advocates for a particular approach have presented their school of psychiatric thought as definitive and exclusive of all others. This attitude is now archaic and potentially harmful to the patient. The modern psychiatric clinician must be familiar with all of the fundamental "approaches of the mind" (Havens, 1973) and be prepared to use whichever is most helpful to the patient.

Conceptual Models
Aaron Lazare (1973) has noted that clinical psychiatry today routinely employs four conceptual models: medical, psychological, behavioral, and social. These models are the outcomes of historically distinct research and treatment approaches mentioned previously.

MEDICAL MODEL
The medical model emphasizes the similarity between psychiatric disorders and nonpsychiatric medical illnesses. There is a strong emphasis on detached observation and description of symptoms, etiology, pathogenesis, differential diagnosis, prescribed treatment, and prognosis. The medical model assumes that psychiatric disorders result from brain function disturbed by physical pathology. If the specific syndrome can be determined, therefore, there should be a corresponding treatment, often of a somatic type (for example, psychopharmacologic treatment). The goal of such intervention is relief of symptoms and restoration of function.

The contemporary medical model has its foundation in the late nineteenth century work of Emil Kraepelin. It was Kraepelin who effectively employed the disease concept of mental disorders to define the core classification of severe psychiatric disorders. This classification endures essentially intact to the present. By correlating observable clusters of signs and symptoms with known etiologies, Kraepelin was able to separate out numerous specific illnesses. He stressed longitudinal observation on the assumption that different outcomes probably indicated different diseases. With this approach, Kraepelin also achieved his greatest single finding—the distinction between "manic depression" and "dementia praecox" (soon after to be called "schizophrenia" by Bleuler). Although Kraepelin never established the etiology of these two psychoses, he did describe critical signs and symptoms sufficiently to correlate with the very different outcomes of these illnesses. Ever since Kraepelin, most researchers and clinicians involved with manic depressive illness and schizophrenia have continued to employ the medical model to a great degree. Advances in knowledge about brain chemistry and in psychopharmacology have given this approach new prominence in the last decade.

PSYCHOLOGICAL MODEL
The psychological model has also been of great importance in both research and treatment of psychiatric disorders. In this model, mental disturbances result from early life experience. Developmental trauma, emotional deprivation, disturbed early relationships, and abnormal parent-child communications are considered to be fundamental causes of these disturbances. The model is most often applied to the neuroses, personality disorders, and problems in interpersonal relationships. Treatment emphasizes a much more involved, dynamic interaction between doctor and patient. This interaction serves to revive the presumed etiologic situations and relationships, leading to an emotional relearning.

The psychological model has evolved from the work of a number of great investigators, the most prominent of whom, of course, were Sigmund Freud and his followers. As Havens (1973) has noted, Freud, like Kraepelin, placed an emphasis on careful observation and description, but with a new focus on inner mental processes; there was a new emphasis on the dynamic force of emotions and the transformations of these emotions by various functional components of the mind. Freud hypothesized the existence of an active unconscious and a division of the mind into id (instinctual drives), superego (internalized ideas and values), and ego (the regulatory center). He believed that symptoms were only manifestations of more fundamental events. The psychiatrist's role was to assist the patient in tracing the course of mental activity backward from symptoms to the underlying conflict, which Freud argued always originated in infantile sexual urges. In this therapeutic process, the psychiatrist has become more passive and the patient more active. The interaction between the two, however, is much more crucial than in the medical model. In Freudian psychoanalysis, the patient is expected to reproduce his or her core etiologic conflicts in the therapeutic sessions; this "transference" of previous experiences to the doctor becomes a key therapeutic opportunity for corrective learning.

Another variant of the psychological model derives from the work of a brilliant American psychiatrist, Harry Stack Sullivan. Like Freud, Sullivan emphasized the psychological etiology of mental disorders. He believed that each individual develops unique ways of experiencing and communicating with the world around him or her. Expectations and perceptions of others shape personality and interpersonal relationships. When these fundamental expectations and perceptions become distorted in early life, psychiatric symptoms or syndromes could result. Because Sullivan emphasized the interaction between the patient and others, his theories were called *interpersonal psychiatry*. Treatment required the psychiatrist to enter into interactions with the patient and work to correct distortions contributing to the patient's illness.

BEHAVIORAL MODEL
The behavioral model emphasizes attention to symptoms as learned patterns. There is no assumption of underlying organic disease or unconscious emotional conflict. A psychiatric disorder, then, is the result of previous environmental events that induced an enduring response pattern in the patient. This pattern has been maintained by continued positive reenforcement or avoidance of painful consequences.

Much of the pioneering work with this model was done by experimental psychologists, not psychiatrists. Pavlov elegantly demonstrated the phenomenon of a *conditioned response* by an animal to a previously neutral stimulus. J.B. Watson actually created a phobic reaction in Little Albert by pairing the sight of a rat with a sudden, loud noise. Joseph Wolpe later developed a specific therapeutic intervention to counteract the pathologic reation (symptom) by inducing a physiologic state incompatible with the symptoms. The term *reciprocal inhibition* refers to the approach in which the patient is taught to relax even in the presence of a distressing stimulus. When that inhibition is achieved during gradual introduction of the phobic stimulus, the process is called *systematic desensitization.*

As can be seen from the preceding discussion, the behavioral model emphasizes careful definition of the behavior to be changed and the conditions that have maintained it. The therapist must then arrange a new set of stimuli and a schedule of delivering these stimuli to modify or replace the target behavior.

Today, assertiveness training, modeling, systematic desensitization, and flooding are often employed to alter target behavioral and symptom patterns. These techniques have greatly broadened the applicability of the behavioral model.

SOCIAL MODEL

The social model includes not only the identified patient but also the social system in which he lives. Psychiatric disorders are considered to derive from the interaction of the person with his environment. Disturbances in the social milieu can generate symptoms in the individual. The focus, therefore, is on the family, work, or other social group. Key factors are the stresses and supports the group provides to the individual and any change in the ratio. Treatment seeks to alter the patient's interaction with the social system. This is achieved either by changing the patient's approach to his or her milieu or by altering key factors within the milieu which affect the patient.

The social model has evolved from research in widely differing social systems. Sullivan's work, already described in the discussion of the psychological model, obviously included the most fundamental social system—the family. Family systems have received increasing attention from the work of Bowen, Jackson, Satir, and Minuchin. The impact of the larger society was of concern to another of the pioneers of American psychiatry, Adolf Meyer. Meyer sought to understand the individual patient's total life adaptation within the community. He believed that clinical psychiatric disorders significantly reflected the interaction between the person and his or her environment. Because Meyer failed to systematize his understanding of these interactions, however, he is not well-known today.

The work of Hollingshead and Redlich in New Haven had a major impact on the social model when it revealed a correlation between social class and specific psychiatric disorders. While it was eventually recognized that class position is not causal, the clustering of more severely impaired patients in the less affluent social classes had enormous influence on the community psychiatry movement of the 1960s.

Finally, it should be noted that one social system in particular—the psychiatric hospital—has received special attention. From Pinel to Stanton and Schwartz, those concerned with mental illness have sought to understand and improve the social conditions imposed on the most severely disturbed. All too often the same knowledge has had to be relearned repeatedly; however, each renewed appreciation and discovery in these areas has yielded major therapeutic gains.

Application of the Models

The four conceptual models that have been described allow for selection of which clinical data are to be considered primary and for very different treatment techniques. There has been a tendency for individual psychiatric practitioners to align themselves with one of the models and to utilize it exclusively. Lazare (1973) referred to this tendency as the "ideology of the therapist," noting that a particular model may be applied more often on the basis of specific diagnosis, availability of a somatic treatment, social class of the patient, or the availability of clinical services.

It is increasingly apparent, however, that most patients will benefit from application of several conceptual models to their disorders. Treatment should most often involve techniques associated with two or more models, utilized concurrently or sequentially. Progress in diagnostic methods now permit more precise description of psychiatric disorders and more specific prescription of treatments. There are now many more pharmacologic and psychological therapies than had previously been available, and psychiatric and substance abuse hospital programs are now widespread. More than ever before, the understanding and interventions needed by ill patients are available to the practitioner. In order to make effective use of these advances, however, the practitioner must be familiar with a larger body of knowledge than was previously necessary. It is the purpose of this textbook to provide this knowledge in a systematic and coherent form.

A Guide to the Use of This Text

Textbook of Contemporary Psychiatry intends only to be a "clinically useful" introduction to psychiatric disorders and treatments. The book is intentionally structured along the lines of the *Diagnostic and Statistical Manual of Mental Disorders,* Third Edition (DSM-III), published in 1980 by the American Psychiatric Association. DSM-III, through its logical organization and emphasis on observable phenomena, has brought improved order and coherence to standard psychiatric nosology. Whatever its drawbacks, this approach at least attempts to remain within our current knowledge and avoids confusing theory with fundamental understanding. What is not yet fully understood can at least be identified. This textbook, which is meant to be used in conjunction with DSM-III, seeks that same clarity for newcomers to the field of clinical psychiatry. It is organized along the lines of nonpsychiatric medical texts in a manner not usual before DSM-III. Terminology will be consistent with DSM-III usage, though older, more familiar language will occasionally appear.

This book is divided into three sections: Evaluation, Clinical Disorders, and Treatment. For several reasons, there is no distinct section on psychiatric theory or psychological development. Each subject is much too extensive and complex to be abbreviated into single chapters compatible with the length of this book, and there are numerous excellent works available that cover these subjects. Furthermore, diverse psychiatric disorders cannot be reduced to a single, all-encompassing theory or seen as following directly from a unitary developmental concept. When theoretical and developmental issues are crucial to understanding a specific disorder, these issues are discussed in the relevant chapter or cross-referenced within this book (for example, a section on ego defenses is included in Chapter 13, Personality Disorders).

Finally, this book attempts to be realistic about how students use clinical textbooks. Rarely, it seems to me, is such a book read from front to back as a course of study. Rather, after encountering a patient with specific problems, the student reaches for this reference to read on the relevant disorder. It is hoped that this textbook's emphasis on evaluation, diagnosis, and problem-specific treatment will be of greatest use in this real-life situation.

References and Further Reading

Diagnostic and Statistical Manual of Mental Disorders, Third Edition. Washington, D.C.: American Psychiatric Association, 1980.

Havens, L. *Approaches to the Mind.* Boston: Little, Brown, 1973.

Lazare, A. Hidden conceptual models in clinical psychiatry. *N. Engl. J. Med.* 288:345–350, 1973.

Evaluation

The Psychiatric Evaluation
CHERYL T. DUNN, M.D.

The psychiatric evaluation, which is a specialized adaptation of the general medical evaluation, represents a complete data base of the patient's psychiatric condition. It is used as the basis for diagnosis, for treatment, and as a record for reference in the future. The psychiatric evaluation must allow for inclusion of relevant basic medical information while elaborating those aspects of the patient's personal and family histories, manifest behavior, and mental functioning known to be essential in evaluating psychiatric health or disturbance. The psychiatric report is organized to facilitate a coherent, standardized communication of the data obtained and to present it in a usable fashion. This report and its component parts will be reviewed later in this chapter (p. 6).

A report, of course, can be no more valuable than permitted by the quality of data contained therein. Gathering accurate psychiatric data is an especially challenging task for several reasons. Even emotionally healthy patients may be unaware of or actually uncomfortable with the inner emotions that the evaluation seeks to understand. The patient's mind may filter out (defend against) the emergence of certain impulses, desires, or reactions that could be of real significance to the evaluation. As the level of emotional health decreases, this filtering process may intensify and the data become even more difficult to obtain. Second, the evaluator may feel inundated with information and have difficulty making sense of the seemingly endless stream of facts, complaints, and emotions. The chief task of the psychiatric evaluation can be seen as one of separating out the essential from the nonessential; this is true for all medical evaluations, of course, but in psychiatry the process may prove more difficult. Not only are the data "softer" and more open to distortion by either patient or evaluator but also emotional reactions on both sides tend to cloud the clinical picture as it emerges.

Information for the psychiatric evaluation can be obtained from numerous sources. There may be crucial collateral sources of history such as family members, friends, or employer. Previous medical records should never be overlooked, and there are an increasing number of laboratory, psychometric, and radiologic investigations that can prove essential to understanding mental disturbances. In the great majority of cases, however—and in nearly all situations initially—the basic data will be obtained through the patient interview. Any approach to the psychiatric evaluation, then, must begin with an understanding of the interview process.

Interviewing Techniques

There is only one tool for obtaining the psychiatric evaluation: the doctor-patient relationship. In psychiatry, as well as in other aspects of medicine, the doctor-patient relationship is critical. It is essential for positive consequences and a major cause of negative results, including negative clinical outcomes, administrative problems, and malpractice suits.

The physician can usually obtain the psychiatric evaluation only with the patient's cooperation. The degree of cooperation will to a great extent depend on the feeling, or rapport, between the doctor and patient. From the first moment that the patient makes a decision to seek care, he or she is beginning to fantasize about the doctor who will be the helping figure. From the time the doctor's name is presented to the patient until the moment the doctor is introduced, the patient begins to form all sorts of images about feelings that will be experienced during the interview.

For the medical student, other immediately identifying information may also be obvious to the patient, such as the appearance of youth and inexperience, as well as other emotionally charged material, such as race, sex, and ethnicity. Of course, these factors are true for every physician, but the novice may experience them even more acutely; thus the emphasis on doctor-patient relationship must be even greater in order to accomplish the objectives.

Occasionally a patient will start the evaluation session with a critical personal remark about the doctor—for example, "How young you look." There are several ways that this kind of opening remark can be handled by the medical student. Often a bantering, but not hostile, comment may diffuse the patient's anger entirely and make way for a speedy entry into the evaluation process. If the patient's level of anger interferes with the clinician's ability to begin the evaluation, then a more serious look at that anger will be necessary. For example, if the patient is extremely angry that the doctor is late for the evaluation, and he or she is clearly being quite guarded and withholding about information, then the clinician may say something such as: "You sound really quite angry and I wonder if you could say a bit about that." Alternatively, one can begin by taking responsibility for being late, "I apologize for keeping you waiting 40 minutes. I know how it feels to be waiting for your turn." An acknowledgment of the patient's feelings and an opportunity for the patient to let the clinician know exactly how he or she feels will usually clear the way for the evaluation work of the session to proceed.

If the patient looks stricken with terror in the early part of the evaluation and the obvious fright is leaving the patient monosyllabic, the interviewer should deal with that terror first, thus helping the patient relax and speak more freely. For example: "Mrs. Smith, you look so frightened that I am sure it must be very difficult for you to talk about the reason you are here." This kind of comment is called *accurate empathy* and will frequently lead the patient to talk about that fear and the reason for it. Another follow-up comment may be needed to help the patient along, such as, "Can you talk a bit about why you may be feeling so frightened at this moment?" Accurate empathy involves a correct observation of the patient's feelings and a spoken acknowledgment of that observation; this is done in such a way that the patient is clearly aware that his or her feelings have been recognized. This kind of comment also lets the patient know that the interviewer is interested not only in the work at hand, but also in him or her as a human being with feelings. Such an acknowledgment will often change that person's attitude dramatically and facilitate further communication without delay.

Another important technique for helping to establish rapport involves the use of "universal statements"—statements that acknowledge feelings the patient has as being feelings that we all have in similar circumstances at one time or another. One such statement might be, "Mrs. Smith, you look awfully frightened. Most of us are scared when we go to a new doctor." Another example is, "Everyone feels depressed now and then; have you been feeling depressed over the last several weeks?" The universal statement lets the patient know that one is not being critical or judgmental about the feelings the patient is revealing—in fact these feelings are part of the human experience that everyone goes through at one time or another. Accurate empathy and universal statements are two tools that the interviewer can use to help the patient establish a feeling of trust that not only will facilitate obtaining the psychiatric evaluation, but also will increase rapport between the doctor and the patient for any further contact.

More than a word should be said about politeness and courtesy. (Treat the patient the way you would like to be treated by your own doctor.) The interviewer should begin the contact with the patient by introducing himself and saying, "We will be working together during this evaluation," or some such acknowledgment of helping status. The interviewer should then lead the patient to the examining room and motion for the patient to be seated. A remark to help the patient feel comfortable in the new surroundings would also be a courteous way of letting the patient know that you are aware of the stress on the patient entering this cluttered emergency room or this cold, bleak room with two chairs in it, or whatever the circumstance may be. Often the interviewer is too busy, confused, or anxious that his or her self-preoccupation is the only feeling that is communicated to the patient.

It is almost impossible for a patient to erase the feeling of being treated disrespectfully. If you as an interviewer have begun contact with the patient in a discourteous manner, at some point you should take the responsibility for being honest about it, apologizing for it, and then proceeding with a renewed attitude of polite regard for the patient. This obvious observation about human interaction is often flagrantly disregarded, particularly when the clinician feels tired or overworked. Displacing anger onto the patient is not an appropriate way of dealing with feelings of being harried.

Skillful interviewing will greatly facilitate the psychiatric evaluation. The interview must be open enough to allow the patient free expression while being specific enough to help delineate the data base necessary to formulate the evaluation. The interviewer needs to learn to pace himself or herself by keeping in mind how much time is allotted for the information to be obtained from the patient. With repeated experiences, you soon gain a sense of timing and can know how long to allow the patient to speak freely and when to be more specific with questioning.

Very briefly, good interviewing skills require attentive listening, silence when appropriate, and open-ended questions as well as specific questions determined by the data needed. Facilitating statements, universal statements, accurate empathy, and paraphrasing remarks or summary statements are all examples of good interviewing techniques. No matter what has preceded the clinician's interview with a particular patient, and no matter what is to follow, the patient should be made to feel that the interviewer's attention is entirely on him or her at this moment in time. (See Chapter 20 for specific techniques of interviewing.)

In closing the interview, it is best to let the patient know a few minutes ahead of time that the interview is going to close. "We are going to have to stop in a few minutes. Do you have any questions?" This prepares the patient for what may seem to be a rather unnatural closing, because the patient usually has a great deal more to add, but will not be allowed to do so at this appointment. Finally, the interviewer says that the time is up; it is best to make a gesture in that direction, such as standing up and walking toward the door. In this manner the closing will naturally follow one's statement a few minutes earlier.

As in all types of therapy, it is important in brief contact, such as the initial psychiatric evaluation, for you as an interviewer to be aware of the feelings that may arise within yourself, as well as the feelings that the patient may have during the interview. Anger, frustration, caring, flirtatiousness, seductive feelings, sadness—these and other feelings may all occur. It is important for you to recognize what kind of affect is going on inside you. A clinician who is not aware of these feelings may unconsciously lead the interview into inappropriate areas. At the end of the interview, the data base might then be incomplete or inaccurate because of the unobserved feelings that the clinician experienced during the time of contact.

At times, the interview must necessarily be accomplished in an uncomfortable room or in one that is simply not set up for interviewing. One should enter the room and survey it for any possible easy changes. Just moving two chairs appropriately or some other small gesture will allow the interview to be conducted in a more relaxed and comfortable manner.

The Psychiatric Evaluation

The psychiatric evaluation is traditionally organized under several headings. These headings collect all relevant information (positives and negatives) regardless of the sources, which should be specified when there is any discrepancy or doubt as to accuracy. The evaluation is usually organized under the following categories: identifying data, the present illness, past psychiatric and medical history, developmental and family history, mental status examination, other diagnostic information (physical examination, laboratory testing, neurologic data, psychological testing, or other available information), and diagnostic formulation and treatment plan (see Table 1-1).

IDENTIFYING DATA

In the section on identifying data, certain specific information about the patient must be recorded, traditionally including age, sex, marital status, occupation, referring source, and reasons for coming to evaluation—for example, "The patient is a 34-year-old married white male supermarket manager, referred by his family practitioner, Dr. Frank." If the information is not already on record, you should obtain the patient's exact birth date, address, spouse, children, as well as telephone numbers for the patient and the closest responsible person in case of emergency.

The *chief complaint* is the patient's statement about the exact reason that he or she has come for evaluation. If at all possible, the patient should be quoted exactly. If not, a summary statement should be made as close as possible to the patient's definition of the problem. Examples include "I have been thinking about suicide," or "I am an alcoholic," or "My family thinks I need help."

PRESENT ILLNESS

The section about the present illness is an organized delineation of the reasons for the patient's evaluation. The patient will often tell his or her story in a rather scattered, disjointed way, leaving out and inserting information of various import throughout the interview. In the reporting of the present illness, one must take responsibility for collating this information in a coherent manner as indicated in the five divisions described below.

This section should include five specific areas of information: (1) brief, orienting statement about the patient's psychiatric status, (2) onset of the present illness, (3) precipitants or obvious contributors, (4) course of illness since the onset, and (5) effects of the illness on significant areas of functioning.

Brief Statement About the Psychiatric Status

There should be a one-sentence summary of the patient's contact with formal psychiatric treatment, such as, "This is the patient's first psychiatric contact," or "Patient has a long-standing psychiatric history," or "This is the patient's fourth hospital admission." This brief statement will orient the reader to the patient's background very quickly in order to integrate the new information that is about to follow.

Onset of the Present Illness

An attempt should be made to delineate as clearly as possible the onset of the symptoms that bring the patient to the evaluation. One way to begin is to ask the patient when he or she was last well. Another way is to say, "When, specifically, did you notice the symptoms beginning?" Patients will sometimes say, "This problem has been going on for years," but the evaluator must help clarify when the problem became significant. Sometimes asking in just that manner will be sufficient to elicit a closer time frame or inflection point in

Table 1-1. The Psychiatric Evaluation and Report Outline

Identifying data
Present illness
Past psychiatric and medical history
Developmental and family history
Mental status examination
Diagnostic information
Diagnostic formulation and treatment plan

severity of symptoms. The interviewer may wish to use the following kinds of clarifying questions: "What made you decide to come for evaluation now? What made you decide to seek help at this time? Was there a specific event that made you feel that now is the time to seek help?" The interviewer should try to help the patient describe whether these symptoms were of acute onset or of more insidious nature.

It would be important to ask about the patient's "neurovegetative" (biologic) changes at this time. These biologic changes include sleep patterns, appetite, energy level, interest in sex, and diurnal mood variation. You can ask, for example, "Do you experience difficulty falling asleep or staying asleep, or do you wake up early in the morning? Do you sleep more than you used to?" Trying to clarify the sleep disturbance is an important part of the present illness. Comparable questions can be asked about appetite and energy level. Ask the patient if he or she notices any change in appetite, and when the problem began. Similarly, question the patient about any perceived change in energy level and approximately when it began. There should also routinely be questions about interest in sex or ability to perform: "Have you noticed that your interest in sex has changed since the problem began?" At this time it might be helpful to use a universal statement such as, "Many people notice that their interest in sex declines when they are feeling depressed. Have you noticed that in yourself?"

Precipitants
The interviewer should try to elicit specific precipitants or accumulating stresses that may have occurred at the onset of this problem. One question might be, "Do you know why this problem began at the time that it did?" More specifically, inquiry might be made as to, "Were there any major changes in you or your family or friends around this time? Was there a change in your job? Are there any specific events that you can point to around the time of this change?" It is important to ask about alcohol and drugs as potential precipitants or contributors, possibly by saying, "Many people notice that they drink more during times of stress. Has this been a problem for you? Or drugs?" If the answer is "yes," then a specific statement as to how much of which drugs should be included here. Many people minimize the extent of their drug use (or deny any such use) as part of the present illness, and the interviewer should try to determine whether this is going on.

Course of Illness Since the Onset
The interviewer should try to determine how severely the symptoms have progressed since the onset. The patient may begin by saying that at first the symptoms were negligible, but over the last several weeks they have become of major proportion. It would be important to know whether, since the appointment was scheduled, the symptoms have lessened, and whether the patient, in fact, seems to be getting better.

Effect of Illness on Significant Areas of Functioning
It is important to assess the effect of the illness on significant areas of functioning because this aspect of the evaluation can help the interviewer establish the severity of the illness and subsequently make useful treatment recommendations. One might ask, "How much has the illness affected your ability to go to school or work? How much has it affected your relationships with your family or other people close to you? Has your problem involved you in trouble with the law?"

COLLATION OF DATA
ABOUT THE PRESENT ILLNESS
After the data concerning the present illness has been obtained, it must be collated, as in the following example.

Case 1. This is the third psychiatric evaluation for this patient with a 10-year history of bipolar affective disorder. She reports the onset of feeling "high" about three weeks ago after stopping her lithium carbonate one month earlier (or seven weeks ago). She stated that she found a new boyfriend and was afraid of his reaction if he learned that she was "manic depressive." She subsequently stopped her lithium carbonate. Over the past three weeks she has noticed racing thoughts, pressured rapid speech, difficulty falling asleep and staying asleep, decreased appetite with five-pound weight loss, and marked increase in energy level. She notes increase in spending and many long-distance telephone calls. Patient reports that these are the same symptoms as "last time" she became ill. She states that she is now afraid that she will lose both her boyfriend and her job due to her erratic behavior over the last three weeks, and she wishes to enter treatment again.

PAST PSYCHIATRIC AND MEDICAL HISTORY
The next part of the psychiatric evaluation is the past psychiatric and medical history of the patient. The record should include names and dates of any psychiatric outpatient or inpatient care, noting specific treatment, such as names of medications, duration, and any other relevant details. The information should also report the patient's assessment of the effectiveness of these treatments and reason for ending treatment (recovered, frustrated with lack of progress, and so on). The clinician should ask the patient if he or she has ever been given a diagnosis and, if so, what it means to the patient.

The medical history should include any past major illnesses or complications of common illnesses, operations, other interventions, and allergic reactions to medication.

DEVELOPMENTAL AND FAMILY HISTORY
The developmental history includes details of the patient's growth and development from conception to the present. It obviously may require outside sources of information, but the patient may be well aware of even prenatal complications from information shared within the family. Information sought here includes any deviations from the normal processes of gestation, delivery, and physical and social maturation. The earlier any trauma, or other insult has occurred, the greater may be its impact on psychiatric function.

The developmental history can be divided easily into four sections: childhood, adolescence, adulthood, and marital history.

Childhood
A history of the patient's childhood should include the following kinds of information: A history of the mother's difficulty with the pregnancy (particularly with delivery) should be obtained. Was the labor prolonged, or were forceps needed, and was there any history of delayed development, or of respiratory or other severe problems at the time of delivery? Were there any major medical illnesses during the first few years of life? Does the patient know about any developmental difficulties, such as with feeding, toilet training, or learning to walk or talk? These stages are called developmental milestones, and questions about them can be asked quickly. The patient should be asked specifically whether he or she was at any time thought to be a "hyperactive child" and, in particular, whether there were symptoms of bed-wetting, fire-setting, or cruelty to animals—behavior that might support that diagnosis. The patient should be asked whether any other particular psychological problems occurred during the early childhood years. Ask the patient to describe his or her relationship with peers during childhood, using such questions as, "Were you shy?" or "Were you a leader?"

The early separation history (that is, details about when the patient was first left with someone other than the mother or regular caretaker, and similar situations) should be taken at this time. In particular the patient should be asked whether any significant difficulties were experienced going off to school for the first time in kindergarten or first grade. Does the patient recall particular temper tantrums, playing ill, or difficulties at school that might provide evidence of early significant separation anxieties. Learning or school adjustment problems should be pursued in detail when identified.

Adolescence

The history of the patient's adolescence can be divided into psychological, social, and academic areas. Psychological problems should be discussed by asking whether the patient ever saw a therapist during this stage of life; specific reasons should be sought. One should also ask whether the religious thinking of the family affected the patient during this period. Did the patient experience any particular difficulties with sexual development or with psychological issues of sexuality; these difficulties should be specified. How was the patient taught about sexual development and the social issues of sexuality? The patient should be asked about problems in relating to persons of the same sex as well as those of the opposite sex, and about unusual sexual practices. The interviewer should assess the patient's maturity in dealing with issues of separation and individuation from the family. An academic history should be obtained by asking the patient to give a brief description of his or her performance in school, noting any particular strengths or weaknesses.

Adulthood

The section covering adulthood can be approached from three basic divisions of the psychological, the social, and the academic or occupational parameters in a person's life. Psychological issues of adulthood involve (1) early independent, autonomous functioning, (2) dealing with issues of intimate relationships and sexuality, and (3) negotiating career development. The patient should be asked if any psychological disturbance has been experienced during adulthood. Social development is evaluated by asking the patient to assess his or her interaction with peers in terms of both intimate relationships and friendships. Interests other than job or school should be briefly noted. The patient should describe academic and occupational performance through the adult years. If the patient received special training that should be noted. Sexuality should be discussed in this section as well, in terms of patient's heterosexual or homosexual adjustment or deviant sexual functioning that may be of concern to the patient.

Marital History

A specific marital history should be taken, including a detailed assessment of the current marital status. This section should include number of marriages, patient's feeling about the resolution of marriages, and information about the children from the marriages.

Family History

The nuclear family into which the patient was born should be briefly sketched, including details about the number of siblings in the family and the patient's order among those siblings, as well as the occupational, medical, and psychological status of mother and father. A statement about current relationships with these family members is also pertinent.

The patient should be asked specifically whether either biologic parent experienced any psychiatric illness, alcoholism, or drug abuse. Any affirmative responses should be explored in detail. Then the patient should be questioned if any other blood relatives (including siblings, children, grandparents, and immediate collateral relatives) have experienced psychiatric difficulties. It may be necessary to describe the problems being sought in order to gather meaningful information. Certain neurologic disorders should be considered potentially important such as seizure disorder, dementing illnesses, or genetically transmitted problems. If any family member has had a psychiatric illness, the evaluator should then seek details of the course, treatment, and outcome of treatment.

MENTAL STATUS EXAMINATION

The phrase *mental status examination* is the traditional label for a comprehensive systematic examination of the patient's mood, cognition, and manifest behavior. Almost all human functioning can be categorized into these areas. The mental status examination is a detailed way of characterizing and recording each of these three aspects of functioning.

The purpose of the mental status examination is to record the patient's exact condition at the time that the physician is with him or her. It is a "snapshot" that is analogous to the physical examination recording the patient's specific condition at the moment the doctor is with him. The major functions of the mental status examination are to obtain and record the data base systematically, and to provide a baseline record for future evaluation, comparison, and assistance in differential diagnosis. As with the physical examination, both the interviewer and those who care for the patient in the future will use the examination for many purposes.

The mental status examination includes the following areas of assessment:

1. General appearance
2. Attitude
3. Motor behavior
4. Speech
5. Thoughts, including process and content
6. Perception
7. Mood and affect
8. Sensorium and orientation
9. Cognitive functioning
10. Insight

General Appearance
The patient's presentation during the interview should be described, specifically noting whether the patient looks significantly older or younger than the patient's chronological age; a remark about the patient's expression, dress, unusual features, and physical state (such as obesity or being obviously medically ill); patient's posture if unusual, state of cooperativeness, and location if unusual (such as lying in a hospital bed).

Attitude
A brief statement about the patient's attitude during the interview should indicate the level of patient's cooperativeness during examination, as well as any change during the session (for example, resistance or hostility).

Motor Behavior
The section about motor behavior should indicate whether the patient is showing increased movements (hypermotoric) or decreased movements (hypomotoric), or is unremarkable in this area. It should indicate whether the patient is fidgeting a great deal, moving around in unusual ways, or showing posturing of any sort. If the patient clearly needs assistance in ambulation, this should be noted.

Speech
There are several attributes of speech that should be described—its rate (increased, decreased, or unremarkable), loudness or softness, and any unusual qualities, such as slurring, particular speech defects, or noticeable accents, that may distinguish the patient. Provocative language should be listed here as well.

Thoughts
The section about thoughts includes both processes and content of thought.

Processes. Thought processes are described in terms of the order and rate of the thoughts. If the patient's thoughts do not follow in logical order, one after the other, then a *thought disorder* should be noted. If the connections between one thought and another are tenuous or absent, the description *loosening of associations* is applied. Thought processes can also be described in terms of being *tangential* or *circumstantial*. A thought is described as tangential when it relates peripherally to the subject, but not directly to it; clinically it appears as if the patient is missing the point. Circumstantiality is a description of a series of thought processes that do not follow directly from the main idea, but rather lead away from it or around it into unrelated details, eventually returning to the subject. The *rate* of the patient's thoughts can be described as increased or decreased as compared to normal. For example, one patient's assessment might read, "The patient's thoughts were extremely fast and pressured." For one with decreased thought rate, "The patient's thoughts were slow, with long latency in between statements."

Content. Thought content disorders can be divided into four basic categories: incoherence, marked poverty of content, repetitive ideas, and bizarre or unusual ideas. *Incoherence* means disconnected thoughts. *Marked poverty of content* refers to a notable absence of meaning, or a vagueness.

Repetitive ideas, into which the patient has some insight, include obsessions, phobias, or repeated experiences of depersonalization or derealization. An obsession is a thought that repeatedly forces itself into awareness and cannot be easily eliminated from the thought processes. A phobia is a persistent irrational specific fear. Depersonalization refers to the thought that one is unreal or that one's body parts are not real or are unfamiliar, bizarre, or detached from one's mind. Derealization refers to the thought that familiar, real objects or places are unreal, unfamiliar, or bizarre.

Bizarre or unusual ideas include ideas of reference (that talk or actions have special reference to the patient), delusions (a belief accepted by the patient as real but not validated by others—delusions include paranoid or grandiose ideas), intense somatic preoccupations, religious fixations, and thought broadcasting, thought insertion, or thought withdrawal. The definitions of these ideas are as follows: *Paranoia* refers to ideas of exaggerated suspicion of persecution. *Grandiosity* refers to ideas of exaggerated self-importance and abilities. *Somatic delusions* have to do with the false fixed belief involving the body or body parts or body illness. *Thought broadcasting* is a symptom in which the person hears his own thoughts aloud in his head or thinks that his thoughts are broadcast so that others can actually hear them. To determine the presence of this symptom, ask, "Do you ever seem to hear your own thoughts spoken aloud in your head, so that someone standing near might be able to hear them?" or, "Are your thoughts broadcast so that other people know what you are thinking?" *Thought insertion* is the symptom in which a person experiences alien thoughts as being put into his head, such as by x-rays or by radar. One can ask, for example, "Are thoughts put into your head that you know are not your own?" *Thought withdrawal* refers to the idea that one's thoughts are being taken out of one's head. A relevant question for this disorder is, "Do your thoughts ever seem to be taken out of your head, as though some external person or force were removing them?"

Perception

Perceptual problems involve the presence of hallucinations or illusions. A *hallucination* is a perception of a stimulus in the absence of one—for example, auditory hallucinations (such as hearing voices), visual hallucinations (such as seeing objects that are not actually present), and any other type of hallucination, such as tactile or olfactory. An *illusion,* on the other hand, is a misinterpretation of an actual stimulus. An example of an illusion is the misperception of water pooling at the end of a very hot highway, when actually there is no water at all.

If the patient is experiencing auditory hallucinations, he or she should be questioned as to whether the voices are telling the patient to act. This kind of hallucination is called a *command hallucination* and is particularly severe because a seriously ill person may act on the command that is being presented in the hallucination. For example, the patient may be a danger to himself if the voices are telling him to kill himself. Command hallucinations should be specifically noted in the mental status examination.

Mood and Affect

The patient's predominant mood during the interview and appropriateness of manifest feeling should be noted. For example, if the patient speaks in a depressed and sad manner throughout the interview when speaking about her husband's death, the clinician should note that the patient's predominant mood was depressed and her affect was appropriate to the content. In addition, mood can also be described in terms of its being elevated or euphoric or irritable. Intense feelings during the interview—such as anger, hostility, anxiety, or marked fears—should be described. Note should be made of any inappropriate affect, such as laughing at a time that would normally bring about sad feelings. Rapid changes from one feeling state to another area described as *emotional lability*. The patient's thoughts and feelings about suicide should always be stated in the mental status examination as either being present or absent; and if such thoughts are present, details should be given. Feelings about hurting someone else (homicidal thoughts) should also be noted as present (and if so, to whom they are directed) or absent. The documentation as to the patient's suicidality or homicidality is a legal statement as well as a medical one and must never be omitted from the mental status examination. In some formats it may be recorded under a separate heading in the mental status examination.

Sensorium and Orientation

The patient's sensorium should be noted in terms of the exact state of consciousness, such as alert, drowsy, somnolent, semi-comatose, comatose, or variable. Orientation has to do with the patient's being accurate as to person, place, and time; that is, the evaluation should include an assessment of the patient's awareness of himself and his surroundings. Disorientation has degrees of severity. The first function to be impaired is the sense of time. The patient will first lose the ability to sequence events correctly; then he may lose the ability to remember the month of the year, the day of the week, or the year itself. As severity increases, the patient will then lose his ability to be aware of his surroundings, or orientation to place. Initially, he may be disoriented in an unfamiliar place only. As this problem increases the patient will become disoriented even in a familiar location. In even more severe disorientation, the patient will lose the ability to identify people around him with whom he is familiar; ultimately the patient will have difficulty identifying himself or remembering his name. This is a very late occurrence.

Cognitive Functioning

Cognitive functioning is a general category having to do with a number of intellectual capabilities, including specific memory functions, calculations, abstract reasoning, and judgment. Assessment of the fund of knowledge, which is also included in this category, provides an approximate indication of the patient's overall level of intelligence.

Memory function is usually divided into three categories: immediate, recent past, and remote memory. *Immediate memory* is tested with the digit span test. The patient is asked to repeat after the examiner a set of digits beginning with two or three and then increasing by one, with each set up to seven digits in a row. The unimpaired individual can usually remember six digits forward and at least four digits backward in this test for immediate recall. Immediate memory generally refers to memory held for 10 seconds up to several minutes in time.

Recent memory has to do with memory lasting for 24 hours up to the last several months. This function is tested by having the patient recount the history of the present illness and remember specific events prior to the hospitalization or since admission.

Remote memory identifies the ability to recall events prior to several months from the moment. Again, history-taking can help test this type of memory by asking the patient to relate past illnesses and their approximate occurrence in time. Alternatively, the patient may be asked to identify dates of marriage or birth of children or other significant events in his or her life.

Calculations refer to a person's ability to think with numbers, without any assistance. Any simple arithmetic problem may be administered, but the most generally accepted is to ask the patient to subtract 7s serially from 100 (100 minus 7, 93 minus 7, and so on). This tests the patient's ability to work with numbers, to concentrate, and to maintain attention span.

Abstract reasoning involves the ability to generalize ideas from specific information. If a person is not able to generalize, then his thinking will usually be concrete; that is, he will speak about the particular information in terms of the information itself instead of forming a more global conclusion. For example, a proverb such as "a stitch in time saves nine," will be interpreted in terms of sewing cloth.

Fund of knowledge has to do with the patient's retention and use of information as compared with his socioeconomic level and other such revealing parameters. Often, one can assess a patient's general fund of knowledge by just listening to the patient's description of his present illness and past history. However, specific questions can be asked to test sample areas; for example, one can ask patients to recall answers to questions in politics, in geography, in similarities and differences, or in understanding everyday items and everyday activities (such as, "Who is the governor of this state?").

Insight
The section about insight deals with the subject's ability to assess himself and the problems facing him. In the most narrow sense, the interviewer interprets the patient's understanding of his illness, the severity of his illness, and its impact on those around him. In a more broad sense, insight involves the patient's capacity to understand events going on in his life and make appropriate decisions regarding these events. It is actually a complex function involving several mental processes but is a valuable parameter to note on its own.

A severe impairment in any category of the mental status examination is significant and will provide evidence for a differential diagnosis of the problem. For example, a major difficulty with affect can provide evidence for a diagnosis of bipolar affective disorder. Impairment in thought processing may provide some evidence of schizophrenia. Impairment in sensorium and orientation may lead one to suspect substance abuse or withdrawal, or metabolic or other major medical problems. Impairment in memory may provide evidence of dementia or substance abuse. Many such examples are possible, but one must note that a single piece of information does not make a diagnosis; there is a need for the complete mental status examination and the remainder of the psychiatric evaluation.

DIAGNOSTIC INFORMATION
The next section of the psychiatric evaluation, termed *diagnostic information,* includes the following additional studies in order to complete the psychiatric evaluation: (1) complete physical examination and any diagnostic procedures; (2) the consideration of a battery of psychological testing; (3) consideration of interviews with family members or other primary persons in the patient's life; and (4) further specialized procedures such as electroencephalogram, neurologic evaluation, or specific additional time for further interviewing.

History and Physical Examination
The medical history and physical examination of the patient should be done either by the interviewer or by another physician to whom the patient is referred. If the patient has had a history and physical examination within the last six to twelve months, the records from that may be sufficient. If the interviewer has questions about a new problem, however, the patient should be asked to set up another ap-

pointment with his or her physician, specifically requesting a search for any medical basis of the presenting problem. The interviewer may wish to call the physician directly in order to discuss the diagnostic possibilities. Because there is a medical basis for a large number of psychiatric disorders—including problems of hypothyroidism or hyperthyroidism, metabolic problems, and effects of drug abuse—a physical examination should never be left out of the psychiatric evaluation. If there is any consideration whatsoever that the patient may be treated with psychiatric medications, then a physical examination, baseline laboratory values, and an electrocardiogram are absolutely essential.

Psychological Tests
Specific psychological testing may be helpful in providing evidence useful in the differential diagnosis, particularly in the consideration of organic brain disease or underlying major medical illness (see Chapter 2 for a full discussion of psychological testing).

Further Testing
At times the clinician may want to rule out diagnoses such as temporal lobe epilepsy or other specific medical problems and will need to refer the patient for workup. Both psychiatric and medical problems can be present concomitantly and would need to be treated simultaneously for successful outcome.

DIAGNOSTIC FORMULATION
The last part of the psychiatric evaluation, the diagnostic formulation, includes the following four sections: (1) summary of psychiatric and medical findings, (2) the psychodynamic formulation, (3) the diagnosis or the differential diagnosis using the classification of the *Diagnostic and Statistical Manual of Mental Disorders,* Third Edition (DSM-III), and (4) recommendations for treatment. It is, then a process of both *synthesis* and *inference.*

Summary of Findings
The summary of findings should include a systematic summary of the psychiatric findings including the major points of the presenting illness, the mental status examination, history, and so on. It should also include a summary of the positive medical findings; if there are none, then this should be specifically stated.

Psychodynamic Formulation
The psychological, social, and other stresses contributing to the patient's current problem should be fully discussed, tracing the issues historically from early on in the patient's life until the present. The section on psychodynamic formulation reveals the interviewer's understanding of the patient from a comprehensive point of view and emphasizes how the patient's personality structure and function influence the processing of present supports and demands on the individual.

Diagnosis or Differential Diagnosis According to DSM-III
The diagnosis should be stated if it appears to be well substantiated. If the diagnosis is not clear-cut, then a differential diagnosis should be listed according to the DSM-III, the current classification used by psychiatrists. The multiaxial system allows for the concurrent presentation of (1) acute disorders, (2) personality or developmental disorders, (3) medical illness, and (4) psychosocial stressors and level of functioning.

Recommendations for Treatment
The exact recommendations for treatment should include one of the following alternatives: no further treatment, further treatment of a specific type on an outpatient basis, further treatment on an inpatient basis with reasons stated, or alternative recommendations for treatment (which should be specified).

Psychometric Evaluation
NORMAN J. KARL, Ph.D.

Purposes of Psychological Tests

Psychometric evaluation is useful in responding to many questions that might be raised in the clinical setting. It is often critically important to make determinations about such issues as suicide potential, severity of depression, or the presence of a thought disorder or of organic brain damage, to name a few. Answers to diagnostic questions raised by psychiatrists have major implications for treatment, including the use of medication and the possibility of hospitalization. Psychological tests can often shed light on the type or severity of a disorder for which a treatment plan must be derived.

Historically, medical diagnosis has had as its purpose the identification of disease so that the patient could be treated. This disease orientation, or medical model, still prevails as the major one by which many psychologists and psychiatrists work. Psychological tests represent part of this process of identification, classification, and treatment. They can often be quite helpful in reducing the amount of time taken to effect relief from mental disorders through their prompt identification of the specific difficulty. Tests may also be used during treatment to assess the progress being made, and one can use them to help identify problem areas that are not immediately apparent through more typical interview or observational procedures.

Psychological tests have been derived from two main roots: (1) those having to do with objective and standardized measures of personality and intelligence, and (2) those dealing with the unconscious aspects of personality function—that is, projective tests. The standardized tests of personality and intelligence represent a rating of the extent to which an individual conforms to cultural norms. Projective tests, on the other hand, yield unique responses that reflect the personal and idiosyncratic aspects of meaning and organization for that particular person. These tests are especially sensitive to motivations of which the person may be unaware. The projective tests seek to determine these underlying and unconscious motives by providing material of limited structure out of which the individual "projects" his needs, wishes, and motives, so that the underlying defensive organization is revealed.

PREDICTIVE VALUE
OF PSYCHOLOGICAL TESTS

An important requirement for both standardized and projective tests is that they have heuristic value in terms of their ability to enable one to predict and understand behavior (Bellack and Fielding, 1978). Further, they must also provide indications and inferences regarding treatment. Many problems in validation exist, partly because psychiatric diagnoses are unreliable, and partly because personality theory does not provide adequate guidance. Statistical methods and other appropriate methods that can be applied to analyzing projective techniques are also still inadequate.

A psychological test should be an objective and standardized measure of behavior. Its predictive value depends on its ability to indicate a broad area of behavior while using uniform procedures of administration and scoring. The *reliability* of a test refers to the consistency of scores that are obtained by a person when retested with the same test at a later date or when tested with an equivalent form of the test. The *validity* represents the degree to which the test measures what it says it does. The determination of the validity of a test generally requires an independent measure of what the test is seeking to measure. As an example, if a medical aptitude test is used to select applicants, success in medical school is a criterion for validity. Psychological tests—especially projective techniques—have long suffered from great difficulty in both reliability and validity. Test batteries using several instruments give a more comprehensive picture and increase total accuracy compared with results obtained with any single test.

ADVANTAGES AND DISADVANTAGES OF PSYCHOLOGICAL TESTS

Sundberg and Tyler (1962) point to some other advantages and disadvantages of psychometric tests. On the positive side, they suggest that (1) tests are better than alternative methods of evaluation, (2) the results can be communicated with ease, (3) they are free from examiner bias, (4) many tests can be analyzed statistically, and (5) they are more economical than extensive individual interviews. On the negative side, they indicate that (1) results can be influenced by the attitude of the test-taker; (2) their value is dependent on the skill of the examiner; (3) they may be overly relied on and relegate observation and interviewing to a secondary role; (4) the relationship may be structured in undesirable ways by tests; (5) people with special skills or defects may not be appropriately measured; (6) tests place too much emphasis on the individual and overlook important life circumstances; and (7) validity is seldom as high as would be desired.

Despite these difficulties, tests are clearly used in making significant decisions regarding people's lives, and they are useful adjuncts in the decision-making process. Tests can provide important information in questions of diagnosis, disposition, and determination of treatment methods and assessment of their effectiveness.

Perhaps the most important point to be made is that the clinical skill, insight, and experience of the person who administers, scores, and interprets the tests is crucial in psychodiagnostic evaluation. Scoring a test, for example, is merely a way of reducing behavioral samples to a level at which they can be analyzed. Tests record these behavioral features but it is ultimately through the inference of the clinician that a comprehensive picture is achieved. That clinician must be thoroughly familiar with the tests and also with the principles of personality theory.

Intelligence Testing

Intelligence tests result from two different trends in the history of psychology. First, greater attention was paid to differences between individuals as interest in the theory of evolution developed during the latter half of the nineteenth century. Second, there was increasing interest and concern with the practical problems of classification and placement of children in school. Both of these forces led to the work of Binet, who constructed a scale that became the model for later intelligence tests. All intelligence tests correlate well with academic performance and are mainly measures of verbal ability. The Stanford-Binet test has fallen more into disuse because it is complex to administer and score; it is increasingly being replaced by the Wechsler Intelligence Scale for Children, which has simpler requirements. A separate test for the measurement of adult intelligence was also devised.

WECHSLER ADULT
INTELLIGENCE SCALE (WAIS)

The first adult form of the Wechsler test, known as the Wechsler-Bellevue Scale, had as its chief weakness the nonrepresentativeness of its normative sample. The Wechsler Adult Intelligence Scale (WAIS), published in 1955, rests on the observation that mean scores decline with age, and thus defines a score in terms of the adult's position among people of his or her own age.

The WAIS is made of eleven subtests, divided into a verbal scale and a performance scale. The raw scores on the subtests are translated into standard scores that permit the comparison of these subtests for a given individual, thus allowing identification of the relative ease or difficulty of different types of tasks. It is an efficiently designed and interesting test that has good predictive validity.

Wechsler (1958) described intelligence as goal-directed behavior that represents the overall ability of the individual to act purposefully, think rationally, and relate effectively to his or her environment. This global definition of intelligence viewed it as more than a sum of various intellectual parts; however, Wechsler did believe that intelligence can only be evaluated quantitatively by measuring different aspects of these abilities. The test measures the interaction among these factors, and the intelligence quotient (IQ) is seen as a more or less permanent identification of that individual's brightness or capacity. Wechsler contended that an individual's IQ remained generally the same through life relative to his or her own age group.

The WAIS remains one of the most sensitive indicators of cognitive and emotional functioning. The test is composed of six verbal subtests and five performance subtests.

Verbal Subtests
The verbal subtests measure general information, abstracting ability, comprehension of social norms, arithmetic, and short-term memory skills. The subtest skills may give a good estimate of premorbid functioning because such skills may be quite resistant to impairment due to emotional disturbance. The subtest dealing with interpretation of social acculturation is, on the other hand, quite sensitive to bizarre and antisocial functioning. The logical associative thinking measured by the similarities subtest is particularly affected by thought disorders such as schizophrenia, as well as by organic disorders.

Performance Subtests
The performance subtests measure visual and motor coordination, planning in social relationships, and attention to the outside world. These are frequently affected by emotional instability, distractibility, brain damage, and schizophrenia.

WECHSLER INTELLIGENCE SCALE FOR CHILDREN

The Wechsler Intelligence Scale for Children (WISC) is a test used for children under 16 years of age. It has several advantages over the Stanford-Binet test: (1) the subtest format helps ameliorate the frustration required to establish a "ceiling" as in the Binet, (2) its diversity maintains high motivation, and (3) the verbal-performance differentiation helps in the testing of physically handicapped (Glasser and Zimmerman, 1967). It uses essentially the same subtests as those in the adult scale. The WISC reveals adaptiveness, ridigity of thinking, and the extent to which cognitive functions are being deleteriously influenced by emotional factors. Children are considerably more vulnerable to impairment of intellectual efficiency caused by emotional upsets.

INTERPRETATION OF INTELLIGENCE TESTS

Wechsler scales (WAIS and WISC) are used primarily for diagnosing intellectual impairment related to brain damage, psychosis, and anxiety. Wechsler suggested that when there is a *difference* of 15 or more points between the scores on the verbal and performance IQ scales this should be considered statistically significant and indicative of some type of impairment. Another important concept, *scatter,* refers to the extent of variation of performance among the eleven subtests (intertest scatter) or within individual subtests when easier items are failed while more difficult ones are passed (intratest scatter). In severe psychopathology, scatter of both types is usually great.

A verbal score markedly greater than performance score (15 points or more) is frequently suggestive of right hemisphere brain damage. Wechsler (1958) pointed out, however, that there is also typically a decrement in the performance scale in most mental disorders, which simply serves to remind us that one indication of a process is never sufficient.

Diagnostic Applications

Specific diagnostic categories may be identified through Wechsler performance—for example, many schizophrenics will perform poorly on the comprehension subtest, whereas they will do well on other parts of the test. Compulsive personalities will emphasize detail and exhibit a precise, technical quality to cognition; this population typically does well on the information subtest and exhibits a generally high IQ. Antisocial personalities are likely to show a higher performance score than verbal score, and they characteristically perform better on certain of the subtests, such as picture arrangement.

Cetain subtests are quite sensitive to organic brain disease. Gross central nervous system dysfunction often results in difficulties in concept formation, memory, and in visual, motor, and perceptual activity. Concept formation becomes less abstract and more concrete, the ability to shift from one thought or activity to another is diminished, and analytic and synthesizing abilities are affected. Confusion, uncertainty and perseveration of responses may occur. As a result of the difficulty with abstract thinking, the subject is most likely to do poorly on the similarities and block design subtests. Marked interference with attention and concentration may also be indicative.

Effects of Cultural Deprivation

Test are constructed and interpreted with the assumption that an individual being tested is similar to the standardization group. It is difficult to tell whether these tests are fair when given to members of certain cultures or classes. While the scores of an underprivileged person may be lowered because of his or her circumstances, such scores are nevertheless useful indicators of the person's immediate functioning. Clinicians need to be cognizant of the effects of cultural deprivation, however. Many minority group children have test performances affected by the lack of appropriate standardization and by the fact that they are less verbal and perhaps less self-confident.

In general, intelligence tests present standard circumstances under which people can be observed. Such tests yield a very useful picture of current mental functioning. While some doubt has been expressed about predictive ability, IQ tests certainly yield many important clues with regard to emotional disturbance and mental efficiency or defect, and they have served as a good measure of improvement in patients.

MINNESOTA MULTIPHASIC PERSONALITY INVENTORY

The Minnesota Multiphasic Personality Inventory (MMPI) belongs to a class of psychometric devices classified as *structured inventory* tests. The MMPI consists of 566 items in response to which a patient must determine whether the items apply to him or her. While many of the items are obviously tapping into psychological, phsyical, and neurologic symptoms, the test includes many less obvious "innocuous" items that contribute heavily to the overall psychiatric scales (Marks and Seeman, 1963).

The impetus for the development of the MMPI came from the need for a personality inventory that could be used in a psychiatric facility. It was developed during the late 1930s and early 1940s by Hathaway and McKinley to meet this need.

The MMPI was meant to be an aid in evaluating adult patients and in determining the severity of a psychiatric disorder. While it is the most widely used personality inventory in the United States today, only 60 to 70 percent of the mentally disturbed population taking this test will produce profiles that independent judges consider representative of the type and severity of the applicable disorder. The interpretation of this test is quite subjective, therefore, and constitutes an art form that is very dependent on the skill and training of the examiner.

Validity data indicate, however, that the test is quite valid when compared to other tests. Again, the validity increases when the instrument is used as part of a more thorough evaluation that includes other test information, history, and observations. It is objective in terms of its standard scoring, and its scales provide good summaries of behavioral patterns. There is also a strongly established experience that the MMPI generates reliable psychological interpretations.

Recent data indicate that the MMPI profiles of black patients in various psychiatric diagnostic categories do not significantly differ from those of white patients. The MMPI is useful in identifying alcoholic patients, who typically have some degree of anxiety and depression, and it can reflect characterologic problems as shown by the PD (psychopathic deviate) scale. Drug addicts tend to present a psychopathic profile that includes hostility and impulsive behavior, while the alcoholic manifests more neurotic indices. The MMPI has been found to be quite helpful for screening and selection purposes, for determining the level of impulse control, for differentiation among diagnostic groups, and for assessing treatment potential. A *psychotic tetrad* that has been identified consists of four scales that form patterns in one combination or another; this tetrad is considered indicative of serious disturbance. These four scales are: Pa (paranoia), Pt (psychasthenia), Sc (schizophrenia), and Ma (hypomania).

In an attempt to deal with a major criticism of the test—that is, that there could be faking or intentional distortion—four validity scales were developed to assess test-taking attitudes. The various scales can assess the validity of the profile and also identify personality characteristics and dysfunctions. Included in some of the clinical evaluations are estimates of self-centeredness, somatic concerns, depression, hysteria, and antisocial orientations. More severe forms of behavior are also identified, including paranoia and delusions, and the type of bizarre content typically associated with schizophrenia. Major affective disorders can also be identified, although milder manifestations can readily be missed.

Projective Techniques

The Rorschach test is one of the most important of the unstructured projective techniques. Other projective techniques include the Thematic Apperception Test and sentence completion methods, which are used for evaluation purposes. The Bender Visual Motor Gestalt Test, which is used both projectively and also for the identification of certain types of organic brain dysfunction, provides a transition between the discussion on projective methods and the subsequent topic of neuropsychological evaluation.

THE RORSCHACH TECHNIQUE

The Rorschach test has a long and stormy history of advocates and detractors; my view is that it represents a highly useful tool when it is included within the context of a full test battery. It yields information about an individual's intellectual functioning and affective circumstances as well as helps to reflect the adequacy of emotional control, the spontaneity or emotional constriction present, how introspective or denying the person is, what the effects of anxiety are on personality organization, what conditions seem to precipitate this anxiety, and what defensive operations are employed to deal with very uncomfortable feelings. Additionally, the Rorschach test will give a picture as to whether the defensive operations are working well, or whether there has been decompensation into a more pathologic form of functioning, such as can be found in schizophrenia.

The use of inkblots for diagnostic purposes was generated by the Swiss psychiatrist Hermann Rorschach in 1911. He originally employed 35 inkblots but reduced them to the 10 that are presently used. Several scoring systems were developed from 1936 to 1957; although they are quite different, these systems all use Rorschach's basic ideas in interpreting the data and all are based on an underlying psychoanalytic theoretical framework. The differences that do exist have to do with technical issues of administration, scoring, and interpretation.

Rorschach assumed that an individual's responses to highly ambiguous stimuli would reflect his or her unique way of perceiving the world and would therefore provide an "x-ray" of the personality organization. The test itself consists of 10 inkblots on 6- × 9-inch heavy cardboard cards. The inkblots are symmetrical in shapes; half have one or more colors, while the other half are in black and white or various shades of gray.

Scoring Criteria

Rorschach responses are scored on the basis of many criteria. The location in the blot of the thing seen, the originality of the response, and the various stimulating qualities used (that is, form, color, texture, shading, and human or animal movement) are all interpreted. In addition, the content of the response (for example, animal, human, or inanimate object) is important in the overall analysis of the record. The scores obtained are taken as indices of specific tendencies. For example, a patient, who sees the blots as a whole is regarded as exhibiting an abstract and theoretical orientation, while one who concentrates on small details is thought of as having a more compulsive orientation. Color is related to emotionality in the Rorschach, and human movement responses are related to imagination and creativity. Form is taken to represent the person's ability to take reality into account. Thus, someone who combines form and movement is felt to be accepting of his inner impulses, while a person who rarely reports movement or color is regarded as lacking in imagination. Ratios of the various scores are also seen as having considerable diagnostic value. A high ratio of color to form responses is taken as an indication of strong tendencies to "act out" emotional behavior. A high ratio of human movement to color responses, on the other hand, is interpreted as reflecting withdrawal and introversive tendencies.

Application in Specific Disorders

Borderline personality disorder has become an increasingly important area of study in personality disturbance. Briefly, individuals with this diagnosis are characterized by strong emotions related to hostility or depression, they have a history of impulsive behavior (possibly including suicide attempts and chronic chemical abuse), they have difficulties in establishing more than superficial interpersonal relations, and they experience brief psychotic episodes. This is an interesting group in terms of psychometric evaluation, because some clearly characteristic patterns emerge. The Rorschach tests of these patients typically reveal the same type of thinking disturbance that is found in many psychotic patients. The WAIS, however, yields no evidence of a thought disorder in subjects with borderline personality disturbance. We thus have a relatively good measure for the differential diagnosis of these two groups.

Rorschach has suggested that where there is a predominance of color over movement, combined with other signs of disturbance, the main symptoms are motor. If, on the other hand, human movement responses are greatly in excess of color, symptoms tend to be ideational or mental. Histrionic personalities produce more color than human movement responses. Signs pathognomonic of schizophrenia include contamination (the fusing of two separate responses to an area of the blot into one percept), position responses, and a drop in form quality. There may also be a content that symbolically expresses the nature of the difficulties the person is dealing with.

Criticisms of the Rorschach Test

The Rorschach test has been criticized in many aspects: (1) its failure to produce an objective system of scoring, (2) lack of reliability, (3) difficulty in establishing validity, (4) failure of scoring systems to relate to diagnosis, (5) lack of predictive validity with regard to treatment outcome, (6) inability to discriminate among groups of normal subjects, and (7) failure to establish empirical evidence relating Rorschach scores with intelligence.

THEMATIC APPERCEPTION TEST
The Thematic Apperception Test (TAT) was introduced in 1935 by Morgan and Murray within the context of psychoanalytic theory as a method for investigating unconscious fantasies. It consists of 31 cards, 30 of which have black and white pictures, while one is blank. The subject is asked to make up a story telling what is going on in the picture, what led up to the situation described, and how it will turn out. The interpretation is dependent on the theoretical framework of the examiner. The literature is extensive and presents much contradictory evidence. The form and content are examined for the insight they give into the person's feelings and motivations. Two broad working principles include the frequency of motifs and the degree of uniqueness of the theme. Such areas as parent-child relations, psychosexual functioning, goals, and intellect are inductively observed.

Although the validity of the TAT has been questioned, Harrison (1965) cites many indices of indirect validation, including the following: (1) significant differences have been found between various diagnostic groups, (2) differential descriptions have been obtained for patients with a range of psychosomatic conditions, (3) thematic expression of achievement, aggression, and other motives are related to behavioral manifestations of these needs, and (4) the effects of psychotherapy can be demonstrated (that is, changes in responses are seen in tests repeated after therapy).

SENTENCE COMPLETION TESTS
Tests that ask the subject to finish sentence stems are considered particularly useful in personality evaluation and assessment of adjustment and interpersonal attitudes in adults and children. Sentence completion tests also provide a good measure of anxiety and aggression. There are three such tests in wide use. (1) The *Rohde Sentence Completion Method* consists of 65 items, representing a wide stimulus range. Rohde interprets the responses on overt content and on the personality dynamic inferred from both overt and latent content. Formal aspects (for example, sentence structure) are seen as useful diagnostic tools and may be helpful in diagnosing brain damage and schizophrenia. (2) The *Rotter Incomplete Sentence Blank* consists of 40 items, most of which are short and unstructured. This test is thought of as a basic screening device that would aid in structuring areas of inquiry in further interviews. (3) The *Forer Structured Sentence Completion Test* is a 100-item test that emphasizes speed; the stems are structured to force the patient to deal with material helpful in diagnosis. It is designed to measure attitudes towards interpersonal figures, dominant needs, and aggressive tendencies. Generally, sentence completion tests have been relegated to a screening role and do not represent a major aspect of most test batteries.

Tests for Diagnosis of Organic Disorders
Many of the tests that have been discussed are used for projective purposes and intellectual measurement, but they can also be used to identify organic disorders. Neuropsychological test batteries, however, use quite sophisticated measurement techniques to diagnose neurologic pathology.

Clinical neuropsychology is concerned with the ways in which disorders of the brain express themselves behaviorally. Neuropsychological examination must measure the strengths and the weaknesses of a patient across a broad range of activities. Organic disturbances manifest themselves in the complex interaction of intellect, emotion, and behavioral control.

Intellectual function is generally divided into four major categories, any of which can exhibit disturbances. (1) *Receptive* functions involve the acquisition, classification, and processing of information. (2) *Memory and learn-*

ing represent the process through which information is stored. (3) *Cognition* involves the mental organization of information. (4) *Expressive functions* include the communication and acting on information.

Although there is a tendency for the amount of impairment of these functions to be associated with the extent of brain injury, this is not always the case. Lesions involving certain areas of the cerebral cortex may affect selected functions but not others. Furthermore, certain brain areas are more crucial to mental function than are other, more silent areas. Higher intellectual functions such as thinking, reasoning, concept formation, and abstracting ability are more sensitive to the effects of a generalized brain disorder, but conversely, remain relatively stable in specific receptive, expressive, and even memory disturbances. Impairment of attention and concentration are among the most frequently observed problems seen with organic disorders. Personality changes also occur, and depression and anxiety often result from the individual's reaction to his or her perception of diminished function. Control factors may also be affected, and lability, impulsivity, rigidity and deterioration in grooming are observed. Delusions and hallucinations that mimic schizophrenic disorders may appear. Differential diagnosis can often be made through neuropsychological evaluation. Schizophrenics, for example, typically have performances superior to those of patients with brain tumors or cerebrovascular disease on the trail-making test of the Halstead-Reitan battery.

The WAIS constitutes a major portion of a neuropsychological examination. Lateralized brain injury is primarily manifested as a pattern of differences between verbal functions and visuospatial measures on the WAIS. Concrete thinking, as reflected in the lowered scores of the similarities and picture completion subtests, is also pathognomonic. Organic features may affect an individual's performance on the block design subtest. Information is the least affected subtest in brain injuries, but it does tend to fall with damage to the dominant hemisphere.

The similarities subtest, which measures verbal concept formation, is one of the best predictors of dominant hemisphere disorder, and it tends to reflect left temporal and frontal lobe disturbances. The digit span subtest involves auditory attention; it is sensitive to the presence of brain damage and is generally affected regardless of the locus of the lesion. The picture completion and vocabulary subtests are quite resilient and impervious to organic impairment, and they provide excellent indices of premorbid ability.

BENDER VISUAL MOTOR GESTALT TEST

The Bender test, introduced in the late 1930s as a test of visual/motor coordination, is based on gestalt principles of perception. The test consists of nine geometric figures on individual cards that are presented one at a time. The person is asked to draw or copy each figure. While developed primarily to identify brain damage, the test has come to be employed as a projective test as well, so that collisions of figures can imply disorganization and exact duplication may be indicative of compulsivity. Hasty executions and expansions in size suggest impulsivity, while reductions in the size of the figures frequently reflect withdrawal tendencies, inadequacy, and inhibition. Sequential increase in the size of the figure is indicative of low frustration tolerance. Scattered, expansive arrangements show aggressive tendencies and may also suggest manic conditions. Psychotic patients frequently show confused and chaotic arrangements. Well-adjusted children typically show a greater use of orderly sequence, with less change in curvature, fewer closure difficulties, and fewer rotations than seen in drawings by emotionally disturbed children.

Many signs are indicative of organic impairment, including collision of figures, difficulty in producing angles, rotation of figures, simplifcation and fragmentation, and perseveration and concreteness. The occurrence of four or more of these signs in a record is strongly suggestive of organic impairment. Difficulties in the Bender test are most likely to be seen with right hemisphere, and particularly parietal lobe, dysfunction.

Boll (1978) points to two approaches in psychological evaluation and diagnosis of brain integrity and human abilities. (1) The *medical or neurologic model* assumes that the brain is a unitary organ and that its impairment will have a unitary effect and a single behavioral impact. This approach is binary (for example, presence or absence of brain damage). (2) The *neuropsychological model* has as its goal the understanding of the patient's areas of strength and weakness, and it provides a description of current functioning rather than a diagnosis. The first approach requires symptom occurrence or the presence of impaired performance, whereas the neuropsychological approach permits inferences with regard to health as well.

The neuropsychological examination, therefore, must be able to sample broadly from a large range of brain-related disorders, and it must evaluate a wide array of human functions including stored information, receptive and expressive language, memory and concentration, motor and perceptual skills, and learning and abstracting abilities. Halstead and Reitan developed their well-known test battery with these requirements in mind. They also included several additional procedures in their evaluative process—the age-appropriate Wechsler intelligence scale, an aphasia and sensory perception battery, the trail-making test, a measure of grip strength, and the MMPI.

HALSTEAD-REITAN NEUROPSYCHOLOGICAL TEST BATTERY

The Halstead-Reitan battery (HRB) actually consists of three batteries—one for adults, one for children aged 9 to 14, and one for children 5 to 8. The test is composed of several different parts and may take up to six hours to administer. The tests assess abstracting abilities, tactual performance, perceptual and motor function, coordination, various visual and auditory behaviors, and receptive and expressive language function.

Most neuropsychological batteries include tests of motor or sensory functions, in order to determine the efficiency of functioning on both sides of the body. Tests of aphasia are also commonly included since they are sensitive to left and right hemisphere functions. Reitan and others found that motor and tactile-perceptual measurements are usually significantly different in subjects with cerebral lesions and those without such lesions. They also reported that discrepant relationships between the performance of two hands occur more among brain-damaged than control subjects, and they conclude that motor and somatosensory functions represent a major component of the overall differences between normal and brain-damaged children.

The effect of any lesion depends on whether the lesion is focal, bilateral, or diffuse, and on where it occurs when located in a particular hemisphere. Additionally, the size, rate of growth, length of presence, and patient's age when it began will also influence its effect. Brain damage occuring in the adult tends to impair problem-solving, abstracting ability, and flexibility, while such impairment in children is more likely to affect current learning and ability to solve problems.

Another test of neuropsychological evaluation that has been developed, the Standardized Luria-Nebraska Battery (SLNB), is different from the HRB. The SLNB is derived from a neurologic approach and provides for a rapid administration of pass/fail tests that cover many functions.

It seems that each approach may be appropriate for certain areas of the central nervous system. When cortical projection areas are disrupted, there tends to be an all-or-none distribution; a disturbance of this type might be most appropriately measured by a pass/fail type of test such as the SLNB. Impairment in the associative areas reflects a more continuous distribution, which would make the gradual approach of the HRB a superior measuring device. Further, the SLNB appears less sensitive in identifying the type of borderline damage found in early alcoholic encephalopathy. The

SLNB is seen as not being as sensitive as the HRB in diagnosing diffuse and right hemisphere brain damage.

Other Psychometric Issues

There are three additional areas of importance in psychometric evaluation—assessment of the mentally retarded, testing of the aged, and legal issues.

MENTAL RETARDATION (DEFICIENCY)

The term *deficiency* is not currently being used in the United States because of its negative implications. Retardation encompasses multiple etiologies, including neuropathologic, developmental, and environmental causes. It is intended to define subnormal intellectual functioning combined with generally insufficient adaptive behavior.

Retardation is translated as follows in terms of IQ scores on the Wechsler scales: mild, 53 to 69; moderate, 40 to 52; severe, 25 to 39; profound, 24 and below. Classification on the basis of IQ alone is not sufficient; there must also be an assessment of how well the person is functioning in the community. Intellectual functioning is, however, a major part of such assessment, and subtest scores help identify areas of strength and weaknesses for the purpose of remediation.

The use of projective techniques is questionable with this population. Paucity of responses for retarded individuals is a major drawback with ambiguous stimulus material. The TAT may be superior to the Rorschach in this regard, since it tends to stimulate fantasy and can give clues as to how the subjects evaluate their interpersonal relations and how they generally cope with and defend against anxiety. The Bender test can provide some clues as to visual and motor function, while tests such as the Wide Range Achievement Tests (which measures basic spelling, reading, and mathematics abilities), can shed light on important areas of weakness.

THE AGED

The diagnosis of disorders in the elderly needs to include the specification of the relevant syndrome, its etiology, and a plan for treatment, with an accompanying prognosis. Any number of physical disorders can produce symptoms and need to be identified.

The typical test battery is too time-consuming and demanding for this group; fatigue can have an important influence on test scores. While recent evidence suggests that neuropsychological evaluations can differentiate changes due to aging from those related to brain damage, such evaluations are so lengthy that they may be nearly impossible to complete. Impaired intellectual function is, however, a sensitive index of the effect of many stressors.

The elderly often return to more primitive defenses, including withdrawal, projection, and denial. Psychological testing can be used to identify these mechanisms and might help clarify the person's ability to adapt to life's changes. Test scores also provide a baseline measure for future comparisons, and this data may give some general clues as to the possibilities for adaptation and independent functioning.

LEGAL ISSUES

Our legal system works quite differently for people who are "mentally ill" and thus cannot assist in their defense or understand the proceedings against them. "Illness" may also be used as an excusing factor to exclude legal sanctions against a person, as when someone is judged innocent because of "insanity." Alternatively, psychological data can be used to help determine sanctions (for example, probation, or sentencing to a mental institution).

When someone's competency is questioned (that is, can the person stand trial or make out a will), the capacity at issue is comprehension skills. While it is usually a question of degree of impairment, the requirement is often that a discrete decision be made (that is, whether "mental illness" is absent or present). Current diagnosis employs the techniques described throughout this chapter to arrive at the answer to this question.

The area of psychometric evaluation is complex and fascinating. Some appreciation for the subtlety of the process should have been achieved through the material presented. In closing, a plea is again made for the use of test batteries (rather than single instruments), in the hands of experienced clinicians, as representing the best means to ensure the gathering of reliable and valid data.

References and Further Reading

Anastasi, A. *Psychological Testing,* 2nd ed. New York: Macmillan, 1961.

Bellack, L., Fielding, C. Diagnosing schizophrenia. In B.B. Wolman (ed.), *Clinical Diagnosis of Mental Disorder: A Handbook.* New York: Plenum Press, 1978.

Berg, I.A., Pennington, L.A. (eds.). *An Introduction to Clinical Psychology,* 3rd ed. New York: Ronald Press, 1966.

Boll, T.J. Clinical neuropsychology. *J. Pediatr. Psychol.* 1(3):63–66, 1976.

Boll, T.J. Diagnosing brain impairment. In B.B. Wolman (ed.), *Clinical Diagnosis of Mental Disorders: A Handbook.* New York: Plenum Press, 1978.

Boll, T.J. The Halstead-Reitan neuropsychological battery. In S.B. Filskov, T.J. Boll (eds.), *Handbook of Clinical Neuropsychology.* New York: Wiley (in press).

Boll, T.J. Psychological differentiation of patients with schizophrenia versus lateralized cerebral-vascular neoplastic or traumatic brain damage. *J. Abnorm. Psychol.* 83(4):456–458, 1974.

Boll, T.J. A rationale for neuropsychological evaluation. *Prof. Psychol.* 8(1):64–71, February 1977.

Boll, T.J., Reitan, R.M. Motor and tactile—perceptual deficits in brain-damaged children. *Percept. Mot. Skills* 34:343–350, 1972.

Butcher, J.N., Owen, P.L. Objective personality inventory: recent research and some contemporary issues. In B.B. Wolman (ed.), *Clinical Diagnosis of Mental Disorders: A Handbook.* New York: Plenum Press, 1978.

Byrd, E. The clinical validity of the Bender-Gestalt Test with children: a developmental comparison of children in need of psychotherapy and children judged well-adjusted. In B.I. Murstein (ed.), *Handbook of Projective Techniques.* New York: Basic Books, 1965.

Carr, A.C., et al. Psychological tests and borderline patients. *J. Pers. Assess.* 43:6, 1979.

Cronback, L.J. *Essentials of Psychological Testing,* 2nd ed. New York: Harper & Row, 1965.

Dreger, R.M. Objective personality tests and computer processing of personality data. In I.A. Berg, L.A. Pennington (eds.), *An Introduction to Clinical Psychology,* 3rd ed. New York: Ronald Press, 1966.

Garner, A.M. Intelligence testing and clinical practice. In I.A. Berg, L.A. Pennington (eds.), *An Introduction to Clinical Psychology,* 3rd ed. New York: Ronald Press, 1966.

Glasser, A.J., Zimmerman, I.L. *Clinical Interpretation of the Wechsler Intelligence Scale for Children (WISC).* New York: Grune & Stratton, 1967.

Graham, J.R. The Minnesota Multiphasic Personality Inventory (MMPI). In B.B. Wolman (ed.), *Clinical Diagnosis of Mental Disorders: A Handbook.* New York: Plenum Press, 1978.

Harrison, R. Thematic apperception methods. In B.B. Wolman (ed.), *Handbook of Clinical Psychology.* New York: McGraw-Hill, 1965.

Hathaway, S.R. Personality inventories. In B.B. Wolman (ed.), *Handbook of Clinical Psychology.* New York: McGraw-Hill, 1965.

Holtzberg, J.D. Projective techniques. In I.A. Berg, L.A. Pennington (eds.), *An Introduction to Clinical Psychology,* 3rd ed. New York: Ronald Press, 1966.

Holtzman, W.H. Holtzman inkblot techniques. In B.B. Wolman (ed.), *Clinical Diagnosis of Mental Disorders: A Handbook.* New York: Plenum Press, 1978.

Hutt, M.L. The Hutt adaptation of the Bender-Gestalt Test: diagnostic and therapeutic implications. In B.B. Wolman (ed.), *Clinical Diagnosis of Mental Disorders: A Handbook.* New York: Plenum Press, 1978.

Karp, E., et al. Diagnosing mental deficiency. In B.B. Wolman (ed.), *Clinical Diagnosis of Mental Disorders. A Handbook.* New York: Plenum Press, 1978.

Korner, A.F. Theoretical considerations concerning the scope and limitations of projective techniques. In B.I. Murstein (ed.), *Handbook of Projective Techniques.* New York: Basic Books, 1965.

Krech, D., Crutchfield, R.S. *Elements of Psychology.* New York: Alfred Knopf, 1969.

Lezak, M.D. *Neuropsychological Assessment.* New York: Oxford University Press, 1976.

Marks, P.S., Seeman, W. *Actuarial Description of Abnormal Personality.* Baltimore: Williams & Wilkins, 1963.

Murstein, B. I. (ed.). *Handbook of Projective Techniques.* New York: Basic Books, 1965.

Ogdon, D.P. *Psychodiagnostics and Personality Assessment: A Handbook,* 2nd ed. Los Angeles: Western Psychological Services, 1979.

Pesetsky, F.J., Rabin, A.I. Diagnostic procedures in the clinical justice system. In B.B. Wolman (ed.), *Clinical Diagnosis of Mental Disorders: A Handbook.* New York: Plenum Press, 1978.

Piotrowski, Z.A. The Rorschach inkblot method. In B.B. Wolman (ed.), *Handbook of Clinical Psychology.* New York: McGraw-Hill, 1965.

Shneidman, E.S. Projective techniques. In B.B. Wolman (ed.), *Handbook of Clinical Psychology.* New York: McGraw-Hill, 1965.

Sundberg, N.D., Tyler, L.A. *Clinical Psychology.* New York: Appleton-Century-Crofts, 1962.

Watson, R.I. The sentence completion method. In B.B. Wolman (ed.), *Clinical Diagnosis of Mental Disorders: A Handbook.* New York: Plenum Press, 1978.

Wechsler, D. *The Measurement and Appraisal of Adult Intelligence,* 4th ed. Baltimore: Williams & Wilkins, 1958.

Wilensky, H. Diagnosis in old age. In B.B. Wolman (ed.), *Clinical Diagnosis of Mental Disorders: A Handbook.* New York: Plenum Press, 1978.

Wolman, B.B. (ed.). *Clinical Diagnosis of Mental Disorders: A Handbook.* New York: Plenum Press, 1978.

Zimmerman, I.L., Woo-San, J.M. *Clinical Interpretations of the Wechsler Adult Intelligence Scale.* New York: Grune & Stratton, 1973.

Psychobiologic Evaluation of Psychiatric Disorders

STEVEN D. TARGUM, M.D.

The diagnosis and treatment of psychiatric disorders has historically relied on the description of overt symptoms, a consideration of the patient's past history, and the clinical judgment of the therapist. Until recently, there have been no objective laboratory tests that would help the psychiatrist in making an accurate diagnosis of patients with major psychiatric disorders like schizophrenia or major depressive disorder. Over the last quarter of a century, the rapid expansion of psychobiologic research has made the laboratory evaluation of psychiatric disorders possible and is likely to change the nature of psychiatric practice in the coming years. Neurochemists, psychophysiologists, endocrinologists, and neurobiologists, among others, have provided basic scientific advances that challenge clinicians to seek an integration with their clinical understanding of the patient.

In this chapter an attempt will be made to focus on some areas of psychobiologic investigation in order to demonstrate the clinical significance that these methodologies have today. It is the intention of this chapter to provide an introduction to psychobiologic methods and to their potential application within clinical practice, rather than to provide a comprehensive review of the field of psychobiology. The field of psychobiology is evolving so quickly that many of the techniques described within this chapter may be outdated or replaced by more precise tools within the next few years.

Psychobiology and Clinical Assessment

The development of any psychobiologic technique requires both standardization and validation prior to any claim that it has clinical utility and reliability. There are some psychoneuroendocrine and psychophysiologic techniques that have met these rigorous criteria for clinical reliability and validity. These techniques have particular value in the differential diagnosis of patients with major psychiatric disorders, as well as in the delineation of patients with underlying biologic syndromes from those with more reactive-environmental problems. These techniques may be especially valuable in patients who have become psychotic for the first time (first break) who are described in the criteria of the *Diagnostic and Statistical Manual of Mental Disorders,* Third Edition (DSM-III) as having schizophreniform disorder.

The neuroendocrine challenge studies described in this chapter were used by endocrinologists long before they were found to be useful in a psychiatric population. However, it is understandable that there might be an association between neuroendocrine abnormalities and depressive disorders. The depressive syndrome is associated with several symptoms that are directly related to hypothalamic function: disturbances in mood, disturbances in sexual interest, sleep disorder, appetite disorder, autonomic function, and circadian rhythms. Further, the same neurotransmitters that have been implicated in the psychobiology of mood disorders (catecholamines and serotonin) are also involved in the regulation of the hypothalamic neuroendocrine cells. Thus, deficiencies in the receptor function or neurotransmitter function of the hypothalamus may be reflective of a central disturbance that is related to the mood disorder.

THE DEXAMETHASONE SUPPRESSION TEST
Several studies have demonstrated that patients suffering from major depressive disorders have abnormally elevated levels of serum cortisol compared with those found in the general population. Further, many of these depressed patients do not respond to exogenous

challenges of steroid drugs as would normal individuals or those with other types of psychiatric disorders, such as schizophrenia. The dexamethasone suppression test (DST) has been shown to be a safe and extremely interesting tool for the evaluation of patients with major depressive disorders. In some, but not all studies, an abnormal DST has been reported in as many as 50 percent of patients with major depression; a 90 to 95 percent specificity was found.

The DST measures the response of the hypothalamic-pituitary-adrenal (HPA) axis to an exogenous dose of the steroid drug dexamethasone. Patients are given a 1 mg oral dose of dexamethasone before midnight (11:00 to 11:30 P.M.), and plasma cortisol concentrations are measured over the next 24 hours. In normal individuals, the dexamethasone dose is sufficient to suppress the release of adrenocorticotropic hormone (ACTH) from the pituitary gland, thereby reducing the circulating levels of plasma cortisol below 5 μg/dl for the next 24 to 28 hours. There may be a failure of cortisol suppression in many endogenously depressed patients (40 to 50%) who do not have primary endocrine disorders. These patients apparently have a neuroendocrine dysregulation that results in the failure of the HPA axis to respond adequately to the dexamethasone challenge. The neuroendocrine dysregulation in depressed patients appears to be state dependent, which means that when the patients are acutely depressed, they will reveal a failure to suppress plasma cortisol following the dose of dexamethasone, but when they are clinically improved there should be a normalization (biologic recovery) of their DST test results. In this way, the DST may be useful as an identification technique for underlying biologic depressive syndromes as well as a serial monitoring instrument for the clinical management of psychiatric patients. The use of the DST in clinical practice must still be considered a potential rather than a confirmed tool.

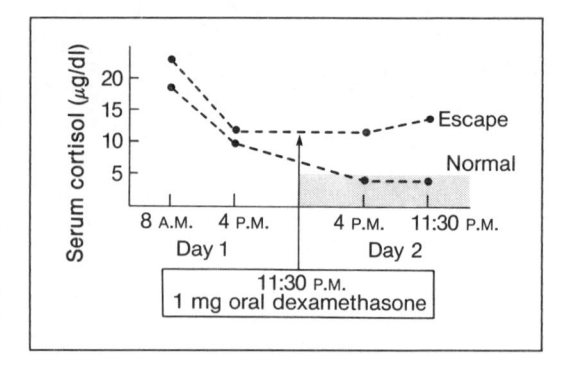

Figure 3-1. Dexamethasone suppression test.

In clinical practice, the test can be administered quite simply and is relatively inexpensive. Baseline measurements of plasma cortisol are collected on the day before the administration of dexamethasone at 8 A.M. and 4 P.M. Patients are given a 1 mg tablet of dexamethasone to take at 11:30 P.M. on that evening. Two additional blood specimens are collected the following day at 4 P.M. and 11:30 P.M. In outpatient practice, the collection of a single 4 P.M. specimen is usually sufficient. Thus, the test can actually be used as an office procedure as an adjunct to the clinical assessment of psychiatric patients. Currently, a plasma cortisol level of greater than 5 μg/dl at either 4 P.M. or 11:30 P.M. after administration of dexamethasone is considered a failure of suppression, or an abnormal DST result. This threshold criterion, however, is an arbitrary value that may vary from laboratory to laboratory. Cortisol levels between 3 and 7 μg/dl after a dose of dexamethasone may be considered a gray zone between normal and clearly abnormal DST results.

THYROTROPIN-RELEASING HORMONE STIMULATION TEST

The thyrotropin-releasing hormone (TRH) stimulation test is another neuroendocrine challenge study. This procedure has been shown to be effective in delineating patients with major depressive disorders from those with schizophrenia, as well as identifying underlying biologic syndromes in psychiatric patients. Endogenous TRH is secreted from the hypothalamus into the portal capillary plexus and stimulates both the production and the secretion of thyroid-stimulating hormone (TSH). The measurement of the release of TSH by the pituitary after the intravenous injection of TRH is an established endocrinologic procedure in the diagnosis of thyroid disease and recently in psychiatric evaluations as well. Numerous studies have shown that the TSH response to TRH injection may be impaired in patients with major depressive disorders in the absence of primary endocrine dysfunctions. A decreased (blunted) or absent TSH response to TRH has been reported in 25 to 35 percent of patients with major depression. This report has been confirmed by a large number of independent studies in both the United States and Europe. As in the case of the DST, the blunted TSH response has been reported to be 90 to 95 percent specific in some settings, depending on the threshold criterion chosen. Some investigators have reported an augmented TSH response to TRH, well above the anticipated increment, in some patients with major depression as well. It is possible that the TRH test may be capable of distinguishing between primary and secondary depression and between unipolar and bipolar depression, as well as discriminating between patients with major depressive disorders and schizophrenics.

This wide variability of TSH responses to TRH injection in depressed patients is a reflection of an impaired neuroendocrine adaptability to challenge during acute illness. As in the DST described above, the impaired TSH response to TRH injection may return to normal (biologic recovery) when the patient has recovered. It has been reported that patients with persistently impaired TSH responses to TRH injection tend to suffer clinical relapse within six months despite apparent clinical recovery. Thus, the finding of a biologic return to normal may be an important prognostic factor in determining the clinical management of these depressed patients. The TRH stimulation test may also be useful for the identification of underlying biologic psychiatric syndromes as well as in the serial monitoring of these patients over time. One application of the procedure has been to distinguish acutely manic patients from schizophrenic patients. Manic patients frequently have blunted TSH responses to TRH injection whereas schizophrenic patients usually have normal responses. Thus, a schizophreniform patient (first-break psychosis) who manifests a blunted TSH response to TRH injection may eventually be reclassified as having a depressive disorder rather than being a schizophrenic.

Thyroid-stimulating hormone undergoes a circadian variation, as do other endocrine hormones; thus test procedures must be standardized. Basal TSH values are greatest at midnight and lowest at noon or early afternoon, and the TSH response to TRH injection is higher at midnight than in the morning. The test is generally conducted in the morning. While small changes in response may occur during the menstrual cycle or in pregnancy, these changes do not appear to affect the interpretation of test results. Further, there is some sex difference (women have a somewhat greater response than men), and advancing age appears to impair the TSH response to TRH injection as well. TSH response is also affected by malnutrition, chronic liver disease, hemodialysis, and endocrine dysfunction (as in Cushing's disease as well as primary thyroid disease). Many drugs can influence the TSH response as well. Thus, it is best to perform the TRH test in the morning in drug-free patients who are at rest and in relatively good physical condition.

The TRH test is performed as an intravenous procedure. A 500-μg dose of the synthetic peptide TRH is infused over 30 seconds in an antecubital vein, and blood specimens are collected at 15-minute intervals following this infusion. Some patients experience a mild nausea for about a minute or two following infusion of the hormone, but in general there have been no serious side effects reported from this procedure. Laboratories can measure the TSH in the serum by radioimmunoassay with fair reliability and consistency. The change in TSH levels from the the baseline that was recorded prior to the TRH injection is the basis for interpretation of test results. Aberrant TSH responses are determined on the basis of threshold criteria, which differ among institutions. TSH changes from a baseline of less than 5 μU/ml would be considered a conservative threshold for a blunted response, and some centers have reported that a change of less than 7 μU/ml is a useful threshold criterion in their setting. The interpretations of augmented responses have been even more variable, but generally responses of greater than 23 to 25 μU/ml from baseline may be considered augmented or high-normal TSH responses to TRH injection.

In clinical practice, the psychiatrist may want to administer both the DST and TRH stimulation tests to many newly admitted patients. Neuroendocrine dysfunction may be found in as many as 60 to 70 percent of newly hospitalized depressed patients meeting DSM-III criteria for major depressive disorder with melancholic features. The tests appear to elicit independent phenomena in that a patient may reveal dysfunction on either test but generally not on both.

It is important to note that the response to neuroendocrine challenge studies can be influenced by a patient's nutritional state. In fact, some recent reports have noted abnormal DSTs in normal individuals who have abrupt weight loss. This finding merely highlights the importance of conservatism in the utilization of psychobiology in psychiatric practice.

ELECTROENCEPHALOGRAPHIC SLEEP ANALYSIS

Several studies have examined the electroencephalographic (EEG) sleep patterns of psychiatric patients, particularly depressed patients requiring hospitalization. These studies have noted marked sleep continuity disturbances characterized by intermittent wakefulness and early morning awakening, low delta (stages 3 and 4) sleep, and a clear preponderance of the lighter stages of sleep (stages 1 and 2). In addition, these studies have reported a reduction in the latency period before the onset of rapid eye movement (REM) sleep in comparison with findings in normal patients and an inverse correlation of the shortened REM latency with the severity of illness. In patients meeting DSM-III criteria for major depressive disorder with melancholic features, more than 30 percent of the time spent trying to sleep may be spent in fretful wakefulness.

Research studies suggest that shortened REM latency points to a strong affective component in a patient's illness. In one study, patients meeting DSM-III criteria for major depressive disorder or schizoaffective disorder, as well as certain schizophrenic patients who later responded to tricyclic antidepressants revealed shortened REM latency in comparison with nonaffectively ill patients. As was true for the psychoneuroendocrine challenge studies, the shortened REM latency time appears to be

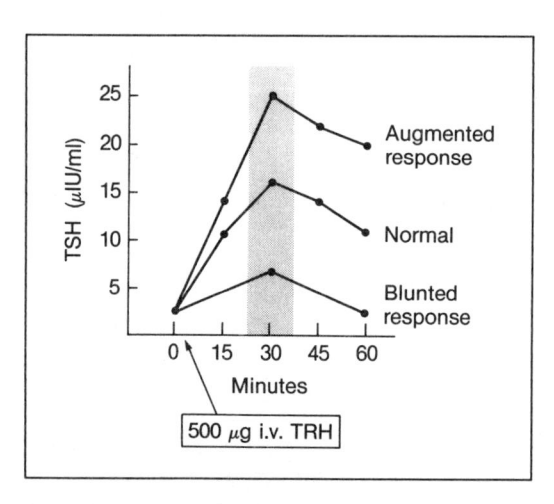

Figure 3-2. Thyrotropin-releasing hormone (TRH) stimulation test. TSH = thyroid-stimulating hormone.

state dependent and recovers when the patient's clinical state improves. REM latency measurements appear to be independent of age, drug use, and changes in other sleep measurements; appear to be refractory to adaptation to the sleep laboratory; and are found in virtually all drug-free patients suffering from a primary depression. Thus, it is a valid and reliable psychobiologic marker of the endogenous feature of depressive illness.

VISUAL AVERAGE
EVOKED RESPONSE STUDIES
Some electrophysiologists have developed an assessment measurement that examines the cortical evoked responses to stimuli; this technique may have clinical value. The average evoked response (AER) provides a specific measure of brain electrophysiology in a noninvasive manner and gets closer to measuring brain functioning than any other current biochemical or physiologic measure. These studies measure the cortical response to repeated visual or auditory stimuli as measured by electrodes attached to the patient's head. Using visual AER studies in which stimulus intensity is gradually increased, individual differences have been found. In some patients (called reducers) the amplitude of the evoked response decreases with increasing stimulus intensity while in others (augmenters) the amplitude increases with increasing stimulus intensity. It is interesting that men tend to be reducers whereas women tend to be augmenters. Further, schizophrenic patients tend to be reducers, whereas patients with bipolar major depressive disorders tend to be augmenters. Further, there tend to be differences between the amplitude/intensity slope of schizophrenics and that of affectively ill patients. Unlike the markers described previously, the visual AER responses appear to be heritable and replicable measurements that are not state dependent. Using multivariate discriminant analysis, and a second biologic marker (platelet monoamine oxidase), one research group was able to make correct classifications of 61 percent of bipolar, unipolar, schizophrenic, and normal control subjects from each other. Thus, the adjunctive value of electrophysiologic measurement of cortical response in differential diagnosis is clear.

SUMMARY
As already described, the use of certain psychoneuroendocrine challenge studies and psychophysiologic measurement procedures can be valuable adjuncts in the differential diagnosis of psychiatric disorders. An important caveat to note, however, is that these procedures must be used in the clinical context in which the patient is presented. Therefore, simply using these psychobiologic tools in an isolated fashion to make diagnoses would be incorrect and unjustified. It is imperative that the clinical judgment of the psychiatric clinician take precedence in the interpretation and integration of these psychobiologic tools as part of the overall clinical assessment of a psychiatric patient.

Psychobiology in Clinical Treatment

The psychobiologic laboratory can have value in the clinical management and treatment of psychiatric patients as well as in deepening the diagnostic understanding of patients as described in the preceding section. The development of assay techniques to measure the circulating plasma levels of psychotropic drugs accurately has enhanced the understanding of individual pharmacokinetics; the use of these medications in clinical practice has also been augmented. Further, the serial use of psychoneuroendocrine procedures as described in the preceding section can facilitate the clinical management of patients and provide premonitory warning signs of impending relapse as well. Thus, it is possible to make an objective evaluation of the clinical efficacy of a psychotropic medication, to monitor a patient's biologic responsiveness, and to correlate these measurements with that patient's clinical condition.

PLASMA LEVELS OF TRICYCLIC ANTIDEPRESSANTS

It is common practice in many areas of medicine to measure plasma levels of precribed medications. This type of routine measurement provides some assurance of clinical efficacy and tends to reduce the incidence of toxicity and minimize side effects. Recently, standardized techniques that have become commercially available allow accurate measurements of plasma levels of psychotropic drugs, particularly the tricyclic antidepressant medications. Plasma levels have been correlated with clinical efficacy and are known to be affected by an individual's age, sex, race, polygenetically determined factors, diagnosis, and concurrent interacting medications; patient compliance with taking the medication is also a factor related to plasma level. The derivatives of many tricyclic antidepressants are also psychoactive (desipramine is a metabolite of imipramine), and they must also be assayed as part of the plasma level measurement. Monitoring of plasma levels of the tricyclic agents can help the clinician determine whether the patient is receiving suboptimal therapeutic dosages of a drug because the steady state plasma levels are insufficient. For instance, one study gave 30 depressed female inpatients 150 mg per day of nortriptyline for 4 weeks and then assayed their plasma levels of nortriptyline. Levels ranged from 48 to 238 ng/ml among these patients. One of the reasons for this wide variation may be that the tricyclic antidepressants differ in the amount of protein binding that occurs, resulting in variable amounts of unbound pharmacologically active agent.

Several studies have sought to determine optimum drug dosages for each of the tricyclic antidepressants as a function of plasma level. One of the earliest and best studies noted a so-called therapeutic window relationship between nortriptyline plasma levels and therapeutic efficacy such that patients with nortriptypline plasma levels below 50 ng/ml or above 150 ng/ml were less improved than patients with levels that fell between those limits. Some studies have reported a similar curvilinear relationship between plasma levels of desmethylclomipramine (the major metabolite of clomipramine) and therapeutic responsiveness. On the other hand, a linear direct relationship has been found with imipramine and its major metabolite desipramine and clinical response. In one study, after 4 weeks of treatment, 22 of 31 clinical responders to imipramine had plasma levels of imipramine plus desipramine exceeding 180 ng/ml as contrasted with 21 of 29 nonresponders who had levels below this limit ($p < 0.01$). Thus, there did not appear to be a therapeutic window among patients receiving imipramine or desipramine. Studies with the other tricyclic antidepressants (protriptyline, amitriptyline, doxepin) and the tetracyclic antidepressant maprotiline have been few and inconclusive, and they await further clarification from future studies. It should be noted that these studies have included only patients with depression sufficient to meet critieria for melancholia, and have not been conducted with nonendogenously depressed patients (characterologic, delusional, or acute situational depressions). Further, the clinical value of these assays will depend in large part on the quality of the assay itself, and the commercial laboratory that completes the work. The assay's sensitivity and specificity may vary from center to center, and the actual value of the therapeutic level may vary as well.

Currently, it makes good clinical sense to monitor plasma levels after steady state has been reached. For most tricyclic agents, steady state is achieved in one to two weeks, with wide differences in plasma levels due mainly to genetic or drug-affected differences in the activity of liver microsomal enzymes. Because the therapeutic concentrations of the tricyclic drugs in plasma are very low, gas liquid chromatographic techniques are used for measurement. Generally, accepted plasma ranges for imipramine and its metabolite desipramine is any level greater than 150 ng/ml, and most patients respond when concentrations exceed 240 ng/ml. On the other hand, nortriptyline, which has a clear curvilinear relationship, is most effective when plasma levels are between 50 ng/ml and 150 ng/ml. Therapeutic levels with other tricyclic antidepressant medications are not as yet well established.

SERIAL PSYCHONEUROENDOCRINE CHALLENGE TESTS

As described earlier, the psychoneuroendocrine techniques of DST and TRH stimulation tests have been applied for the differentiation of affective from schizophrenic disorders. These procedures appear to be state dependent—the neuroendocrine dysfunction that was seen when the patient was depressed may return to normal (biologic recovery) when the patient's clinical state returns to normal. Thus, the serial measurement of DST and TRH tests can provide a measure of normalization of neuroendocrine dysfunctions and serve as a biologic marker of the clinical condition.

In several studies, it has been shown that normalization of a previous endocrine dysregulation is correlated with clinical improvement in most patients. Kierkegaard and Carroll have used the TRH stimulation test in Europe and have found that normalization of blunted TSH responses to TRH is correlated with clinical improvement following electroconvulsive therapy (ECT). In their latest series they reported on 78 patients who had apparently recovered after ECT; they were followed for six months without antidepressant treatment. There were 31 of these patients who did not reveal a normalization of TSH response to TRH injection (an increase in maximum TSH change from baseline studies of $> 2 \mu U/ml$), and 27 of those 31 had relapsed within the period of observation. Thus, the increase in maximum change of TSH after treatment compared to that before treatment was able to predict outcome in greater than 90 percent of the patients studied.

In another study, treatment with antidepressant drugs failed to prevent a relapse in patients who had not revealed normalization of their TSH response to TRH injection. Thus, the TRH test has been demonstrated to be an effective prognosticator of future clinical state.

Similar findings have been reported for normalization of the DST. Thus, patients who failed to suppress the serum cortisol response following dexamethasone despite clinical recovery were at greatest risk for relapse.

Psychobiology and Family Predisposition

Several studies have suggested a genetic predisposition in the development of the major psychiatric disorders such as schizophrenia, schizoaffective disorder, and the major depressive disorders. It is conceivable that a psychobiologic disorder, manifested as a psychiatric syndrome, would have a genetic basis and therefore be transmissible within the family. If this were the case, then biologic relatives of an affected individual would be at risk for the development of a similar psychiatric disorder. In fact, this concept has invariably been supported by psychiatric genetic studies that have been conducted throughout the world. This information may be useful in the evaluation, counseling, and treatment of individuals who are biologically related to patients with one of these illnesses.

PSYCHIATRIC GENETICS

The idea that certain psychiatric disorders might have genetic predispositions was generated before this century, and even Kraepelin noted a "hereditary" taint in many of his patients suffering from dementia praecox (later called schizophrenia) and circular insanity (later called bipolar disorder, mixed). Studies done early in this century noted an increased incidence of mental disorders in the families of the patients with schizophrenia or depression; according to some psychiatrists, a specific biochemical abnormality that could be transmitted from generation to generation increased one's vulnerability to the development of a psychiatric disorder. In the past 20 years, the refined research methods and diagnostic classifications have improved on these earlier studies and confirmed the belief that genetic predispositions may yield psychiatric disorders in some cases. Notably, schizophrenia and the major depressive disorders have been reported as having genetic factors contributing to their overt manifestation.

Twin, family, and adoption studies have demonstrated a positive correlation between the degree of biologic (genetic) relatedness and the manifestation of psychiatric disorder. Twin studies examine the degree of similarity for traits between identical (monozygotic) and fraternal (dizygotic) twins. The underlying assumption is that a true genetic predisposition will result in greater concordance (similarity) in monozygotic compared to dizygotic twins. Numerous studies have shown a greater concordance for major depressive disorder as well as schizophrenia in monozygotic compared to dizygotic twins. For instance, if one monozygotic twin is diagnosed as having a bipolar disorder, there is an 85 percent chance that the other twin will also develop that disorder, while that likelihood would be only 13 percent in dizygotic twins. Similarly, there is a 40 to 50 percent chance of such concordant schizophrenia occurring in a pair of monozygotic twins compared with 10 to 15% in dizygotic twins. Thus, twin studies support the hypothesis that genetic factors are significant in the development of these major psychiatric disorders. There remains some discordance between monozygotic twins, which suggests that other factors (environmental and psychosocial) are also important in the ultimate overt manifestation of the underlying genetic predisposition for the development of these illnesses.

Family studies have documented that the degree of biologic relatedness is correlated with the risk for development of psychiatric disorder (Tables 3-1, 3-2). The degree of risk appears to be a function of the specific type of psychiatric illness. For instance, the first-degree relatives (parents, siblings, offspring) of patients with bipolar disorders have a 15 to 20 percent risk

Table 3-1. Risk for the Development of Schizophrenia

Schizophrenia	Morbid Risk for Schizophrenia (%)
Monozygotic twin	40–50
Dizygotic twin	10–50
Siblings	
No parent schizophrenic	8–10
Both parents schizophrenic	10–15
Offspring	
One parent schizophrenic	12
Both parents schizophrenic	39
Grandchildren	2.8
Nephews/nieces	2.2
General population	0.86

Table 3-2. Risk for the Development of Major Affective Illness

Major Affective Illness	Morbid Risk for Affective Illness (%)
Monozygotic twin	67 (85% for bipolar illness)
Dizygotic twin	13
Siblings	
One bipolar sibling	15–20
One unipolar sibling	7
Offspring	
One bipolar parent	13–15
One unipolar parent	5
Two bipolar or unipolar parents	20–40
Grandchildren	3
Nephews and nieces	3
General population	
Males	1.8
Females	2.5

for the development of depressive disorder in their lifetime, whereas the first-degree relatives of individuals with unipolar depression (major depressive disorder, depressed type only) have about a 7 percent risk of developing depressive illness in their lifetimes. Within the group of schizophrenic illnesses, there appears to be a three times greater risk for familial schizophrenia in the families of nonparanoid schizophrenics than in the families of paranoid schizophrenics. Family studies have also demonstrated that a spectrum of schizophrenic or depressive syndromes appears to be present in some family systems, in conjunction with the primary illness. For instance, in the families of patients with major depressive disorder, there is often found cyclothymic disorder dysthymic disorder, and schizophreniform disorder. In this last case the occurrence of an acute first-break psychosis (schizophreniform disorder) in the biologic relative of a patient with a bipolar disorder may suggest the eventual diagnosis of major depressive disorder rather than schizophrenia for this individual.

Adoption studies seek to distinguish biologic from environmental factors in the etiology of illness. The adoption studies of schizophrenia and major depressive disorder have been the most convincing evidence to demonstrate genetic predispositions in the development of these psychiatric disorders. One method of adoption study has been to examine the biologic and adoptive (nonbiologic) parents of individuals with psychiatric disorders who had been adopted out of the biologic home early in their lives. These studies have shown a greater incidence of similar psychiatric disorder within the biologic parent group (who had had no involvement in childrearing), and almost no psychiatric disorder within the adoptive nonbiologic parents. Using a different design of adoption study (cross-fostering), Wender and co-workers examined the outcome of the offspring of schizophrenic parentage who had been adopted into apparently normal homes. They found that presumably normal childrearing did not prevent the development of schizophrenia in the children who were biologically predisposed to develop the illness. On the other hand, children from apparently normal biologic parentage who were adopted into the home of a parent who ultimately developed schizophrenia did not develop schizophrenia at a rate greater than that of the general population. Thus, the predisposition for the development of psychiatric disorders appears to be relatively independent of environmental influences. In fact, one review of the incidence of major depressive disorder in monozygotic twins who had been reared apart from each other from birth found that 67 percent were concordant for illness, whereas a similar group of dizygotic twins reared apart revealed only 13 percent concordance for major depressive illness.

All of the preceding investigations have confirmed the belief that a familial tendency for the development of a major psychiatric disorder is an expression of genetic rather than environmental factors. It should be noted, however, that the environment does have a significant impact on the severity of expression of the underlying genetic predisposition. Some investigators believe that the offspring of psychotic parents can emerge quite healthy, and can in fact have excellent interpersonal and academic lives, if the impact of the ill parent is counteracted by an active, presumably well parent. This possibility enlarges the importance of identifying individuals who are at risk for the development of illness, since early intervention and management are necessary and may prevent severe psychopathology.

PSYCHOLOGICAL MARKERS OF VULNERABILITY

Currently, there are no markers that can reliably identify individuals who have a high risk for the ultimate development of a psychiatric disorder. With the advent of neurochemistry and modern psychobiology it has been possible for psychogeneticists to test their hypotheses about genetic predispositions with greater objectivity. Recent studies have sought to ascertain specific physiologic, biologic, or psychosocial functions that could distinguish individuals who have already developed illness from well individuals within the same family.

As diagnostic refinements have become more specific, there have emerged certain diagnostic subgroups within the major categories of schizophrenia and major depressive disorders; these subgroups may have prognostic and therapeutic implications. One group of investigators, for example, distinguished three forms of major depressive disorder, depressed type (unipolar illness) on the basis of historical and biochemical parameters. Familial depressive disease is diagnosed when first-degree relatives have a history of depression; depressive-spectrum disease is diagnosed when first-degree relatives have histories of alcoholism or sociopathy as well as depression; and sporadic depressive disease is diagnosed when there is no family history of psychiatric disorder. It appears that the clinical outcome and treatment objectives vary depending on the subtype of major depressive illness found. Thus, the likelihood of rehospitalization is only 26 percent for patients with depressive-spectrum disease, but 44 percent for patients with familial depressive disease and 33 percent for patients with sporadic depressive disease.

A biochemical distinction has also been claimed within the subgroups of major depressive disorders. Using the dexamethasone suppression test, one group reported abnormalities in 80 percent of familial depressives, 37 percent of sporadic depressives, but only 4 percent of depressive-spectrum disease patients. While other investigators have not confirmed these findings, the attempt to make a psychobiologic distinction within the heterogenous group of depressive patients remains an important and provocative area of psychiatry. It is clear that genetic-biologic subtyping may ultimately improve clinical diagnosis, and it represents a promising area for the clinical application of psychiatric genetics.

One area of active psychobiologic investigation in recent years has been the study of monoamine oxidase. Monoamine oxidase (MAO) is a major oxidative enzyme responsible for the metabolism of the major catechol and indoleamines in the central nervous system. A reduction of MAO, as measured in the blood platelet, has been reported in patients with schizophrenia or major depressive disorder (bipolar subtype) in contrast to the general population. It occurred to some researchers that reduced platelet MAO might be correlated with a predilection to psychopathology in the general population. Buchsbaum and co-workers (1977) screened 375 college student volunteers for platelet MAO activity levels. His group did clinical interviews and collected family history information. The findings were dramatic; there was such a wide range of platelet MAO activity levels that high and low platelet MAO groups could be designated. The study found that those subjects who had the lowest platelet MAO values (the bottom 10 percent of the group) had an increased incidence of personal psychopathology and an eightfold greater rate of suicide or suicide attempts in their families in contrast to those in the high platelet MAO group. Thus, this biologic marker was able to discriminate a group of apparently normal college student volunteers who were at high risk for the development of psychiatric disorders from a general population of college students.

Another group of investigators studied the transmission of platelet MAO activity (which is apparently a heritable function) from one generation to the next within families with major depressive disorder. If low platelet MAO were really correlated with psychiatric disorder, then those family members who had high platelet MAO should be protected from or resistant to the same form of psychiatric disorder. However, family studies that examined the segregation of platelet MAO with psychiatric disorder in the same families have not revealed this correlation.

Recently, psychiatrists have learned that platelet MAO is affected by the drugs that an individual takes. Thus, schizophrenic patients who have begun treatment with antipsychotic medications will, over a period of months, have a gradual lowering of their platelet MAO activity. It is possible that some of the earlier studies of platelet MAO in patients with schizophrenia or bipolar disorder may have been influenced by a drug effect. Currently, studies are being conducted with drug-free patients who meet the same criteria for illness to determine whether the platelet MAO effect is still valid. All the same, the correlation found in the college student population remains a dramatic finding in psychobiology, suggesting that future studies will explain the true relationship of platelet MAO activity to psychiatric disorder.

Another approach being used to identify patients at high risk for the development of psychiatric disorder utilizes known genetic markers (traits that have been recognized on specific regions of specific chromosomes) that might be linked to a major psychiatric disorder although not directly etiologic in the expression of that disorder. In recent years, for instance, one area of psychiatric research has focused on the human leukocyte antigen (HLA) region located on chromosome 6. Several studies have reported associations of specific HLA alleles with either schizophrenia or major depressive disorder. To date, there have been no consistent findings. A family study that examined the segregation of HLA alleles with bipolar disorder in families with multigenerational illness did not find a correlation between the HLA region and the disorder. On the other hand, some investigators have reported that specific HLA alleles A-3 and B-18 may be correlated with faster relapse in patients with major depressive disorders who are receiving lithium carbonate. These reports suggest that psychopharmacologic response may be a function of genetic determinants.

If one assumes that there is a common underlying genetic predisposition within the family for the development of a psychiatric disorder, it is logical to assume that similar psychotropic medications would be useful in related family members. One study reviewed the effects of lithium carbonate in patients with major depressive disorders and compared it with their family histories. In this study, it was found that patients who had a family history of major depressive disorders were more likely to respond to lithium carbonate than were those who had no such family history. In fact, 19 of 21 (90%) patients with positive family histories of bipolar disorder in the first- or second-degree relatives were lithium carbonate responders, in contrast to 5 of 15 (33%) patients with negative family histories for this disorder. Thus, family history findings may be able to predict pharmacologic responsiveness.

Genetic-psychopharmacologic relationships have received limited attention in the research literature. Two studies have examined the relationship of tricyclic antidepressant treatment in biologically related pairs of depressed patients. Both studies reported a tendency of biologically related patients to respond to the same antidepressant medications. In one study of nine patient pairs, each suffering from depressive illness, concordant drug responses were noted in eight of the nine pairs.

In summary, it is clear that the use of the psychobiologic laboratory and examination of psychogenetic relationships can have value in the clinical assessment and treatment of psychiatric disorders. There is a growing interest in genetic counseling for family members who are unaffected but at risk, as will be discussed in the next section.

PSYCHOBIOLOGY AND PREVENTIVE PSYCHIATRY

There are as yet no reliable specific markers that will help in the identification of apparently normal individuals who are likely to develop a psychiatric disorder in their lifetime. The development of such specific tests of psychiatric vulnerability will be simultaneously identifying high-risk individuals and defining a biologic etiology to a specific disorder. The future treatment of the major psychiatric disorders may include diagnostic subtyping along biologic-genetic lines rather than the descriptive-phenomenologic terminologies that are currently utilized. As psychobiology provides clues to the identification of vulnerable individuals, it will also allow psychiatry to enter into the realm of preventive medicine.

Currently, studies are being conducted with the high-risk offspring of patients with schizophrenia or depressive disorders. These studies seek to determine psychosocial, psychological, or psychobiologic factors that might predict the future development of schizophrenia or major depressive disorder in these individuals. Increasing data about cognitive and psychophysiologic parameters suggest that a distinction can be made between children at high risk who will go on to develop psychosis and those who will not develop psychosis. The identification of the specific prognostic variables that are correlated with the ultimate development of a psychiatric disorder will naturally lead to specific therapeutic interventions designed to avert or modify the expression of the disorder.

Neuroradiologic Procedures

A renewed interest in structural morphology of the brain has occurred as a consequence of the development of nuclear medicine and neuroradiology. The computerized tomographic (CT) scan is a noninvasive neuroradiologic procedure that has been applied to the study of psychiatric disorders. In one group of investigations, it was found that enlarged lateral cerebral ventricles were correlated with poor premorbid social and interpersonal histories and poor outcome in schizophrenic patients. Further, it has been suggested that those patients with structural abnormalities of the brain (enlarged ventricles as a marker) may represent a different subtype of schizophrenic disorder than those patients with normal morphology and good premorbid histories. Similar studies have similar findings also yielded in depressive patients. Thus, it may be possible that subgroups of patients with major psychiatric disorders may be delineated on the basis of structural morphologic abnormalities.

The development of a more advanced tool, the positron emission tomographic (PET) scan, may further advance the understanding this area of research. The PET scan examines the metabolic distribution of radiolabeled glucose in the brain. Studies conducted at the Brookhaven National Laboratory in Long Island, New York, have demonstrated marked differences in the PET scan patterns of patients with schizophrenia or mania compared with those in normal patients. In schizophrenics, the PET scans have demonstrated hypofrontality—a marked decrease in radioactive labeled glucose metabolic activity in the frontal lobe. In manic patients, asymmetrical scans revealing glucose consumption at tremendous rates have been demonstrated. Thus, direct evidence of a connection between brain neurophysiology and mental behavior can be recorded by use of this new procedure. The high cost of the PET scan technique limits its current usefulness, but it is clearly a diagnostic tool in the future of psychobiology.

Psychiatric Genetic Counseling

The evaluation of at-risk individuals represents a form of psychiatric genetic counseling. Such evaluations have increased as individuals and their physicians become more aware of the relationship between psychiatric disorders and psychobiologic-genetic processes. It is not uncommon for individuals in psychotherapy to ask about the relationship of hereditary or biologic predisposition to their difficulties. Questions are generally related to an individual's concerns about his or her own risk of developing a psychiatric disorder, or the risk that any offspring might develop a psychiatric disorder. Although specific markers of vulnerability do not exist in the well state, psychiatrists can use the data gained from family studies to determine the risk that an individual will develop a psychiatric disorder in their lifetime (see Table 1-1, p. 6). As described earlier, an individual's risk increases with the degree of biologic relatedness to someone having the disorder. Thus, the individual at greatest risk is one who is the monozygotic twin of a patient with schizophrenia or bipolar affective disorder or who is the offspring of a dual mating. (The term *dual mating* is used to describe the relationship between a man and a woman who have the same disorder and who produce offspring.)

The offspring of dual matings between schizophrenics have a 40 to 50 percent risk of developing overt psychotic disorder, and one may presume that the other 50 percent may have an increased risk for serious character disorders or spectrum disorders. In one study of 32 dual matings, nearly half the children born after the mother's first hospitalization for schizophrenia required the intervention of child care agencies. Only 2 of these marriages were found to have produced home environments that could be classified as unbroken or not chaotic. The avoidance of child bearing in these marriages would therefore be good preventive psychiatry.

Other patients at high risk for marital problems and chaotic relationships include those with rapidly cycling bipolar disorder or chronic schizophrenia. It is not uncommon for these patients to deny or minimize the implications of the illness for themselves or for their family members. In one study of patients with bipolar disorders and their well spouses, 47 percent of the well spouses regreted having had children compared to only 5 percent of the patients themselves ($p < 0.01$). Thus, within the same family, one's attitude about childbearing will differ depending on their personalities and relationship to the illness. In fact, it may be that those individuals who are most in need of psychiatric genetic counseling will be the least likely to acknowledge the information and act on it in an appropriate fashion.

Conclusions

The future of psychiatry promises the integration of psychobiologic tools in the overall practice of the clinician. Therapists may incorporate their interpersonal, psychological, and family-oriented approaches with advances in psychobiology to provide a comprehensive treatment for their patients. At the same time, there will always be an element of interpersonal and intrapsychic relationship that will be necessary in the evaluation of psychiatric disorders and the management of patients with these disorders. Psychobiologic techniques will never diminish the need for assessment of human psychodynamics and limitations; the psychobiologic tools are merely an adjunct to the therapeutic relationship between the patient and the therapist.

It will become possible to use the psychobiologic laboratory as an aid in the assessment and treatment of psychiatric disorders, in the same way that one uses the laboratory to diagnose and treat medical conditions like anemia or infectious diseases. The advent of these psychobiologic techniques will lead to the identification of biologically distinct subgroups of psychiatric patients, and ultimately will lead to specific biologic therapies for these patients. Some day it may be possible to identify a specific psychobiologic deficit (e.g., a receptor disorder) and prescribe a specific treatment designed to modify the specific deficit.

The following case illustrates the current clinical applications of some of the assessment techniques described in this chapter.

Case 1. Mr. G., a 22-year-old graduate student in physics, was brought to the emergency room of a local hospital by friends. They had noted that he had become reckless and fretful for several days and had complained of sleeplessness for weeks before that. On the evening before this visit, Mr. G. had been found wandering around the campus, talking to himself, gesticulating as if there was somebody talking to him, and he appeared unkempt and distraught. The friends assured the examining doctor that Mr. G. never drank or used any illicit drugs. The doctor observed Mr. G., who had seemed to be frightened and dazed, and he sat mute during the examination, staring directly into the doctor's eyes. It was clear that he needed to be hospitalized and treated immediately. Mr. G. was placed in a psychiatric unit, where 5 mg haloperidol was given intramuscularly in four successive hourly doses. By midday, he began to talk. He described hearing a powerful voice telling him that the solar system was being gradually deteriorated by cigarette smoke and that he was responsible for curtailing this process. Subsequently, Mr. G. became jittery and was mute again.

Over the next few days, Mr. G.'s progress waxed and waned. At one point, he attempted to swallow packs of cigarettes in order to avert their use by others. He sometimes appeared to be confused about who he was and whether he was human or humanoid, and displayed identity and boundary confusion. At other times, he seemed to be insightful, expressed great distress about this psychotic episode, and asked about future chances of recurrence. His diagnosis was schizophreniform disorder, because the schizophrenic picture with which he presented was of less than six months' duration.

The psychiatrist requested psychobiologic evaluation. Notwithstanding Mr. G.'s disorganized behavior it was possible to administer a dexamethasone suppression test and TRH stimulation test. On the DST, Mr. G. revealed a normal diurnal variation of serum cortisol and an adequate suppression of the cortisol response following dexamethasone. However, he revealed a blunted TSH response to TRH: his maximum peak elevation of TSH was only 4.3 μIU/ml above the baseline level.

Mr. G. gradually improved while he received antipsychotic medications; he regained his previous composure and capacities, was given maintenance doses of haloperidol, and was discharged from the hospital.

Mr. G. returned to his graduate studies following the psychotic episode and did extremely well. His psychotherapist discontinued maintenance haloperidol after six months of successful treatment and was confident that his patient had essentially recovered. Mr. G. had developed an intense and warm interpersonal relationship and had continued his academic achievements without medication. However, two years after his first episode he began to get restless and sleepless again. He described irregular sleep patterns (sleep-continuity disturbance) and was unable to get back to sleep after 4 A.M. He noticed a loss of appetite and a six pound weight loss in less than two weeks. Most of all, he was worried about having difficulties concentrating on his work, particularly in the morning. This difficulty persisted, and Mr. G. grew increasingly despondent and desperate to complete his assignments. It seemed as if everything was collapsing and that he was out of control. He began to describe himself as worthless as a scientist and talked about wishing he were dead. He had stopped caring for his appearance and began to look the way he had two years earlier in the emergency room. However, on this occasion a different clinical picture emerged. It was clear that Mr. G. met DSM-III criteria for a major depressive disorder with recurrent symptoms. Further, he described a diurnal variation in his mood (which was generally worse in the morning), excessive guilt, and a loss of pleasure and reactivity to the activities he usually enjoyed—he also met the DSM-III criteria for melancholia.

The dexamethasone suppression test conducted at this time revealed a failure of suppression. His cortisol level at 4 P.M. the day after being given dexamethasone was 8 μg/dl, well above the 5 μg/dl criterion for abnormal results. Further, the TSH response was blunted, much as it had been two years earlier.

Mr. G.'s doctor gave him a tricyclic antidepressant, imipramine, in increasing doses up to 200 mg per day. Initially, he began to sleep better and could take better care of himself, but he was still very despondent and complained about memory and concentration difficulties. The imipramine dose was increased to 300 mg per day and continued for four more weeks. Although Mr. G. had returned to class, he could not do his work. He was clearly anxious and discouraged about his unremitting depression. Sometimes this secondary dysphoria has more serious psychosocial sequelae than the primary depressive disorder itself. The psychiatrist ordered studies of plasma levels of imipramine and its metabolic derivative desipramine, and requested repeated DSTs on a weekly basis.

The combined plasma levels of imipramine plus desipramine were 72 ng/ml despite the 300-mg daily dose of imipramine. The psychiatrist chose to increase the imipramine to 400 mg per day, with serial measurements of the plasma level. A repeated plasma level the following week was 160 ng/ml for the combined imipramine plus desipramine levels, which was within the presumed therapeutic range for the drug. In addition, the psychiatrist used a standardized clinical rating instrument, the Hamilton Depression Scale, to assess Mr. G.'s response objectively. Scores increase with the severity of symptoms, and scores above 27 are considered to be consistent with severe depression. Mr. G. showed a gradual lessening of his depressive symptoms as measured by reduced Hamilton scores; this improvement was positively correlated with reduction in cortisol levels after administration of dexamethasone. Three weeks later, his cortisol levels had returned to normal (biologic recovery) and his clinical state had improved.

Mr. G. had responded to high doses of tricyclic antidepressants and had revealed a neuroendocrine dysregulation that was correlated with his clinical state. He was delighted by his positive response and the "biologic" explanation of his problems. He recalled that his grandmother had been known to have episodic depressions throughout her lifetime. It occurred to him that his sister, a frequent sufferer of depression, might benefit from a psychobiologic evaluation since the disorder seemed to run in the family.

References and Further Reading

Buchsbaum, M. Average evoked response augmenting/reducing in schizophrenia and affective disorders. In D.X. Freedman (ed.), *Biology of the Major Psychoses*. Research Publications: Association for Research in Nervous and Mental Disease, vol. 54. New York: Raven Press, 1975, pp. 129–142.

Buchsbaum, M.S., Haier, R.J., Murphy, D.L. Suicide attempts, platelet monoamine oxidase and the average evoked response. *Acta Psychiatr. Scand.* 56:69–79, 1977.

Carroll, B.J., Feinberg, M., Greden, J.F., et al. A specific laboratory test for the diagnosis of melancholia. *Arch. Gen. Psychiatry* 38:15–22, 1981.

Gershon, E.S., Targum, S.D., Kessler, L.R., et al. Genetic studies and biologic strategies in the affective disorders. *Prog. Med. Genet.* 11:101–164, 1977.

Kierkegaard, C., Carroll, B.J. Dissociation of TSH and adrenocortical disturbances in endogenous depression. *Psychiatr. Res.* 3:253–264, 1980.

Kupfer, D.J. REM latency: a psychobiologic marker for primary depressive disease. *Biol. Psychiatry* 11:159–174, 1976.

Loosen, P.T., Prange, A.J., Jr. Thyrotropin releasing hormone (TRH): a useful tool for psychoneuroendocrine investigation. *Psychoneuroendocrinology* 5:63–80, 1980.

Risch, S.C., Huey, L.Y., Janowsky, D.S. Plasma levels of tricyclic antidepressants and clinical efficacy: review of the literature. *J. Clin. Psychiatry.* 40:4–69, 1979.

Targum, S.D., Schulz, S.C. Clinical application of psychiatric genetics. *Am. J. Orthopsychiatry* 51:45–57, 1982.

Targum, S.D., Sullivan, A.C., Byrnes, S.M. Compensatory pituitary thyroid mechanisms in major depressive disorder. *Psychiatr. Res.* 6:85–96, 1982.

Weinberger, D.R., Bigelow, L.B., Kleinman, J.E., et al. Cerebral ventricular enlargement in chronic schizophrenia. *Arch. Gen. Psychiatry* 37: 11–13, 1980.

Wender, P.H., Rosenthal, D., Kety, S.S., et al. Crossfostering: a research strategy for clarifying the role of genetic and experimental factors in the etiology of schizophrenia. *Arch. Gen. Psychiatry* 30:121–128, 1974.

Clinical Disorders

II

Organic Mental Disorders
DANIEL J. O'DONNELL, M.D.

This chapter is divided into two major sections: (1) organic brain syndromes, referring to the cognitive, emotional, and behavioral changes resulting from organic brain dysfunction but without identification of a specific etiology; and (2) organic mental disorders, linking an organic brain syndrome to a specific known or suspected etiology. There is also a third section that examines psychiatric aspects of seizure disorders, an area of significance for understanding human behavior.

Organic Brain Syndromes
There are six categories of organic brain syndrome (OBS) recognized in the *Diagnostic and Statistical Manual of Mental Disorders,* Third Edition (DSM-III):

1. Delirium and dementia, syndromes characterized by global cognitive impairment
2. Amnestic syndrome and organic hallucinosis, in which there is selective impairment of memory or perception, respectively
3. Organic delusional syndrome and organic affective syndrome, which resemble functional schizophrenic or affective disorders, respectively
4. Organic personality syndrome, in which personality features are primarily altered
5. Intoxication, resulting from the ingestion of a substance, and withdrawal, resulting from discontinuance or reduction in use of a substance
6. Atypical or mixed organic brain syndrome, which is a residual category for otherwise unclassifiable OBS

DELIRIUM AND DEMENTIA
Delirium and dementia are conditions in which cognitive abilities are globally impaired because of toxic, biochemical, structural, or electrical disturbances. They correspond roughly to the older terms *acute* and *chronic* brain syndromes although they are used in this text descriptively and do not reflect duration of disturbance or imply prognosis. These syndromes are very common conditions, many cases of which are obvious enough to be taken for granted. Other cases, seemingly mild and subtle, may progress to insidious deterioration of social, business, and self-care skills. Anxiety may mount and depression set in without patient, family, or physicians knowing of the episodic mild delirium secondary to drugs or progressive dementia secondary to Alzheimer's or other diseases.

Delirium
Delirium, the organic brain syndrome perhaps most commonly encountered in general medical practice, is a condition that always is presumed to be organically based; exhaustive and rigorous investigation must be made if necessary to establish an etiology. The clinical picture of delirium is one of a clouded (reduced) state of consciousness, disturbed patterns of sleep and wakefulness, decreased attention, impaired sensory perceptions, disorientation, and memory deficits. Table 4-1 gives the diagnostic criteria.

Typically, delirium results from an acute insult to the brain, and onset is relatively rapid (within minutes to days). It is presumed to be caused by diffuse disruption of brain metabolism. The course can fluctuate, and the clinical picture may change rapidly from one extreme to another, permitting periods of normal intellectual functioning. All of the higher mental functions are altered, including the ability to maintain and regulate alertness; register process; retain and recall information of all types, both old and new; and organize and maintain thinking logically and coherently. Frequently,

Table 4-1. Diagnostic Criteria for Delirium

A. Clouding of consciousness (reduced clarity of awareness of the environment), with reduced capacity to shift, focus, and sustain attention to environmental stimuli.
B. At least two of the following:
   1. perceptual disturbance: misinterpretations, illusions, or hallucinations
   2. speech that is at times incoherent
   3. disturbance of sleep-wakefulness cycle, with insomnia or daytime drowsiness
   4. increased or decreased psychomotor activity
C. Disorientation and memory impairment (if testable).
D. Clinical features that develop over a short period of time (usually hour to days) and tend to fluctuate over the course of the day.
E. Evidence, from the history, physical examination, or laboratory tests, of a specific organic factor judged to be etiologically related to the disturbance.

Reproduced with permission from *Diagnostic and Statistical Manual of Mental Disorders,* 3rd ed., p. 107.

impairment in one area of functioning may be very disturbed, while the patient may retain sufficient cognitive functioning to be a good judge of his or her impairment. Many delirious patients have vivid hallucinations (usually visual, sometimes tactile, less frequently auditory), with fluctuating levels of consciousness, but are able to report that they are hallucinations and that they know the sensation to be hallucinations—that is, not based in reality.

Disturbances of consciousness typically include periods of heightened alertness and even extreme, agitated vigilance. The patient often has difficulty sleeping at night, and the relative sensory deprivation of darkness may reduce sensory perception and contribute to the occurrence of bizarre and frightening hallucinations and misperceptions. Waking experiences that resemble nightmares may combine auditory, visual, visceral, and tactile hallucinations to a terrifying extent.

Thinking and speech are usually disturbed. These patients have difficulty thinking or expressing themselves logically and coherently. They may change subjects rapidly, lose their train of thought, or experience poverty of thoughts. Words, phrases, and ideas may be repeated endlessly, often as if they had great but cryptic meaning. Similar perseveration may be exhibited in repetitive behavior. Mood lability (the rapid change from one mood to another) can be striking. Sudden laughing, which may quickly turn into anguished crying, is common. Pacing, hand-wringing, assaultive behavior, and unpredictable outbursts are disturbing to the patients' families, staff, and others and are often difficult to manage.

Dementia

Dementia is an organic brain syndrome characterized by a "loss of intellectual abilities of sufficient severity to interfere with social or occupation functioning. The deficit is multifaceted and involves memory, judgment, abstract thought, and a variety of other higher cortical functions. Changes in personality and behavior also occur. The diagnosis is not made if these features are due to clouding of consciousness, as in Delirium. However, Delirium and Dementia may coexist" (DSM-III, p. 107).

While dementia is diagnosed most often in the elderly, earlier onset caused by specific underlying disease processes is not uncommon. The course of most dementia is one of gradual deterioration over years, but functional worsening can appear relatively suddenly. Of course, specific etiologic factors may cause sudden and permanent impairment. Table 4-2 gives the diagnostic criteria for dementia.

The clinical syndrome of dementia resembles delirium in that it is presumed to be caused by organic disease diffusely affecting the function of brain tissue. The hallmark of the illness is decreasing intellectual function, not merely deficient intellectual function as in stable mental retardation (see Case 1, p. 58).

Intellectual deterioration may be marked and obvious in some of its manifestations or more subtle when only secondary behavioral changes cause the patient or, more typically, the family to seek help. Patients with dementiform syndromes, more often than those with delirium, ignore or deny or even conceal deficits and are more likely to be resistant or hostile in response to examination.

Table 4-2. Diagnostic Criteria for Dementia

A. A loss of intellectual abilities of sufficient severity to interfere with social or occupational functioning.
B. Memory impairment.
C. At least one of the following:
   1. impairment of abstract thinking, as manifested by concrete interpretation of proverbs, inability to find similarities and differences between related words, difficulty in defining words and concepts, and other similar tasks
   2. impaired judgment
   3. other disturbances of higher cortical function, such as aphasia (disorder of language due to brain dysfunction), apraxia (inability to carry out motor activities despite intact comprehension and motor function), agnosia (failure to recognize or identify objects despite intact sensory function), "constructional difficulty" (e.g., inability to copy three-dimensional figures, assemble blocks, or arrange sticks in specific designs)
   4. personality change, i.e., alteration or accentuation of premorbid traits
D. State of consciousness not clouded (i.e., does not meet the criteria for delirium or intoxication, although these may be superimposed).
E. Either 1 or 2:
   1. evidence from the history, physical examination, or laboratory tests, of a specific organic factor that is judged to be etiologically related to the disturbance
   2. in the absence of such evidence, an organic factor necessary for the development of the syndrome can be presumed if conditions other than organic mental disorders have been reasonably excluded and if the behavioral change represents cognitive impairment in a variety of areas

Reproduced with permission from DSM-III, pp. 111–112.

The most common early complaint is memory impairment of insidious development. It is difficult to date the onset accurately, particularly with the progressive dementias, and early signs may be mild absent-mindedness. Memory and information processing deficits may range from a barely noticeable need to reread material to an inability to care for one's own hygiene and health. Patients with moderate or severe dementia can be harmful to themselves by neglect of self-care and of the immediate environment. Changes in personality and judgment may lead to loss of friends, business skills, and family relationships. Loss of function, reaction to progressive failure, alienation from previously supportive friends, and increased impulsivity can in turn lead to increasing anxiety, frustration, depression, and even suicide.

Changes in personality are common. The types of changes vary and can involve completely atypical behavior or exaggerations of long-standing personality traits. A reserved, orderly, self-controlled man may become loud and rowdy, making crude sexual advances with seemingly little appreciation of his behavior or its social consequences. Extreme but not uncommon examples include disrobing, urinating, or masturbating in public. Exacerbations of premorbid personality traits are often not considered very unusual until they become severe or are accompanied by clearly organic symptoms, such as increasing memory or language dysfunction. There is no definite pattern to personality changes in dementia, but friends and family usually perceive that at least "something is wrong" or the person is "not quite himself." The finer points of social skills are usually the first to be lost.

Language difficulty, difficulty finding proper words, misusing words, rambling to avoid forgotten words, and other similar problems are common. Patients also often have a decreased ability to tolerate stress and frustration. On the other hand, they may be curiously indifferent to events that previously would have caused a clear emotional response. Irritability, argumentativeness, compulsiveness, and even paranoia may be responses to decreasing abilities and increasing failures. Patients commonly blame others for these difficulties. The internal sense of loss of control is often explained away by accusing others of causing problems and failures. Insight is usually poor, but individuals with dementia often experience marked frustration and embarrassment.

AMNESTIC SYNDROME

The amnestic syndrome is an organic brain syndrome chiefly affecting memory. Both establishment of new learning (anterograde amnesia) and recall of previous memory (retro-

Table 4-3. Diagnostic Criteria for Amnestic Syndrome

A. Both short-term memory impairment (inability to learn new information and long-term memory impairment (inability to remember information that was known in the past) are the predominant clinical features.
B. No clouding of consciousness, as in delirium and intoxication, or general loss of major intellectual abilities, as in dementia.
C. Evidence, from the history, physical examination, or laboratory tests, of a specific organic factor that is judged to be etiologically related to the disturbance.

Reproduced with permission from DSM-III, p. 113.

grade amnesia) are decreased or absent. Immediate recall (a span of 10 to 15 seconds) is intact, however, as it appears to reflect a different mental operation. Remote memory may also be preserved. The defect in memory is relatively circumscribed, and the more global impairment of mental functioning found in delirium and dementia is absent (Table 4-3). There may be significant associated features, however, including confabulation to cover memory gaps, lack of insight, frank denial of the problem, indifference, emotional shallowness, and lack of initiative. This disorder has also been known as Korsakoff's psychosis.

ORGANIC HALLUCINOSIS

Organic hallucinosis is characterized by hallucinations occurring in a clear state of consciousness (full alertness) and attributable to a known or strongly suspected organic etiology. Any of the senses can be involved, and may be determined by the site of the etiologic process. The impaired individual may or may not have insight into the nature of the hallucinatory process.

ORGANIC DELUSIONAL SYNDROME

In an organic delusional syndrome, the predominant clinical feature is the occurrence of delusions in a clear state of consciousness. The delusions may or may not be accompanied by hallucinations and may be of any of the various types described in Chapter 1. Etiology may influence the type of delusion, although pre-existing personality pathology may also prove significant.

ORGANIC AFFECTIVE SYNDROME

The organic syndrome is characterized by a persistent change in mood of either a manic or depressive nature resulting from a specific organic cause. As in other circumscribed organic brain syndromes, the symptoms must occur in a normal state of consciousness and without the features that would meet the diagnostic criteria for delirium or dementia. The signs and symptoms of organic affective syndrome are the same as those listed in Chapters 7 and 8 for bipolar disorders and depression.

ORGANIC PERSONALITY SYNDROME

The organic personality syndrome is a rather variable clinical entity primarily demonstrating disinhibition of emotions or impulses resulting from a specific organic disorder (Table 4-4).

Table 4-4. Diagnostic Criteria for Organic Personality Syndrome

A. A marked change in behavior or personality involving at least one of the following:
   1. emotional lability, e.g., explosive temper outbursts, sudden crying
   2. impairment in impulse control, e.g., poor social judgment, sexual indiscretions, shoplifting
   3. marked apathy and indifference, e.g., no interest in usual hobbies
   4. suspiciousness or paranoid ideation
B. No clouding of consciousness, as in delirium; no significant loss of intellectual abilities, as in dementia; no predominant disturbance of mood, as in organic affective syndrome; no predominant delusions or hallucinations, as in organic delusional syndrome or organic hallucinosis.
C. Evidence, from history, physical examination, or laboratory tests, of a specific organic factor that is judged to be etiologically related to the disturbance.
D. This diagnosis is not given to a child or adolescent if the clinical picture is limited to the features that characterize attention deficit disorder.

Reproduced with permission from DSM-III, pp. 119–120.

The presentation is influenced by the nature and location of the etiologic process. In one common clinical picture, there is explosiveness, emotional lability, or sudden, inappropriate tearfulness. Social restrictions may be openly violated without concern. For other patients, a withdrawn apathetic stance is more common. Irritability, suspiciousness, or frank paranoia may develop and become the predominant clinical feature.

INTOXICATION AND WITHDRAWAL

The diagnostic categories of intoxication and withdrawal are residual categories for substance use–related disorders that do not meet the criteria for one of the preceding syndromes. Intoxication obviously refers to a disturbance in mental function and behavior resulting from recent ingestion of an exogenous substance. Withdrawal involves a change in mentation and behavior following decrease in or abstinence from a previously regularly ingested mood-altering chemical. In both disorders, the clinical picture is influenced by the specific substance used, the baseline personality, the social context, and the physical health of the affected person. (Chapter 5 covers substance use disorders in greater detail.)

ATYPICAL OR MIXED
ORGANIC BRAIN SYNDROME

The residual category for syndromes not meeting the diagnostic criteria for any other syndrome but known to be the result of a specific organic factor is termed atypical or mixed organic brain syndrome.

DIFFERENTIAL DIAGNOSIS

The major differential diagnostic problem in organic brain syndrome and organic mental disorders is to assess whether the presenting clinical problem is in fact organic or nonorganic in its etiology. While this might seem to be obvious and straightforward, the task often is difficult. The difficulty arises from the overlap in signs, symptoms, and behaviors between organic and functional disorders. Specifically, there are functional disorders that can resemble an organic brain syndrome, and there are numerous organically based disorders that can mimic functional psychiatric illnesses. Errors can be made in either direction.

Functional Disorders Presenting as Organic Mental Disorders

This is a more limited group than its converse, but correct diagnosis of the etiology can be critical to outcome. Delirium can be mimicked by the functional psychoses (e.g., schizophrenia or mania), especially when sleep deprivation is prominent. The distinction usually becomes obvious quickly, and there is no associated organic pathology. More common is the problem of distinguishing depressive pseudodementia from organically based dementia, especially in the elderly. Depressed individuals frequently complain of memory difficulties, and they tend to score lower on memory testing. Elderly patients may already be showing some decrease in memory function. There typically may be concurrent medical illnesses. In such cases, severe depression (often to the point of inertia and apathy) with prominent memory deficit may be quite hard to recognize. It is essential to obtain a very careful evaluation of the patient's present condition and previous history, family history, and mental status examination. Past depressive episodes, fluctuating memory performance, and any evidence of depressed mood should alert the evaluator to the role of depression. Neuroendocrine testing (for example, the dexamethasone suppression test) may prove useful. Finally, a clinical trial of antidepressant medication or electroconvulsive therapy should be actively undertaken if there is any possibility of response.

A third disorder that can resemble an organic brain syndrome is *factitious disorder with psychological symptoms*. Here the individual voluntarily produces symptoms similar to any mental disorder, including the organic disorders. The motivation is to become a patient. Gross inability to answer simple questions such as "What is your name?" or persistently approximate but inaccurate answers should raise the possibility of a factitious disorder.

Organic Mental Disorders Presenting as Functional Disorders

Many organic processes, with less global effect on brain function than occurs in delirium or dementia, can cause syndromes that are similar in clinical presentation to psychiatric illnesses with no demonstrable organic basis. Disturbances of thinking, reality test, perception, sensation, mood, affect, and personality can be caused by a variety of organic disorders.

Organic Delusional Syndrome. There are numerous organic causes of delusional syndromes that can prove very difficult to distinguish by clinical picture alone from functional schizophrenia, paranoid disorder, or mania. The most frequent cause is substance abuse. Cannabis, hallucinogen, phencyclidine, cocaine, and amphetamine abuse can be virtually identical to functional delusional disorders. Paranoia usually predominates and can persist for days to months. Huntington's chorea and interictal temporal lobe epilepsy may also present with a schizophreniform picture. Finally, various other cerebral lesions, particularly of the nondominant hemisphere, can produce a delusional picture. Corticosteroids can definitely produce or release delusional ideation in a clear sensorium and should always be suspect when identifed as present.

Organic Hallucinosis. The most common diagnostic problems result from substance abuse, especially abuse of alcohol and hallucinogens. Focal seizure states can be difficult to recognize when generating chiefly perceptual effects, whether visual, auditory, or somatic.

Organic Affective Syndrome. The differential diagnosis of affective disorders is probably the most difficult and most often encountered problem of this section. The organic causes of mood disturbance are extensive and prevalent in routine medical practice and contemporary life. Once again, substance abuse leads in being able to produce either a manic or depressive picture. Amphetamine and cocaine intoxication can produce a very manic appearance. Conversely, withdrawal from amphetamines, can result in a profound depression. Withdrawal from alcohol or almost every illicitly used drug can be followed by significantly depressive features. Prescription drugs known to produce mania include anticholinergic drugs, adrenocorticotropic hormone (ACTH), and various corticosteroids. Depression, on the other hand, can be caused by reserpine, methyldopa, other dopaminergic and catecholaminergic medications, and corticosteroids.

Endocrine disturbances of the pituitary, thyroid, and adrenal glands can cause major mood changes. Severe head trauma has been reported to produce manic episodes in individuals with no history of bipolar disorders in themselves or their family.

Organic Personality Syndrome. The diagnostic problem for organic personality syndrome results from the frequent presentation of the patient complaining of personality changes or of the family complaining about the potential patient's personality change. There is no organic label attached. It can be all too easy to fit the personality traits into a psychological framework—for example, a life-adjustment crisis. There is no certain diagnostic formula here, but a good clinician should take a detailed history and baseline personality description.

Previously well-adapted, adjusted patients without a family history of psychiatric disturbance should cause a high degree of suspicion. The potential causes for an organic personality change are vast, and only a complete workup will suffice.

Organic Mental Disorders

There are numerous specific etiologies for each of the organic brain syndromes that have been described. There are, therefore, many different patterns of onset, course, and complications. The following section will review the most commonly encountered etiologies and associated features. It is important to appreciate that OBS and many specific organic mental disorders can occur at any age; they are not confined to the geriatric population. Nearly all of the organic brain syndromes and disorders can be caused by factors either occurring within the central nervous system or acting on the nervous system from a more distant site. The etiology, course, and complications will be discussed in sequence.

DELIRIUM

The possible causes of delirium include acute and chronic diseases of all types of all systems. Appropriate laboratory evaluation is obviously indicated to rule out certain possibilities; the following partial list of which has been adapted from Lipowski (1980b).

1. Intoxication: drugs of abuse, prescribed medications, or polypharmacy even at therapeutic doses; industrial agents; heavy metals
2. Withdrawal syndromes: especially from alcohol, sedatives, and hypnotics
3. Metabolic encephalopathies: hepatic, renal, pulmonary failure, hypoxia, hypoglycemia, vitamin deficiencies, endocrine disorders, fluid and electrolyte imbalance, and errors of metabolism
4. Infections: systemic and intracranial bacterial, viral, protozoal, and parasitic
5. Seizure disorders
6. Systemic illnesses: porphyria, lupus, other collagen vascular diseases, and sickle cell disease
7. Head injury
8. Vascular and cardiovascular diseases, including arrythmias and congestive heart failure
9. Intracranial tumor
10. Cerebral degenerative diseases: multiple sclerosis, Alzheimer's disease, Huntington's chorea, Parkinson's disease, Pick's disease

The course of delirium depends on the underlying etiology and its treatment. Delirium develops rapidly and may fluctuate in intensity of clouding of consciousness and agitation. There is a lengthened risk of falling and secondary injury. Random physical lashing out may occur, and adequate medical treatment may be hindered.

DEMENTIA

The most common forms of dementia, primary degenerative disorders, are usually insidious in onset and progress over a period of years, eventually leading to death. Other forms may be sudden in onset and not progress beyond a certain point (e.g., brain injury due to trauma or surgery). Some forms of dementia may be treated and reversed (e.g., normal pressure hydrocephalus). Dementia is a syndrome, not an etiology, and specific etiologies must always be sought.

In 222 patients evaluated for dementia (Wells, 1978) the diagnoses were:

Atrophy of unknown cause	51%
Vascular disease	8%
Normal pressure hydrocephalus	6%
Dementia in alcoholics	6%
Intracranial masses	5%
Huntington's chorea	5%
Depression	4%
Drug toxicity	3%
Dementia (uncertain)	3%
Other	9%

The category *atrophy of unknown cause* probably represents, for the most part, Alzheimer's disease. Other potential causes are central nervous system infection, including neurosyphilis, and viral, bacterial, or fungal infections; toxic-metabolic disturbance, such as vitamin deficiency, pernicious anemia, or thyroid disease; multiple sclerosis; Parkinson's disease, and anoxia. Dementia is categorized in Table 4-5.

Table 4-5. Common Dementias

A. Primary degenerative dementia, senile onset:
1. Uncomplicated
2. With delirum
3. With delusions
4. With depression
B. Primary degenerative dementia, presenile onset.
C. Multiinfarct dementia.

Primary degenerative dementia is nearly always caused by Alzheimer's disease or, less frequently, by Pick's disease. Alzheimer's and Pick's diseases were described around the turn of the century and had been called presenile dementia. There are no clinical features specific to Alzheimer's and Pick's diseases. Likewise, only age of onset separates senile (age 65 and older) from presenile dementia (under 65). At autopsy, patients with Alzheimer's disease have characteristic histopathologic features: senile plaques and neurofibrillary degeneration, both found in large numbers through the cortex. The rarer Pick's disease is characterized by distinctive lobar atrophy, primarily affecting the frontal and temporal lobes and less extensively the occipital and parietal lobes, with sharp distinction between affected and unaffected lobes. Both diseases involve loss of neurons and glial proliferation. The degree of mental deterioration has been directly correlated to the quantity of lost brain tissue, the density of plaques and neurofibrillary tangles, and degree of ischemic damage. In both conditions computerized tomographic (CT) scan characteristically demonstrates brain atrophy with enlarged sulci and ventricles. Dementia, however, is a clinical condition and not a CT scan finding. There is only a partial correlation between radiologic findings and clinical change. Psychometric evaluation may be more sensitive. Dementia should be diagnosed only when there is deterioration of intellectual abilities severe enough to interfere with social or occupational functioning.

Multiinfarct dementia is the correct term for what has too often and erroneously been called arteriosclerotic organic brain syndrome. The latter has been a common diagnosis in geriatric wards of state hospitals and nursing homes. It has often been made because the patient was found to have hypertension or cardiac illness, presumably secondary to atherosclerois. When thoroughly evaluated, however, fewer than 10 percent of these patients are shown to have dementia caused by vascular disease. Multiinfarct dementia is a clinical entity with demonstrable pathologic changes in cerebral blood vessels and multiple areas of brain softening. Clinically, the dementia has a less uniformly deteriorating course than in Alzheimer's or Pick's disease, and has more of a stepwise progression. There are usually more extensive physical findings on neurologic examination, with focal sensory and motor signs, gait disturbances, and reflex asymmetry. Difficulty in talking and swallowing frequently accompanies dementia symptoms and is presumed to be a result of vascular accidents in areas of the brain other than those controlling higher cortical functions. Other physical findings of vascular disease (e.g., bruits or hypertension) are common.

Other dementias, while less frequent individually, comprise up to 40 percent of those cases diagnosed as demented. While there are many neurologic conditions with dementia as a prominent feature, distinguishing among them requires a proper history, including family history; physical examination, including thorough neurologic examination; appropriate laboratory evaluation, including CT scan, electroencephalogram (EEG), serologic studies, thyroid function tests, and tests for levels of folate and vitamin B_{12}; liver function tests; and, depending on the results, further special tests (e.g., cerebrospinal fluid measles antibody titer, to evaluate for subacute sclerosing panencephalitis resulting from measles; copper metabolism studies to rule out Wilson's disease).

Huntington's chorea is a progressive neurologic illness characterized by chorea, multiple psychiatric symptoms, and progressive dementia, leading to death. It is generally transmitted as an autosomal dominant and onset is usually during mid-adulthood (25 to 50 years old). Presenting complaints may be psychological, with anxiety as a very common first symptom. Early intellectual deterioration may be the presenting symptom problem. There is no effective treatment.

Normal pressure hydrocephalus is caused by disorders of cerebrospinal fluid absorption from any of a number of causes. Cerebrospinal fluid pressure is not elevated, and there are no symptoms (e.g., pain) or signs (e.g., papilledema) of increased cranial pressure. CT scan or pneumoencephalogram reveals enlarged lateral ventricles, widened basilar cisterns and atrophic changes. Clinical presentation may be with symptoms of dementia, gait disturbances, or incontinence (or a combination of these). Personality changes are prominent, with unusual or embarrassing behavior, and marked indifference to social consequences; these can be the first symptoms. Treatment, which involves surgical shunting of the cerebrospinal fluid, is effective in halting the process or reversing some symptoms in approximately half of the cases.

Chronic subdural hematomas, neoplasms, vitamin B_{12} deficiency, multiple sclerosis, thiamine deficiency, and petit mal epilepsy in children are all treatable causes of conditions that resemble dementia. There are rare, progressive, dementing diseases that offer intriguing clues to the development of such illnesses. Slow viruses have been demonstrated to cause or be highly suspected of causing dementias. Subacute sclerosing panencephalitis (SSPE) is a progressive fatal disease that occurs from 2 to 10 years of age after measles infection and has been demonstrated to be caused by the measles virus. Progressive rubella panencephalitis is rarer and thought to be caused by the rubella virus. JD virus, a papovavirus, has been associated with progressive multifocal leukoencephalopathy. Kuru is known to be caused in New Guinea cannibals by the eating of affected human brains. Jakob-Creutzfeldt disease is thought to be transmitted by an as-yet-unidentifiable filterable particle and has been transmitted by corneal transplant.

AMNESTIC SYNDROME

The amnestic syndrome may result from any bilateral damage to certain diencephalic and medical temporal structures (e.g., mamillary bodies, fornix, hippocampal complex). The most common etiology is thiamine deficiency associated with chronic alcohol abuse. Other causes include head trauma, surgery, hypoxia, posterior cerebral artery infarction, and herpes simplex encephalitis. The course is usually a chronic one; however, in the case of thiamine deficiency, rapid and sustained replacement therapy may lead to significant improvement continuing for up to several months. Severe memory impairment produces obvious complications for self-care and independent functioning.

ORGANIC DELUSIONAL SYNDROME, HALLUCINOSIS, AND PERSONALITY SYNDROME

Etiologic factors which are extremely numerous and diverse, are covered in the discussion of differential diagnosis. The course is dependent on the primary etiologic process and its treatment.

Management and Treatment

Management refers to behavioral and symptomatic control and treatment to curative interventions, which are obviously quite different for different pathologic processes. For the primary degenerative disorders, there is no effective treatment to date. For substance-induced intoxications, supportive and behavioral control measures may be indicated. In patients undergoing withdrawal, it may be necessary to replace the recently discontinued alcohol or drug with a medication that has similar actions to allow for stabilization of nervous system functions and controlled detoxification.

In most organic brain syndromes and mental disorders, however, there is an immediate demand to alleviate and control the manifest signs, symptoms, and behaviors. For purposes of this chapter, this immediate intervention will be called management.

DELIRIUM

Management of delirium can be quite challenging. This syndrome can be characterized by wide fluctuations in intensity with periods of marked agitation. Virtually all delirious patients require close observation, intensive nursing care, and general medical support. Maintenance of adequate fluid intake is essential. Effort should be made to decrease excessive stimulation; however, loss of adequate sensory input, such as occurs in isolation or darkness, usually lowers the level of consciousness further and paradoxically leads to an increase in agitation. Pharmacologic intervention should occur only when necessary and with a minimum of overt sedation. The neuroleptics are often employed; haloperidol, which is currently in favor, is given in intramuscular or oral doses of 0.5 to 5 mg. Treatment should always begin at a low dosage until the patient's tolerance and response can be assessed. Hypnotics and sedatives should be avoided and polypharmacy (the use of multiple medications) minimized. Medication is no substitute for human contact, however, and should never be used as such. Simple physical contact and reassurance may prove most effective. Orienting cues such as a calendar, a clock, and adequate lighting are crucial. Comments to the patient should include basic orienting information at short intervals.

DEMENTIA

Treatable causes of dementia or dementiform illnesses are present in a minority of cases but should always be sought. A full review of these etiologies and treatments is beyond the scope of this chapter (see Lipowski, 1980b).

Management of dementia can present its own unique challenges. First of all, it is essential to recall that the individual with this disorder is highly vulnerable to changes and stresses of all types. Environmental familiarity and stability should be sought. A simple change in location can produce a marked clinical deterioration. Medical treatments including medications should be undertaken with the individual's increased central nervous system sensitivity always under consideration. It is quite easy to produce a delirium superimposed on the dementia. As in delirium, careful supervision, orienting cues, and reassurances can prove invaluable. Pharmacologic intervention, again, tends to focus on the neuroleptics; haloperidol and thioridazine (for its low extrapyramidal effects) are used quite often.

In dementias, time is an important factor to consider. The gradual deterioration that is frequently encountered can be extremely difficult for family members and close friends. There may be unresolved sadness, frustration, and anger about the patient. Anger, when unacknowledged, can lead to much guilt in response to the desire to be rid of this person, who may no longer resemble the long-beloved one. A good clinician will be available to family and encourage an open recognition of and practical adaptation to the strains involved.

AMNESTIC SYNDROME

Treatment of amnestic syndrome, of course, depends on etiology. Management is chiefly an exercise in long-term supervision and protection.

ORGANIC DELUSIONAL SYNDROME AND HALLUCINOSIS

Neuroleptic medication, it should be recalled, is nonspecific in terms of the etiology of the disorder and is effective in organic as well as functional psychotic states. The effectiveness may eventually be undermined by the primary disease process but this is a late phenomenon.

Response to neuroleptic medication, then, should be seen as a practical, not a diagnostic, event.

ORGANIC AFFECTIVE SYNDROME
Treatment and management of organic affective syndrome are similar to those of the primary affective disorders discussed in Chapters 7 and 8. If any etiologic factor can be removed or counteracted, of course, those steps should be taken.

ORGANIC PERSONALITY SYNDROME
Management of organic personality syndrome attempts to minimize demands placed on the patient, to provide a highly structured environment, and to decrease irritability and impulsivity with low-dose neuroleptic medication.

Psychiatric Manifestations of Seizure Disorders
Seizure disorders can have serious psychological and behavioral features that can be of such a nature and intensity as to lead to psychiatric evaluation and treatment. This evaluation and treatment can be sought even without a recognition of the underlying seizure problem. It is the purpose of this section to emphasize the psychiatric aspects of epilepsy (seizure disorders) so as to facilitate (1) accurate recognition of epileptic disorders contributing to the manifest psychiatric disorder, and (2) proper management and treatment of the combined disorders.

Temporal lobe and focal epilepsy were referred to previously under the differential diagnosis of organic delusional syndrome and hallucinosis. It is also important to recognize the potential etiologic significance of seizure states in diverse behavioral and psychiatric disturbances. The term *epilepsy* refers to the clinical aberrations of mood, cognition, sensation, consciousness, and behavior caused by neuronal hyperactivity and hypersynchronous discharge. Cortical electrical manifestations of the discharge can often, but not always, be detected by EEG recordings of the impulses that manage to extend through meninges, skull, and scalp. There are many varieties of epilepsy, the most familiar being grand mal seizures and focal seizures. Grand mal seizures are of subcortical origin and cause rapid loss of consciousness and onset of violent tonic and clonic striated muscle contractions. Focal seizures affect limited areas of the brain and have a wide variety of behavioral effects. In one example, Jacksonian seizures, the patient is conscious and aware of the progression of seizure activity over the area of the body; at any one time, the seizure may affect only the single limb controlled by the area of the brain to which the abnormal electrical discharge has spread. Even a general discussion of the wide varieties of epilepsies and their anatomic and physiologic causes, treatments, and sequelae is beyond the scope of this chapter, and the reader can refer to standard neurology texts for further study.

The identification and treatment of epilepsy are important in psychiatry and general medicine for many reasons. Certain types of epilepsy cause symptoms that are primarily behavioral or mood altering and are often mistaken for functional psychiatric conditions, such as schizophrenia or hysterical episodes. Readily recognized epileptic conditions (such as grand mal seizures) may have strong emotional complications or personality effects. Patients and families may live in dread of attacks or may futilely deny the reality of the illness, thereby making proper medical help very difficult or impossible.

There are many causes of epilepsy: trauma, infections, vascular accidents, tumors, degenerative neurologic disorders, drugs and toxins, metabolic disorders, and birth trauma or congenital malformations. There is evidence for a genetic contribution in some cases. Everyone has the potential for seizure activity, and the threshold for response to a seizure-inducing stimulus varies widely from person to person.

In general, epilepsy can be caused by any disorder of brain metabolism that promotes the development and spread of abnormal impulses. Recurrent attacks are presumed to be related to the development of an *epileptogenic focus* causing brain tissue irritation; one possible cause is scar tissue secondary to trauma, stroke, tumor, or abscess. The clinical manifestation of the epilepsy depends on the area of the brain immediately affected and the pattern of spread.

Epilepsy is most commonly misdiagnosed as being a functional psychiatric disorder when it takes the form of petit mal or psychomotor seizures.

PETIT MAL SEIZURES
Petit mal seizures usually affect only children and younger adolescents and are rarely seen in adults. The most common form is *petit mal absence,* a brief (seconds long) loss of contact with the environment. The child appears to stare blankly and there may be brief muscle twitches (three per second) around the eyes and bilateral symmetrical movement of the limbs. The child is unaware of the absence and may resume activity or conversation as if nothing had happened. The attacks can occur with great frequency (up to hundreds per day), although a rate of five to ten per day is more common. The EEG pattern is very characteristic and consists of sudden interruption of the normal pattern with generalized, bilaterally synchronous spike and wave patterns of high amplitude, at a rate of three per second (Kiloh et al., 1972). Patients are often referred for psychiatric treatment for day dreaming, poor school performance, abnormal peer relations and social adjustment, and other emotional problems. Children with frequent episodes may suffer marked academic and social consequences and secondary psychological problems. Treatment with the anticonvulsant succinimides and oxazolidines is usually successful, and episodes generally decrease markedly by early or middle adolescence. The etiology is not known. Up to 40 percent of children with petit mal epilepsy develop grand mal seizures (Detre and Jarecki, 1975).

PSYCHOMOTOR SEIZURES
Psychomotor seizures "are the complex behavioral and experiential manifestations of ongoing epileptic discharge" (Lishman, 1978). They cause a large variety of complex, unusual, and sometimes bizarre perceptions, mood changes and behavioral patterns, many of which can be mistaken for purely psychological problems. Other terms used include complex partial seizures, fugues, temporal lobe epilepsy, and twilight states. Many of these patients have a temporal lobe focus but 10 to 20 percent of patients with a demonstrable temporal lobe focus (such as a tumor) have only grand mal seizures. In most of the attacks (80 to 90 percent), the origin is in a temporal lobe, particularly involving the amygdala, Ammon's horn, insula, or temporal pole.

Diagnosis
Patients with psychomotor seizures experience a number of symptoms that may not be recognized as epileptic. Autonomic effects and visceral sensations may include dizziness, churning sensations in the stomach and throat, and vague pain. Unusual perceptual experiences, such as sensation of déjà vu (familiarity) or jamais vu (strangeness), the feeling that events may have special significance, and the sense of being removed from reality as well as feelings of derealization and depersonalization are common. A frequent complaint is the feeling of being outside of one's self and looking down at the self and others as if watching a play. One patient described feeling suddenly as if he and the people he was with were two-dimensional figures on a postcard while he was watching with detachment. Unusual hallucinations, particularly of taste and smell, may be accompanied by lip smacking, shouting, grimacing or unusual grunting, growling, or making animallike vocalizations. Cognition may

be severely affected, with transient thought confusion, racing, or incoherence. Some patients experience time distortions, during which events may seem to be occurring with extreme slowness, feel "out of sync," or appear to be racing. Strong, sudden, rapidly changing emotions—fear, joy, crying, euphoria, depression, guilt, and others—may be experienced. Psychomotor seizures can also cause complex, automatic behavior patterns. There may be repetitive actions, subtle or bizarre, and potentially grossly inappropriate (such as undressing in public).

These unusual symptoms should be specifically sought when evaluating patients for possible psychiatric illness. Many symptoms are embarrassing or frightening; often patients do not remember an entire sequence of events, and the seizurelike behavior may be reported only by family members or friends.

Aberrant behavior related to cerebral dysrhythmias and ameliorated by anticonvulsants can be very complex; such behavior may strongly resemble not only psychiatric illness but also antisocial behavior.

Epileptic illnesses are sometimes misdiagnosed as functional psychiatric disorders. Common misconceptions are probably responsible in some instances. Many seizure disorders *do not* cause unconsciousness, memory loss, incontinence, or grand mal tonic-clonic movement. EEG changes may not be found, and the EEG may need to be repeated many times in patients with highly suspect behaviors. Hysterical seizures or behavior *do not* rule out a true seizure disorder. Many patients with hysterical or feigned attacks have clear-cut EEG seizure patterns during some of their episodes. Seizures are dramatic events that cause a great deal of attention, and the "secondary gain" may be sufficient to lead to hysterical seizures as well. (In a similar way, myocardial infarction patients may have cardiac symptoms that are not organically based.)

The clinician should suspect the presence of a seizure disorder in a patient whose symptoms develop and recede suddenly when: (1) symptoms are similar or identical from one episode to the next; (2) there is a family or personal history of seizure disorder, motor fits, or unexplained episodes of unconsciousness; (3) the patient describes a sense of premonition or *aura* that precedes each episode; (4) there are focal motor manifestations, particularly stereotyped ones, during the episodes; (5) the patient seems vague and confused for a brief time after the episode subsides; and (6) at the conclusion of the episode, the patient is unable to remember what his or her behavior was like during its course (Detre and Jarecki, 1971).

Management

The treatment of choice for psychomotor seizures is carbamazepine, an anticonvulsant that is related chemically to the tricyclic antidepressants. The initial dose is 200 mg twice per day, increasing if needed to 1,200 mg per day. If carbamazepine is not tolerated, phenytoin and phenobarbital may be used.

Psychiatric complications of seizure disorders are numerous. Personality disorders have been reported in up to 50 percent of patients with temporal lobe epilepsy and in many patients with grand mal and other types of epilepsy. It is not known whether the personality disorders and changes are a result of the psychological and social stress connected with epilepsy, the effects of seizure activity on brain function and tissue, or the organic factors that have contributed to the seizure disorder. Psychological effects of the anticipation and consequences of seizures may include anxiety, frustration, social inhibitions, disturbed relationships, and other emotional losses. Patients with seizure disorders should be supported and treated with sensitivity to their justifiable and imagined concerns. Effective psychiatric intervention may prove possible only when there has been more complete control of the seizure activity. On the other hand, successful emotional and behavioral assistance may promote better seizure control.

Case 1. A 58-year-old overweight patient with congestive heart failure, hypertension that was difficult to control, mild adult-onset diabetes, rheumatoid arthritis, asthma, and peripheral neuropathies had been a patient at a medical clinic for many years. Each of her medical problems was being treated with at least one and up to three prescribed medications. In her early 40s she developed slowly progressive symptoms of dementia of unknown etiology, and she was treated in a state hospital for five to six years until released to live in a transitional living facility designed to reintegrate chronic mental patients to community living. The living facility was loosely supervised but the patient had not caused trouble and the staff and ever-changing residents at the medical clinic gradually accommodated to her cognitive impairments and paid little attention to them as the years went by. Medical students involved in her case changed every three months while the patient came nearly every week, usually without appointment, with varying complaints and with nearly all of her multiple medical problems at least mildly out of control. Review of her voluminous medical record revealed that for more than 10 years resident after resident had started fresh with new medication adjustments, hoping to improve on the obvious failure of the preceding resident, only to end the tour of duty as frustrated as the next was doomed to be. The patient was always pleasant and would chat for hours with the receptionist and other patients. The staff at her group home always accompanied her to the pharmacy to pay her bill and turned the medications over to the patient. A psychiatric intern on a medication rotation conducted a brief mental status examination and discovered anew that the patient could not do simple, one-figure addition, could not name the president (answered "FDR" in 1976), did not know the year, could not follow a three-stage direction, could not cross the midline in terms of left-right discriminations, and had other symptoms of marked cognitive impairment. When asked how she knew what medications to take she said that she took them from a jar. Further investigation revealed that for years the patient had taken each of her carefully thought out and dutifully filled prescriptions and mixed them all in one large jar in her room. She took some of the pills four times a day. Thereafter the staff directly supervised her medication taking, resulting in slight but measurable improvement in most of her medical problems, less frustration among the residents, and no change in frequency of clinic visits, which she continued to enjoy.

References and Further Reading

Benson, F.D., Blumer, D. *Psychiatric Aspects of Neurologic Disease.* New York: Grune & Stratton, 1975.

Detre, T.P., and Jarecki, H.G. *Modern Psychiatric Treatment.* New York: Grune & Stratton, 1975.

Freedman, A.M., Kaplan, H., Sadock, B. (eds.). *Comprehensive Textbook of Psychiatry,* 3rd ed. Baltimore: Williams & Wilkins, 1980.

Kiloh, L.G., McComas, A.J., Osselton, J.W. *Clinical Electroencephalography,* 3rd. ed. London: Butterworths, 1972.

Lipowski, Z.J. A new look at organic brain syndromes. *Am. J. Psychiatry,* 137:674–678, 1980a.

Lipowski, Z.J. Organic Mental Disorders: Introduction and Review of Syndromes. In A.M. Freedman, H. Kaplan, B. Sadock (eds.), *Comprehensive Textbook of Psychiatry,* 3rd ed., Baltimore: Williams & Wilkins, 1980b.

Lishman, W.A. *Organic Psychiatry: The Psychological Consequences of Cerebral Disorders.* Oxford: Blackwell Scientific Publications, 1978.

Mulder, D.W. Organic Mental Disorders Associated with Diseases of Unknown Causes. In A.M. Freedman, H. Kaplan, B. Sadock (eds.), *Comprehensive Textbook of Psychiatry,* 3rd ed., Baltimore: Williams & Wilkins, 1980.

Weiss, G., Hechtman, L., Perlman, T., et al. Hyperactives as young adults. *Arch. Gen. Psychiatry* 36:675–681, 1979.

Wells, C.E. Chronic brain disease: an overview. *Am. J. Psychiatry* 135:1–12, 1978.

Wender, P.H., Reimherr, F.W., Wood, D.R. Attention deficit disorder ("minimal brain dysfunction") in adults. *Arch. Gen. Psychiatry* 38:449–456, 1981.

Substance Use Disorders
C. GIBSON DUNN, M.D.

The substance use disorders discussed in this chapter include the pathologic mood and behavioral changes resulting from abuse of or dependence on chemical substances acting on the central nervous system. Such abuse or dependence is considered pathologic when it alters mood or behavior in a culturally unacceptable way. In the *Diagnostic and Statistical Manual of Mental Disorders,* Third Edition (DSM-III), the substance use disorders and the substance-induced organic mental disorders constitute separate diagnostic categories; aspects of both are discussed in this chapter. The substance use disorders in DSM-III include five classes of chemicals—alcohol, barbiturates and other sedatives and hypnotics, opioids, amphetamines and related sympathomimetics, and cannabis (and derivatives). By far the most widely used and abused chemical is alcohol (ethanol). Alcoholism, the excessive use of or dependence on alcohol, is truly one of the most ancient and painful of mankind's self-inflicted diseases. Nearly one-half of the United States population uses alcohol; of these 100 million or more individuals, as many as 9 to 14 million may be addicted to the point that they can be diagnosed as alcoholic. One in five alcoholics will also abuse one or more drugs from the other four categories. Many thousands in addition will abuse one of these other substances without pathologic alcohol use pattern. It is now estimated that between 3 and 5 percent of males and 0.1 to 1 percent of females have a substance use disorder of some type. These are undoubtedly underestimates, possibly substantial ones. The financial cost of such a massive illness is now estimated to exceed $40 billion per year. The human cost in terms of individual suffering, impaired physical health, broken marriages, damaged children, and premature death is incalculable. It is estimated that nearly one-half of all fatal traffic accidents, murders, suicides, child abuse, and violent crime involve abuse of alcohol or drug, or both.

Historically, men have been diagnosed as suffering from one of these disorders three to five times more frequently than have women. This ratio is now seen to be declining, unfortunately not because the rate for men has dropped but because the incidence in women has increased. The onset of alcoholism has generally been estimated to occur in the late teens to the late twenties in men and in the late twenties through the thirties in women. Unfortunately, this pattern is also changing, and there is a strong tendency toward earlier onset. It is not at all uncommon in clinical practice today to encounter adolescents in their middle teenage years (14 to 16 years old) who give a history of well-established substance abuse disorder since the age of 8 years. Despite these overwhelming facts, our society continually denies the significance of the problem, while claiming that the disorders are hopeless. Both attitudes are erroneous: substance abuse disorders of all types exist and are treatable.

This chapter is divided broadly into two sections. The first section, Medical Descriptive Model, covers the diagnostic and symptomatic patterns of the substance use disorders including withdrawal states and their management. The second section, Rehabilitative Model, includes a broader look at the course of the substance use illnesses, their treatment, and the total recovery process. This approach, while used less frequently in psychiatric and medical textbooks, is by far the more valuable as a basis for providing significant long-term help to a person suffering from one of these disorders. Optimal understanding and management should depend on both approaches.

Medical Descriptive Model

CONCEPTS OF SUBSTANCE ABUSE AND DEPENDENCE

An initial distinction should be made between the concept of abuse and that of dependence. The term *substance abuse* as employed in DSM-III involves the following aspects: (1) a pattern of pathologic use, (2) impairment in social or occupational functioning due to substance use, and (3) minimum duration of disturbance of at least one month. Pathologic use can be difficult to distinguish from the more extreme end of socially sanctioned use. For practical purposes, however, pathologic use refers to one or more of the following: prolonged periods of intoxication, repeated unsuccessful efforts to control use, inability to stop use despite disturbed behavior or social reasons to do so, the need for frequent use in order to function, and repeated episodes of complications caused by substance use. Impairment in social or occupational functioning resulting from substance use can include any of the major areas of normal day-to-day functioning, including the family, work, social contacts, other interpersonal behavior, or legal difficulties. Work difficulties usually involve decreasing performance, tardiness, absences, or failure to advance relative to inherent abilities. Family complications run the gamut from increased irritability to explosive anger, abusiveness, unreliability, and emotional unavailability. Physical or psychological deterioration can also occur, leading to impairment in one or more of the areas defined above. Mood lability, impaired judgment, depression, paranoia, or globally decreased cognitive functioning also have an adverse effect on any or all of the core areas of basic function. The requirement for a duration of one month may be met by the repeated rather than continuous appearance of the abuse pattern, and daily impairment is not essential for the diagnosis.

Substance dependence in DSM-III refers to the physiologic dependence demonstrated by physical tolerance and withdrawal. *Tolerance* refers to a physiologic change in which increasing amounts of the substance are required to achieve a typical effect of the substance or a given amount of the substance has a decreasing effect on the individual. The *withdrawal syndromes*, which vary widely among the five classes of substances of abuse, will be discussed under individual headings.

An additional important concept is that of *cross-dependence*—the ability to obtain a similar physical mood-altering effect from substances in different categories. Most typically, individuals can substitute alcohol and one of the barbiturate/sedative drugs for one another. Individuals dependent on one or another substance may take advantage of this interchangeability, and the substances are often combined to achieve a synergistic effect. It is less well appreciated by physicians now generally practicing in this area that opioids and other substances that depress the central nervous system are often interchanged. This concept of cross-dependence, then, has major implications for treatment, since rehabilitating an individual from dependence on one substance then implies that abstinence from substances in the other categories is necessary to prevent the illness pattern from recurring or worsening.

A final note on terminology should include the concept of *addiction*. This term is rather carelessly utilized to refer to substance abuse, to substance dependence (either psychological or physical), or to a substance-seeking behavior that can be quite compulsive. In this chapter the term addiction will be employed to refer to any disorder in which the affected individual feels compelled to seek a substance in order to maintain a sense of well-being. It is, therefore, a behavioral concept rather than one that describes actual physical dependence.

SPECIFIC SUBSTANCES OF ABUSE AND DEPENDENCE

DSM-III focuses on five classes of substances known to be abused and produce physical dependence, as well as three categories of substances known to be abused without leading to dependence. The five substances of abuse and dependence, as noted at the beginning of the chapter, are (1) alcohol, (2) barbiturates and similarly acting sedatives and hypnotics, (3) opiates, (4) amphetamines and similarly acting sympathomimetics, and (5) cannabis and derivatives. The three categories known to be abused without physical dependence are (1) hallucinogens, (2) phencyclidine, and (3) cocaine. Tobacco dependence is recognized, although tobacco abuse is not.

Alcohol Abuse and Dependence

Alcohol abuse and dependence, globally referred to as alcoholism, are the most common substance use disorders. The pervasiveness of this abuse disorder is almost unimaginable to individuals who do not work in the field. In the United States, misuse of alcohol may affect as many as one in four people, some of whom may be adversely affected by alcoholism within their families. Alcohol abuse may follow quite variable patterns. There have been elaborate efforts, most notably by Jellinek, to classify alcoholic disorders into definable categories. Most easily observed, as emphasized in DSM-III, are those of chronic daily alcohol abuse, episodic binge drinking, and heavy weekend drinking. The diagnostic criteria for alcohol abuse, which were generally outlined in the discussion of substance abuse, are presented in Table 5-1. The criteria for alcohol dependence include those for alcohol abuse together with the added factor of tolerance or withdrawal (see Table 5-2).

Table 5-1. Diagnostic Criteria for Alcohol Abuse

A. *Pattern of pathological alcohol use:* need for daily use of alcohol for adequate functioning; inability to cut down or stop drinking; repeated efforts to control or reduce excess drinking by "going on the wagon" (periods of temporary abstinence) or restricting drinking to certain times of the day; binges (remaining intoxicated throughout the day for at least two days); occasional consumption of a fifth of spirits (or its equivalent in wine or beer); amnesic periods for events occurring while intoxicated (blackouts); continuation of drinking despite a serious physical disorder that the individual knows is exacerbated by alcohol use; drinking of nonbeverage alcohol.

B. *Impairment in social or occupational functioning due to alcohol use:* e.g., violence while intoxicated, absence from work, loss of job, legal difficulties (e.g., arrest for intoxicated behavior, traffic accidents while intoxicated), arguments or difficulties with family or friends because of excessive alcohol use.

C. Duration of disturbance of at least one month.

Reproduced with permission from *Diagnostic and Statistical Manual of Mental Disorders,* 3rd ed. Washington, D.C.: American Psychiatric Association, 1980, pp. 169–170.

Table 5-2. Diagnostic Criteria for Alcohol Dependence

A. Either a pattern of pathological alcohol use or impairment in social or occupational functioning due to alcohol use:

Pattern of pathological alcohol use: need for daily use of alcohol for adequate functioning; inability to cut down or stop drinking; repeated efforts to control or reduce excess drinking by "going on the wagon" (periods of temporary abstinence) or restricting drinking to certain times of the day; binges (remaining intoxicated throughout the day for at least two days); occasional consumption of a fifth of spirits (or its equivalent in wine or beer); amnesic periods for events occurring while intoxicated (blackouts); continuation of drinking despite a serious physical disorder that the individual knows is exacerbated by alcohol use; drinking of nonbeverage alcohol.

Impairment in social or occupational functioning due to alcohol use: e.g., violence while intoxicated, absence from work, loss of job, legal difficulties (e.g., arrest for intoxicated behavior, traffic accidents while intoxicated), arguments or difficulties with family or friends because of excessive alcohol use.

B. Either tolerance or withdrawal:

Tolerance: need for markedly increased amounts of alcohol to achieve the desired effect, or markedly diminished effect with regular use of the same amount.

Withdrawal: development of alcohol withdrawal (e.g., morning "shakes" and malaise relieved by drinking) after cessation of or reduction in drinking.

Reproduced with permission from DSM-III, p. 170.

The National Council on Alcoholism has addressed the diagnostic problem of alcoholism by establishing major and minor criteria.*

I. Major criteria
   A. Physiological and clinical signs
      1. Physical dependence, revealed by withdrawal symptoms when alcohol consumption is decreased—shaking; hearing, seeing, or feeling unreal sensations; delirium tremens with confusion.
      2. Tolerance to alcohol—the mind or body is not as affected by large alcohol intake as it normally would be.
      3. "Blackouts"—the person loses all memory for periods of drinking.
      4. Major alcohol-related physical illnesses, including diseases of the liver, pancreas, stomach, blood, and nervous system.
   B. Behavioral, psychological, and attitudinal signs
      1. Drinking despite strong medical advice against it.
      2. Drinking despite strong obvious social pressure from spouse, other family members, or work associates, or despite being arrested.
      3. The drinker's own awareness of loss of control over alcohol consumption.
II. Minor criteria, which are also highly significant and require several together for a diagnosis of alcoholism
   A. Physiological and clinical signs
      1. Direct effects of alcohol on bodily function, such as heart irregularities, changes in blood vessels, or disorders of the nerves in hands and feet.
      2. Indirect effects, such as night sweats, bruising and cigarette burns from carelessness when intoxicated, or loss of earlier tolerance for large intake.
      3. Laboratory evidence of physical damage from alcohol.

*Criteria taken from *Am. J. Psychiatry* 129(2):127–135, 1977.

   B. Behavioral, psychological, and attitudinal signs
      1. Abnormal drinking pattern, including gulping drinks, hidden drinking, morning drinking, failure to stop, or totally uncontrolled drinking.
      2. Work and social problems secondary to drinking, such as frequently missed work, hanging out with heavy drinkers or in bars, loss of interest in nondrinking friends and activities, multiple car accidents, or job loss.
      3. Use of alcohol to relieve anxiety, sleeplessness, anger, fatigue, depression, or social discomfort.
      4. Family problems related to alcohol abuse, including marital conflict, rage outbursts or even physical attacks on spouse or children, separation or divorce, excessive suspiciousness or jealousy, or withdrawal from normal family life.

This outline is not exhaustive, but it clearly demonstrates that alcoholism can eventually affect every area of life. On the other hand, in the early to middle stages a particular alcoholic may show only some of the signs and symptoms and may easily delude himself or herself by looking only at the unaffected areas of life. Signs of alcoholism may at first appear in any area and should be taken seriously at the start. The basic characteristic throughout all of the diagnostic criteria is the inability to live and function without resorting to alcohol in large quantities despite its destructive effects.

Alcohol Intoxication. As the result of alcohol abuse and dependence, several syndromes of altered central nervous system function may occur. The most obvious and frequent is that of *acute alcohol intoxication*. Alcohol is a central nervous system depressant that is rapidly absorbed through the mucosa of the gastrointestinal tract, although the presence of food or other absorbent substances in the stomach may slow this process. It is eliminated to a small degree through the kidneys and lungs, with the great majority being oxidized in the liver. The average adult may eliminate only one-half to one ounce of liquor per hour. It is quite easy, then, to exceed the body's capacity to detoxify itself from the acute accumulation of ethanol.

Alcohol acts in a sequential fashion on the central nervous system, affecting first the higher cognitive functions and progressing eventually to depress even the basic neurovegetative operations of respiration and cardiovascular function. At a very low blood level, or 0.05 percent, alcohol adversely alters intellectual operations, conscience, judgment, and other socially determined guides to behavior (in fact, frontal lobe brain functions have been defined as those functions soluble in alcohol). As the blood alcohol increases, motor control and coordination deteriorate. At a blood level of greater than 0.10 percent, an increasing proportion of individuals can be considered acutely intoxicated, and most legal definitions of intoxication fall within the range 0.10 to 0.20 percent blood alcohol. When the blood alcohol level is above 0.5 percent, the individual is not only unconscious but in danger of death from suppression of vital functions. Alcohol intoxication then is global in its effect on the central nervous system, ranging from the highest abstract operations to the most basic vegetative functions including sexuality, sleep, breathing, and circulation.

A variation of acute intoxication previously called pathologic intoxication is now designated *alcohol idiosyncratic intoxication*. Typically this disorder involves an excessive behavioral change induced by a relatively small amount of alcohol ingested. Behavioral change is usually one of excessive aggressiveness or overt violence. There may be amnesia for the period of intoxication.

The *alcohol withdrawal syndrome* is one with which every practicing physician should be thoroughly familiar since he or she is certain to encounter it repeatedly. The characteristic features are those of central nervous system rebound or overreaction from prolonged depression resulting from chronic alcohol ingestion.

Table 5-3. Diagnostic Criteria for Alcohol Withdrawal

A. Cessation of or reduction in heavy prolonged (several days or longer) ingestion of alcohol, followed within several hours by coarse tremor of hands, tongue, and eyelids and at least one of the following:
 1. nausea and vomiting
 2. malaise or weakness
 3. autonomic hyperactivity, e.g., tachycardia, sweating, elevated blood pressure
 4. anxiety
 5. depressed mood or irritability
 6. orthostatic hypotension

B. Not due to any other physical or mental disorder such as alcohol withdrawal delirium.

Reproduced with permission from DSM-III, pp. 133–134.

The main symptoms, those of autonomic nervous system hyperactivity, may begin within hours of cessation or even reduction in drinking; a good clinician will always inquire as to the time of an individual's last drink in order to determine the probability that this disorder will develop. The diagnostic criteria are listed in Table 5-3.

The central nervous system overactivity in the alcohol withdrawal syndrome may build to the point of seizures within hours. The peak period for seizures is between 12 and 48 hours following the cessation of drinking; however, seizures may occur up to several days after significant reduction in or total abstinence from alcohol.

In addition to seizures, *alcohol withdrawal delirium* may also develop, usually two or more days after significant or total reduction in alcohol intake. This syndrome may occur up to 5 to 10 days after the start of abstinence. The delirium of alcohol withdrawal, previously called delirium tremens or DTs, includes a lower level of consciousness, disorientation, paranoid or other types of delusions, vivid hallucinations (auditory-visual or somatic), and agitated behavior. Visual and somatic hallucinations are especially common, with the somatic hallucinations classically taking the form of a sense that bugs or snakes are crawling on the skin. Individuals so affected may excoriate themselves severely as they attempt to be rid of the perceived pest. Alcohol hallucinosis, another variation of the alcohol withdrawal state, refers more specifically to a syndrome of auditory hallucinations in a relatively clear state of consciousness. The individuals affected with these hallucinations report hearing voices with varying degrees of clarity and often with a persecutory content. The threat seems quite convincing to those hearing the voices, and the impact of such hallucinations must not be underestimated. It is said that occasionally this condition may progress to become fairly a chronic disorder.

These alcohol withdrawal disorders may vary considerably from individual to individual; their presence and intensity do not seem to correlate solely with quantity or chronicity of alcohol ingestion. There does seem to be a significant individual physiologic variation, and many papers have suggested that poor nutrition may contribute to the severity of the withdrawal state. It is a grave error to dismiss the importance of an alcohol abuse disorder because of the relative mildness of the withdrawal state.

Results of Prolonged Alcohol Abuse. The most severe central nervous system effects of prolonged alcohol abuse include the alcohol amnestic disorder and dementia associated with alcoholism. The amnestic syndrome, previously called Korsakoff's disease, is now known to result from thiamine deficiency. While Korsakoff's disease may result from thiamine deficiency of any cause, chronic alcohol abuse and dependence is by far the main cause of this illness in our society. Preceding the development of the amnestic syndrome, there may be an initial withdrawal delirium, which has been characterized as Wernicke-Korsakoff disorder. The acute features of Wernicke's encephalopathy include confusion, ataxia, and gaze palsies. When these acute features subside, the amnestic disorder (Korsakoff's disorder) may remain. Large doses of supplemental thiamine should be administered; this treatment may reduce or minimize the resulting amnestic disorder. It is important to realize that the course may be a gradually improving one over weeks to months, although serious impairment can be life-long. The clinical features of dementia resulting from chronic alcohol abuse and associated poor nutrition are similar to those of dementia described earlier; this dementia varies from mild to severe, and it is the most chronic of the disorders associated with alcohol abuse. This disorder also may be additive with other factors impairing cognitive function, including atherosclerosis or primary dementing illnesses; this combination may account for the fact that its effect in certain individuals seems greater than would be accounted for by the quantity of alcohol ingested.

Abuse of and Dependence on Barbiturates, Sedatives, and Hypnotics

All of the drugs classified as barbiturates, sedatives, and hypnotics resemble alcohol in that they are depressants of central nervous system function. Virtually all are available by prescription, and many are readily obtainable on the street market. The relative frequencies of abuse vary considerably depending on the availability of the specific drugs in any given area at a particular time. All are definitely abused frequently, however, and all are also capable of inducing a state of physical dependence. For many of these drugs, increasing tolerance can occur with sustained use, and all can produce a withdrawal syndrome on their discontinuance.

Barbiturates. The barbiturates have long been heavily used and abused drugs. Any of the numerous available barbiturates produce similar tolerance and dependence. Short-acting and intermediate-acting barbiturates such as pentobarbital and secobarbital seem to be the preferred drugs of abuse when they are obtainable, as compared with the longer acting phenobarbital. Individuals obtaining their drugs illicitly without prescription appear most often to become dependent on those drugs in their teens or twenties. Often, abuse of barbiturates is part of a mixed drug abuse picture, and the drug user is initially seeking the euphoria associated with these drugs. Some people, however, become dependent on barbiturates through prescription medications—often headache treatments that include a short-acting barbiturate. In these cases, patients may begin using the barbiturate for treatment of a specific medical complaint and gradually become dependent on the associated relaxation or on drug-induced sleep.

Other Sedatives and Hypnotics. In addition to the barbiturates, other sedatives and hypnotics are frequently abused. Meprobamate, which is psychologically similar in its effects to the intermediate-acting barbiturates, is a drug previously in wider circulation than it is today, but individuals continue to use and abuse it. It produces a state of physical dependence very similar to that of the barbiturates and poses the same difficulties for detoxification (see p. 71). Hypnotics that are widely abused include glutethimide, methaqualone, ethchlorvynol, and, to a lesser extent, flurazepam.

Benzodiazepines. The benzodiazepines have also come to be frequently abused. It is quite common today to find individuals suffering from a mixed dependence on alcohol and one or the other of the numerous benzodiazepines available on the commerical market. Chlordiazepoxide and diazepam are the most commonly used and most widely available for abuse. While short-term use of these drugs will not produce a state of physical dependence, sustained ingestion of the benzodiazepines produces a quite significant physical dependence. Sudden cessation of intake can result in an extremely uncomfortable, although not so dangerous, abstinence syndrome.

Withdrawal from Barbiturates and Related Drugs. The withdrawal syndrome from barbiturates and similar drugs is similar in its basic symptom pattern to withdrawal from alcohol dependence (that section should be reviewed for familiarity with this specific syndrome). Withdrawal from any of the barbiturates or closely related drugs can be life-threatening and should be managed with great caution in a hospital setting. Seizures, respiratory failure, and cardiovascular collapse are very real dangers. Withdrawal from the benzodiazepines is much less severe in terms of a threat to basic life function, but psychotic withdrawal states can occur, and withdrawing individuals may remain extremely uncomfortable for many weeks after cessation of these medications. It is likely that the longer half-life of the benzodiazepines accounts for the relative safety of the withdrawal syndrome but also the prolongation of the related discomfort.

Opioid Abuse and Dependence

Opioid abuse and dependence, most specifically that involving heroin, have for many years been the most publicized and dramatized of the substance abuse disorders. Far from being confined to heroin and restricted to a specific urban, lower-class population, opioid abuse and dependence are common and widespread in society. As with the barbiturates and sedatives, opioid abuse and dependence occur in one of two basic patterns: reliance on illicitly obtained street drugs, or use of multiple prescriptions, often from many sources, for identical or similar drugs. The second pattern may begin with a serious medical disorder involving sustained pain, such as after a traumatic injury or surgery, or with chronic headache. The most widely abused street opioid remains heroin, but dihydromorphone (Dilaudid), codeine, propoxyphene (Darvon), and others are also available. Prescription opioid abuse most often involves orally active opioids or related compounds such as Percodan (active agent oxycodone), codeine, meperidine (Demerol), or combination medications that include one of the previous agents—for example, acetaminophen with codeine (Tylenol 1, 2, or 3), or Fiorinal-Plus. Individuals may, in fact, develop dual substance dependencies through medications such as Fiorinal-Plus, which contains both a barbiturate and an opioid. Pentazocine (Talwin), while structurally quite different from the previous drugs, is also frequently abused, especially by those in medical positions. Abuse of morphine does occur but is relatively infrequent because it requires intravenous or intramuscular injection. For all these medications, abuse seems to result not only from the "high" of intravenous injection, but also from the analgesic, sedative, and hypnotic qualities of all these agents. Dosage tends to be progressive as tolerance develops. Individuals may switch from oral to intramuscular or intravenous abuse as the disorder progresses.

The signs of opioid intoxication and withdrawal are somewhat different from those of alcohol and central nervous system depressant sedatives and hypnotics. *Intoxication* is characterized progressively by flushing pruritus, myosis (an especially available and objective sign), drowsiness, a mild but increasing respiratory depression, lowered blood pressure and pulse, and a dropping body temperature. *Withdrawal* begins with a craving for drugs and a subjective sense of anxiety; this may be followed by yawning, sweating, tearing, rhinorrhea, and a light sleep. This symptom picture is succeeded by mydriasis, pilomotor erection, muscle twitching, chills, aching bones and muscles, and loss of appetite. Nausea, vomiting, and diarrhea ensue, accompanied by increased restlessness, general discomfort, and usually insomnia. A severe withdrawal state may be characterized by fever, hyperventilation, tachycardia, hypertension, and orgasm. Opioid withdrawal, however, is usually not life-threatening; despite the great subjective discomfort, it is not one of the more dangerous withdrawal syndromes.

Cocaine Abuse

Cocaine is currently one of the most frequently abused stimulant-euphoriant drugs in this country. Physical dependence is not so often seen, possibly because cocaine is very expensive and its effect has a short duration. It is subject to abuse by intranasal snorting or intravenous injection. Subjectively, the drug produces a highly pleasing "rush," elevated mood, and increased sexual interest. With increasing intoxication, effects may progress to produce anxiety, agitation, disorientation, paranoia, and a true psychotic state. Heart rate, blood pressure, and respiration are increased, and pupils may be dilated. The altered mood state may at times be difficult to distinguish from an amphetamine-induced mood change or functional mania.

Abuse of cocaine is usually part of a mixed drug abuse pattern, typically involving depressant substances such as alcohol or barbiturates at the times when cocaine is not being abused. With cocaine, as with amphetamines, many individuals will use the stimulant drug to feel motivated and active early in the day, followed by alcohol or sedative abuse to slow down and relax in the evening or at night.

Abuse of and Dependence on Amphetamines or Similarly Acting Sympathomimetic Drugs

Amphetamines and related drugs are also widely available and abused in this country. Previously, these drugs were easily obtained by prescription; however, recently the medical availability of these drugs has been markedly decreased, much to everyone's benefit. This reduction is the result of active government intervention in what was obviously the illicit channeling of legally produced stimulants. Consequently, amphetamines today are most commonly abused by individuals in their teens and twenties who obtain the drug from street sources. Recently produced anorectic agents, which are not yet adequately controlled, are beginning to replicate the previous prescription drug abuse pattern, but at a somewhat lower level of frequency and intensity. The most commonly available amphetamine today is dextroamphetamine, although methamphetamine is widely procurable.

The acute effects of amphetamines are quite similar to those of cocaine although they are most frequently used as oral tablets. In sustained and large doses, the amphetamines are quite capable of producing a severe paranoid psychotic picture very difficult to distinguish from paranoid schizophrenia. This is seen more often with the amphetamines than with cocaine, possibly because of the greater dopaminergic activity of this class of drug and also because of the larger dosages available and ingested. Treatment of the acute psychoses and withdrawal states is discussed in the treatment section of this chapter (p. 69). It should be remembered that amphetamines, even more than cocaine, usually seem to be part of a multiple substance disorder, almost always being taken in association with an agent that depresses the central nervous system. Some have questioned whether individuals with undiagnosed primary affective disorder, especially the depressive type, might more often seek self-medication of their depression through the use of stimulant drugs. While such persons certainly are seen clinically, inadequate data prevent specific knowledge about the relationship.

Phencyclidine Abuse

Phencyclidine is a drug increasingly abused among teenagers and young adults. It is sold on the street under many names, including angel dust, killer weed (or KW), hog, and PCP ("peace pill"). Most often the drug is sold as a coating on marijuana, but quite frequently also is substituted for lysergic acid diethylamide (LSD) or other hallucinogens; it is sold under the other drug's name, because phencyclidine is easier and cheaper to produce than are the hallucinogens. Phencyclidine was initially developed in the late 1950s and experimentally evaluated as an anesthetic agent. Because its use caused psychotic complications, the drug was withdrawn from human use, only to appear on the street market in the late 1960s. After a period of relatively little interest, abuse of the drug has resurfaced and increased to epidemic proportions. Its effects are many and potentially devastating. The onset of the effects varies depending on whether the drug is administered orally, sub-cutaneously, or through the respiratory system. In any case, within minutes an individual may feel detached or distanced from the surrounding world; a mild form of depersonalization, a subjective sense of relaxation or calm, or a greater internal preoccupation may be experienced. These effects may last for several hours.

Unfortunately, this relatively mild drug-induced state may be replaced by any of several other more severe conditions. An individual may become quite organically disoriented and impaired. There can be major memory loss and inability to function cognitively. Perceptual distortions of the body or the outer world as well as auditory or visual hallucinations may occur. The user may also display be extreme paranoia, agitation, and violence; the violence is quite unpredictable and may be triggered by even minor environmental stimuli. Physical effects may include generalized analgesia, nystagmus, sleepiness, incoordination, and vomiting. Heart rate, respiratory rate, and blood pressure may fluctuate widely. Catatonia, seizures, and opisthotonic posturing may also occur at higher doses. Prolonged abuse may result in a severe psychotic state that is relatively refractory to current neuroleptic medications. There is also increasing evidence that serious and irreversible brain damage may result from sustained abuse.

Diagnosis can be difficult from simply observing the patient's behavior, since the drug can induce so many different states. A careful history, as well as urine toxicologic studies, may assist in this process. The diagnostic criteria are nonspecific but require repeated abuse over at least one month, and there must be significant impairment in social or occupational functioning related to abuse of this drug.

Hallucinogen Abuse

Hallucinogens are drugs that have a primary effect on normal perceptual functions. The most commonly abused hallucinogens include LSD, psilocybin, dimethyltryptamine (DMT), and mescaline. The usual route of ingestion is oral. While ranking among the most widely publicized and (in certain communities) most often abused drugs of the late 1960s, hallucinogens have been somewhat overshadowed as sources of abuse by the upsurge in phencyclidine's popularity. Nonetheless, these drugs remain available on the illicit market (even though approximately 50 percent of drugs sold as hallucinogens are actually phencyclidine). All of the hallucinogens act to alter perception of the individual's body and the outside world. Consciousness is fully retained while there may be an intensification of auditory, visual, and somatic sensations, depersonalization, and derealization. There may also be visual experiences of bright colors and "tracking" (afterimages seen following visual perception). Attention may be concentrated while contact with the outside world is abandoned in favor of internal preoccupation. Physical symptoms include primarily those of sympathic stimulation, including rapid heart rate, sweating, tremors, and pupillary dilatation. While these objective effects may be quite pleasant, there may also be a reaction of anxiety, panic, or paranoia. Sustained use, as with other drugs, leads to deterioration of social and occupational function.

Once again, hallucinogen abuse tends to be part of the multiple abuse pattern rather than an exclusive one. The acute effects of hallucinogenic drugs may be followed by more sustained and profound disorders of thought processes or mood. While it is apparent that the hallucinogens do not generally induce psychotic disorders, these substances may trigger schizophreniform psychoses or major mood disorders of a depressive or manic type in susceptible individuals. An organic delusional or affective disorder is considered to exist separately from the drug's own effect when the disorder is sustained beyond 24 hours after ingestion of the substance. If the drug itself is responsible for the complete effect (rather than having triggered a more endogenous process), the disorder should be relatively time-limited, most commonly to several days or at most two weeks. Hallucinogen abuse is diagnosed when use has impaired social or occupational functioning for at least one month. Physical dependence does not appear to occur with any of this family of substances.

Cannabis Abuse

Cannabis, or marijuana, is one of the most widely used and abused drugs in the United States. The active ingredient in marijuana is tetrahydrocannabinol, which is also present in hashish and is available in purified form. Hashish itself is several times more potent than marijuana, owing to the increased content of tetrahydrocannabinol. The purified form of tetrahydrocannabinol is obtainable in tablets on the street market. The essential effect of cannabis and related drugs is that of a mild to moderately potent hallucinogen. The psychological and physical symptoms are similar to those noted for hallucinogens, although of considerably less intense nature. There may be more of a sense of euphoria with less frequent and less intense occurrence of the major perceptual alterations. Changes in perception that are commonly experienced include a sense of slowed time and increased acuteness of auditory, visual, and gustatory stimuli. There may be a strong feeling of well-being and relaxation. At increasing dosages and in susceptible individuals there may also be experiences of anxiety, panic, and paranoia. As with the hallucinogens, the social setting appears to be able to modify the drug effects for cannabis. Major psychotic or organic reactions are less frequently observed.

Sustained abuse appears to produce a more chronic apathy, which is often described as an *amotivational syndrome;* this disorder may have particularly negative effects on an individual's social, educational, and occupational functions. In addition, there appears to be a need for increasing dosage to achieve the desired effect with sustained use. While cannabis appears to have a sympathomimetic physical effect, no definable physical withdrawal state has been observed when use is discontinued. Many individuals do become quite evidently dependent on cannabis in daily (or several times daily) use in order to carry on what they consider to be normal function.

Tobacco Dependence

As with alcohol ingestion, tobacco use is generally considered to be socially normal and acceptable behavior. Tobacco dependence is diagnosed under very specific conditions, which are set forth in Table 5-4. Although this disorder is given short attention for the purposes of this textbook, tobacco abuse and dependence rank with alcohol abuse and dependence as major public health problems.

Multiple or Mixed Substance Abuse

Multiple substance abuse and dependence are extremely common today. It is rare that someone suffering from a substance abuse disorder confines himself or herself to a single substance at all times. While individuals may have a preferred chemical, most will substitute one substance for another when necessary. The most commonly observed mixed abuse disorders include a mixture of alcohol and one or more of the sedative drugs, a mixture of opioid and alcohol, and a mixture of sympathomimetic stimulant with a sedative drug and/or alcohol.

Table 5-4. Diagnostic Criteria for Tobacco Dependence

A. Continuous use of tobacco for at least one month.
B. At least one of the following:
   1. Serious attempts to stop or significantly reduce the amount of tobacco use on a permanent basis have been unsuccessful.
   2. Attempts to stop smoking have led to the development of tobacco withdrawal.
   3. The individual continues to use tobacco despite a serious physical disorder (e.g., respiratory or cardiovascular disease) that he or she knows is exacerbated by tobacco use.

Reproduced with permission from DMS-III, p. 178.

In order to assess any substance abuse disorder correctly, the examiner must be careful to determine all of the abuse substances that the affected individual will acknowledge and then to establish the relative frequency of each. This can be quite important for both treatment of withdrawal states and long-term rehabilitative treatment.

MEDICAL TREATMENT OF ACUTE INTOXICATION AND WITHDRAWAL SYNDROMES

The medical management of acute intoxication and withdrawal states is deliberately discussed separately from long-term and eventually more crucial rehabilitative aspects of treatment, which are covered later in this chapter. All too often physicians are willing to be involved solely with the medical management of the intoxication and the withdrawal disorders, and often those who seek help are interested in only this type of treatment. While this focus can be lifesaving and must not be neglected, it should only be preparatory to more fundamental treatment of the addictive illness.

While attention will be given to withdrawal techniques for specific chemicals, certain principles apply to virtually all substances. Individuals who are acutely intoxicated must be presumed to be incompetent to care for themselves or to judge the effect of their actions on others. They should be placed in an environment where they can be monitored constantly for behavior and vital functions. This may involve some form of restraint in a medical facility or even within a seclusion room if agitated and violent behavior is involved. Generally, however, individuals benefit from calm reassurance and an opportunity to allow the acute effects of alcohol or drugs to resolve spontaneously. Blood pressure, pulse, and respiration should be monitored on a regular basis; the precise frequency depends on the physical condition of the individual being treated. Certainly the vital signs of an awake person being treated for acute intoxication or acute withdrawal should be checked no less frequently than every two hours. In the following sections discussing treatment of withdrawal syndromes, it should be appreciated that the techniques advocated are only some of the medically acceptable methods that are available. Each method described, however, is clinically practical and reliable.

Alcohol Withdrawal Syndrome
Alcohol withdrawal syndrome, which can be quite severe (as mentioned in the discussion of the alcohol abuse and dependence disorders), is basically treated by substituting a controllable, quantifiable central nervous system depressant medication for the alcohol from which the individual is withdrawing. Historically a combination of chloral hydrate and paraldehyde was the most frequently used; it may, even today, remain the most effective drug regimen. For convenience, however, the benzodiazepines have come to be substituted for these older medications. Chlordiazepoxide (Librium) and diazepam (Valium) are probably the most frequently used benzodiazepines, and either will do quite well. Oxazepam has been used by some centers because of its short duration of action and the depressed likelihood of excessive medication accumulation in the affected individual, who often has quite impaired hepatic function. When assessing a patient's need for treatment of an alcohol withdrawal syndrome, the clinician should ask about previous withdrawal experiences. Often such individuals can provide a fairly accurate picture as to the quantities of chlordiazepoxide that are required and the frequency in timing with which they have experienced seizures or delirium tremens.

Despite this assistance, however, the clinician should rely on some objective evidence that withdrawal syndrome is present, since many individuals can have minimal signs and symptoms of physical withdrawal, even after prolonged intake of large quantities of alcohol. It follows then that the severity of the withdrawal state is not necessarily in direct correlation with the actual abuse pattern. The most reliable signs of the onset of a physical withdrawal syndrome include physical tremulousness (most easily observed in extended upper extremities and digits), restlessness, flushing, subjective discomfort, and elevated vital signs (rising blood pressure and tachycardia). Even before the onset of these symptoms, parenteral B vitamins, especially thiamine, should be administered if there is any question at all as to the patient's nutritional state; these vitamins can avoid the onset of a Wernicke's encephalopathy and subsequent Korsakoff's psychosis. Once physical evidence of withdrawal exists, the clinician should begin treatment with one of the benzodiazepines. In this textbook, chlordiazepoxide will be the medication used for illustration. If the physical symptoms of withdrawal are mild, chlordiazepoxide can be started at 25 mg orally; the maximum dosage of 100 mg orally is reserved for cases that are already well advanced. Rather than setting a frequency for repeated doses, written orders and oral instructions to the nursing staff should state that the patient must be monitored on an hourly basis. Frequently it is observed that a patient will need multiple doses in the first 12 to 24 hours in order to gain control of the withdrawal state; however, the daily dosage can be decreased quite rapidly thereafter. The majority of patients withdrawing from alcohol do not appear to require sedative medication after the first three to four days.

In patients with particularly severe symptoms and in those whose physical state is quite impaired, the rate of decrease may be more gradual over a one- to two-week period. It should be emphasized that this is the exceptional requirement rather than the rule. The formula that calls for a 10 percent decrease per day is simply not necessary in most individuals detoxifying from alcohol. Sleeping medication, preferably flurazepam, may be useful in the first one or two days of treatment.

The above course of treatment generally should be carried out in a hospital setting for two reasons. (1) It is important to prevent the addicted person from mixing his new benzodiazepine medication with his old reliance on alcohol—an all-too-frequent occurrence. (2) In a hospital setting, adjustments in dosage can be made to allow for reasonable physical and subjective comfort but to avoid marked sedation and lethargy. Truly normal sleep may require several weeks to establish in an individual who is dependent on alcohol. A lower limit of four to five hours per night, however, appears important to allow for adequate function during the daytime hours and to enable caretakers to recognize the possible development of a late withdrawal syndrome such as delirium tremens.

The time course for development of withdrawal syndrome varies depending on the syndrome being considered. Withdrawal seizures tend to occur within the first 48 hours after a significant decrease in alcohol ingestion. This occurs rarely enough that institution of anticonvulsant therapy is not generally indicated. In individuals with a strong history of withdrawal seizures or a known seizure disorder, phenytoin can be prescribed from the onset of the withdrawal state. In order to achieve an adequate blood level during the acute seizure period, one can prescribe three or four doses of phenytoin 200 to 300 mg orally over the first 12 hours. After this loading dose has been given, the patient should be given oral doses of phenytoin, 300 mg per day, while the serum level is checked. Delirium tremens, which may occur within the first four to 10 days after a decrease in alcohol intake, can generally be adequately treated with the benzodiazeptines alone. If, however, marked agitation occurs or actual violence develops, a neuroleptic can be prescribed concurrently with the benzodiazepine. Because it is important to avoid lowering the seizure threshold or affecting vital signs more than necessary, haloperidol is an excellent choice. Dosage may vary from 2 to 10 mg orally or 2 to 5 mg intramuscularly, depending on the body weight of the individual and the degree of agitation. Some studies have demonstrated that the combined use of a benzodiazepine and a neuroleptic for withdrawal states may be superior to the use of either alone. This is not generally accepted practice but should be kept in mind for individuals who are agitated and paranoid.

Barbiturate and Other Sedative Drug Withdrawal Syndromes

The principles for treatment of withdrawal from barbiturates and related drugs are quite similar to those for alcohol withdrawal. When an individual is withdrawing from this category of drugs, phenobarbital or pentobarbital is usually the agent selected for the withdrawal process. Phenobarbital has the advantage of a smoother blood level curve and the disadvantage that excessive accumulation of the medication is more likely to occur; pentobarbital has the opposite characteristics. In this chapter a withdrawal technique utilizing pentobarbital is described.

Because individuals dependent on barbiturates or closely related medications may be quite unreliable or unable to describe their dosages, a technique relying primarily on objective observation is preferred. The withdrawal treatment should be carried out only after evidence of an actual abstinence syndrome appears, and it should take place in a hospital setting because of the potential life-threatening severity of barbiturate abstinence syndrome. Once evidence of withdrawal is present, the patient should be given a test dose of pentobarbital, 100 to 200 mg orally. If marked sedation and somnolence occur within one or two hours after the test dose, probably no barbiturate dependence exists. If mild sedation or only adequate relief of withdrawal symptoms takes place, it will probably be necessary to give the patient the test dose four times a day. If withdrawal symptoms persist entirely or in large part, the amount used for each of the patient's four daily doses will probably exceed the test dose.

Treatment orders should allow an increased dosage if objective withdrawal symptoms intensify. On the other hand, dosage should be decreased or the next dose omitted entirely if the patient is markedly sedated or somnolent at the time the next dose would ordinarily be given. Unlike withdrawal from alcohol, withdrawal from barbiturates or similar sedatives or hypnotics should take place on a very gradual and steady basis. Five to 10 percent per day is a reasonable rate of decrease, but orders should be flexible enough that a given dosage can be sustained if the patient appears not to be tolerating the rate of decrease. Many clinicians routinely give phenytoin to persons withdrawing from barbiturates to decrease the risk of seizures.

Withdrawal From Opioids
Withdrawal from opioids, while not life threatening, can be extremely painful. It is generally recommended that methadone be used as the medication for the management of withdrawal from all opioids. Methadone has the advantage that it is taken orally and has a sustained half-life of 15 hours. As a result of this half-life, treatment can be on a twice-daily basis. Once objective signs of an opioid abstinence syndrome have appeared, 10 mg of methadone should be given orally and its effects observed. Usually a reasonable initial dose is 10 mg two times per day; few individuals require more than a total of 40 mg per day. Adjustment of dosage must rely on objective signs, since street narcotics are extremely variable in their concentration, and dosage cannot be estimated from a patient's report. In addition there is a great deal of manipulation frequently associated with the complaints of the narcotic-dependent person. The physician may have to defend and justify a reasonable withdrawal schedule if that schedule is based solely on a subjective report. Dosage should be decreased by approximately 10 to 15 percent per day. If marked complaints of nausea or anxiety appear, the use of phenothiazine such as promazine or chlorpromazine may help relieve anxiety, sleeplessness, and gastrointestinal distress.

Recently clonidine has been reported to be effective for treating an opiate abstinence syndrome. It appears that this drug acts on a presynaptic alpha-receptor to shut off withdrawal symptoms. While this medication is quite promising, it is not at this time licensed for use in treatment of the withdrawal symptoms.

Pentazocine presents a unique problem in that withdrawal from this drug is generally carried out utilizing the drug itself. It is available in oral as well as injectable form, and the former is quite suitable for a withdrawal schedule. Phenytoin may be given since withdrawal seizures can occur with this drug.

Cocaine, Amphetamines, and Other Sympathomimetic Drugs
There is generally no physical withdrawal syndrome from cocaine, amphetamines, and other sympathomimetic drugs. As noted previously, the acute effects of the drugs can produce severe anxiety states or frank paranoid psychoses. In a full-blown psychotic condition, neuroleptic medication may be required in doses equal to those used in the treatment of other acute psychotic states. These drug-induced syndromes may endure for days to weeks, during which time active treatment must be continued. In a withdrawal phase, however, abstinence-related phenomena are generally those of lethargy, hypersomnolence, and depression. This depression may be so severe that it requires active treatment with antidepressant medication. As with other intense withdrawal syndromes, treatment in a secure, protected environment is essential.

Sudden withdrawal from dependence on amphetamines and similar stimulants produces a characteristic and intense withdrawal state. While vital signs are not greatly affected, individuals who have decresed or stopped use of amphetamines frequently demonstrate great fatigue, lethargy, hypersomnolence, and often a profoundly depressed mood. This state can be so severe that suicide is a risk.

Cannabis and Hallucinogens

There is no significant withdrawal syndrome requiring active treatment for cannabis or hallucinogens. Acute effects, including anxiety, panic states, and even transient psychotic disorders, may require antianxiety medication or low to moderate doses of neuroleptic medication, depending on the severity of the disorder. Generally, this treatment can be discontinued within several days.

Phencyclidine

While there is no withdrawal syndrome from phencyclidine, the drug can produce acute effects that are the most difficult to manage of all the drug-induced states. If these effects only involve mild or moderate agitation and anxiety, the patient may be best handled without the use of neuroleptic medication. It is essential, however, to control the environment to minimize sensory input since such stimulation appears to trigger much of the agitation and violence. The use of sedative medication such as diazepam may also be quite helpful. Caretakers must be extremely vigilant because the mental and physical state of someone under the effects of phencyclidine can change rapidly and severely. If agitation becomes extreme, the use of a quiet room and neuroleptic medication may be unavoidable.

If a neuroleptic drug must be used, it is best to avoid those high in anticholinergic effect since phencyclidine itself can have a profoundly anticholinergic action; haloperidol is the agent that is most widely used in the treatment of phencyclidine-induced psychoses. Marked dystonic reactions have been known to occur in treating these disorders, and it appears that there is some potentiating effect between phencyclidine and neuroleptic drug. The severity of the disorder, however, may leave the physician with no alternative to the use of a neuroleptic. The use of the beta-blocker propranolol along with other pharmacologic interventions has recently been recommended in the acutely psychotic phase of phencyclidine intoxication.

DIFFERENTIAL DIAGNOSIS OF THE RELATIONSHIP BETWEEN SUBSTANCE ABUSE AND OTHER PSYCHIATRIC DISORDERS

The relationship between substance abuse and other psychiatric disorders is poorly understood; however, the lack of definitive data has in no way hindered the formation of passionately held opinions. These dogmatic stands have, unfortunately, slowed the progress toward better research and understanding. For many years, psychiatric theory tended to conceptualize substance abuse as derivative from underlying, more fundamental emotional conflicts or disorders. In practice, however, this approach tended to avoid confronting the substance abuse problems with sufficient strength, and treatment outcome was poor. Alcoholics Anonymous, on the other hand, emphasized the primary nature of alcoholism and (by extension) drug abuse. The illness model of alcoholism has had great impact on improving treatment of the substance abuse disorders. Unfortunately, the model has come to be applied simplistically to the exclusion of other psychiatric illnesses that may coexist with substance abuse problems. All too often, the diagnostic and treatment questions raised reflected the beliefs of treatment personnel rather than being based on comprehensive evaluation.

The relationship of substance abuse disorders to other psychiatric disorders can be conceptualized in four ways: (1) substance abuse disorders are derivative from other psychiatric disorders; (2) substance abuse disorders and other psychiatric disorders may coexist in individual patients but there is no etiologic or therapeutic significance to the coexistence; (3) the substance abuse disorders and other psychiatric disorders may coexist, and the coexistence may in certain subgroups of patients have etiologic or therapeutic import; and (4) substance abuse may be capable of generating or exacerbating other psychiatric disorders. At present, information is simply not sufficient to demonstrate when substance abuse is or is not derivative in etiology. One can, however, examine the rates of coexistence of different disorders and some clinical experience in the management of patients with dual diagnoses.

PREVALENCE OF OTHER PSYCHIATRIC SYNDROMES AMONG SUBSTANCE ABUSERS

There is as yet no definitive answer to the question of the prevalence of other psychiatric syndromes among substance abusers. Previous vagueness on diagnostic categories and criteria makes much research of uncertain value. Several recent reports confirm, however, that a large portion of substance abusers meet the criteria for one or more other psychiatric diagnoses at the time of entering treatment. For alcoholics, this proportion may be in the range of 60 percent, and the proportion is equal or higher among opiate addicts.

The most frequently made second diagnosis has consistently been depressive disorder, which usually occurs in more than 40 percent of alcoholics. The relationship of bipolar (manic-depressive) disorder to alcoholism has been more difficult to determine. Inadequate studies abound, leading to every possible conclusion. Several observations seem to have been made in more than one study: (1) there are patients who abuse alcohol preferentially during either phase of bipolar illnesses; (2) there is some diagnostic and genetic overlap of bipolar disorders and alcoholism, and the bipolar alcoholic patients have families with more overlap; and (3) treatment of both disorders may be necessary to achieve successful treatment outcome.

The relationship of schizophrenia to substance abuse appears to be essentially a random one, with no causal connections. As far as anxiety states are concerned, there definitely exists an increased risk of substance abuse and dependence among a subgroup of patients with panic anxiety (phobic anxiety) disorders. This relationship can usually be identified as developing from efforts to medicate severe anxiety. Numerous personality disorders are diagnosed in alcoholics and drug addicts; there are frequently increased paranoid, antisocial, and narcissistic features.

The implications for treatment have yet to be firmly established. Extreme cases are not especially problematic—for example, a florid manic state or disabling panic anxiety obviously must be treated if stable abstinence from addictive chemicals is to be achieved. Suicidal depression demands active intervention regardless of the existence of alcohol abuse. In milder disorders, however, there is more room for uncertainty. Many psychiatric symptoms seem to resolve spontaneously after several weeks of abstinence from alcohol and mood-altering drugs. Psychotropic medications have risks and complications of their own, especially for substance abusers. In addition, the supportive milieu of good alcoholism and drug addiction programs may prove very effective in themselves.

There are no firm rules for treatment. Careful history taking must include a search for preexisting mood swings, pathologic anxiety, and similar problems, together with extensive family interviewing. The clinician may find psychological testing and neuroendocrine studies useful after the patient has been free of alcohol and drugs for two to three weeks. If uncertainty persists, the dilemma should be shared with the patient and the alternatives discussed. Therapeutic trials of nonaddictive psychotropic agents may best be undertaken in a hospital setting, and these measures can serve as a diagnostic procedure as well.

ETIOLOGY OF SUBSTANCE USE DISORDERS

The etiology of the substance use disorders is not known. Considerable research has been devoted to psychological factors, learning theories, and physiologic peculiarities of individuals who become dependent on alcohol or drugs. While there definitely are personality traits and psychological aspects common to many of those who are dependent on alcohol or drugs, there has been no convincing evidence that these factors are in any way causative. Similarly, the application of learning theories and physiologic studies have not definitively demonstrated any single characteristic of a person that can be identified as primary in the etiology of substance abuse. There have been attempts, for example, to show that alcoholics or their children metabolize alcohol differently than do controls, but the findings have not been significant. Variants of alcohol dehydrogenase, the liver enzyme that converts ethanol to acetaldehyde, have been found in Orientals with a high level of atypical enzyme and a low incidence of alcoholism. The meaning of this finding, however, is uncertain.

Nature versus Nature

Perhaps of greatest interest has been the observation that alcoholism runs in families. A family history of alcoholism is the greatest single risk factor for the development of the disorder. The increased risk for both male and female offspring is at least five times that of the population at large. Nearly one-quarter of the sons of alcoholics and one in twenty daughters become alcoholics. There have been numerous studies seeking to separate out genetic from environmental factors in alcoholism. Conclusions from the best and most recent studies can be summarized as follows: (1) for male offspring of an alcoholic parent (father or mother), there is a genetic risk of alcoholism regardless of environment; (2) the risk of developing alcoholism is about four times greater for the sons of alcoholics than it is for controls; (3) the increased risk is confined to alcoholism, not heavy drinking or other psychiatric disorders; (4) it is unproved that daughters of alcoholics run an increased genetic risk; (5) rearing in an alcoholic home, however, may increase the risk of alcoholism in these daughters and definitely increases the risk of depression; and (6) the mode of genetic transmission is not proved, does not seem to be sex-linked, and may approximate a dominant mode of transmission.

The implications of the these findings are uncertain but do point to increased public education and a more cautious, self-observant approach to drinking by the offspring of alcoholics.

At this point, the treatment process must be approached empirically, since etiologic understanding is so uncertain. This is hardly unique to the substance abuse disorders and should not be interpreted as decreasing the chances of successful rehabilitation.

THE ROLE OF THE PHYSICIAN IN TREATMENT

Traditionally the role of the physician in treating alcohol and other substance abuse disorders has been confined to treating acute withdrawal states or the later medical complications of the chemical dependence. This, unfortunately, has resulted in continued long-term complications of the primary illness since detoxification alone does nothing to interrupt the addictive illness. It is essential that the physician conceptualize his or her role in broader terms that involve identifying the existence of the illness, assisting in intervention, and being a coordinator of the larger treatment process.

To begin with, the physician should remember that his or her primary goal is to avoid doing harm. This admonition is included since all too often those who are dependent on alcohol or drugs continue to obtain drugs through manipulating their physicians. Only a high index of suspicion can reduce the frequency of this aspect of the illness. The physician should pay careful attention to requests for potentially addictive analgesic and antianxiety medications. While this caution should not be carried to the extreme of withholding useful and appropriate medical treatment, the physician should note the frequency of requests for these medications and the number of doses ingested by each patient under his or her care. It is quite destructive to maintain the naive belief that by giving adequate doses of medications, the individual no longer has to resort to alcohol or other drug use. This is simply not the case and will only encourage continued progression of the disease.

The physician should also appreciate that he or she is often in a unique position to detect evidence of a substance abuse disorder. Laboratory tests such as liver function studies or red blood cell profiles may give direct evidence of an ongoing problem with alcohol abuse. Likewise, complaints of gastritis, ulcer, gastrointestinal bleeding, or frequent physical injuries may demonstrate the existence of alcoholism. Family members may also come to the physician with evidence of physical or emotional trauma resulting from the behavior of an alcoholic or drug-dependent individual within the family. Once again the physician may be the first to observe this evidence.

All too often physicians have simply not pursued indications of the existence of substance abuse disorder, either out of anxiety over the patient's possible reaction to questioning or out of despair about the availability of any treatment. This attitude of despair has existed among the medical profession because of a lack of understanding of the necessary treatment process. A single physician sitting alone in his or her office will, by and large, fail in an attempt to treat an alcohol or drug abuse disorder. On the other hand, a physician can be tremendously effective by educating and mobilizing the patient and family members or close friends, as well as directing them to appropriate treatment centers or Alcoholics Anonymous. Just as a general physician might refer a patient to a medical specialist for a specific disorder, so too might that physician direct a patient to a specialized treatment program for an alcohol or drug abuse disorder. This is a highly effective part of treatment and should not be minimized just because it requires the involvement of others.

Use of Disulfiram

One additional specific role of the physician may be that of prescribing disulfiram (Antabuse). Disulfiram is a medication that interferes with the enzymatic breakdown of alcohol, causing an accumulation of acetaldehyde in the circulation. Accumulation of acetaldehyde in turn causes symptoms of flushing, conjunctival injection, headaches, nausea, vomiting, palpitations, tachycardia, dyspnea, hyperventilation, sleepiness, and hypotension. Essentially, then, disulfiram creates an uncomfortable disorder, and the anticipation of that disorder leads to avoidance of alcohol ingestion in an individual taking the medication.

There have been negative feelings about the use of disulfiram, but this reaction has been based on a misunderstanding of the uses of this medication. It is not in and of itself a treatment program for alcoholism, but it is a potentially useful adjunct in alcoholic patients who are committed to sobriety. Disulfiram should be prescribed by a physician for a patient only when he or she seems to be significantly committed to sobriety and is participating in a larger recovery program such as Alcoholics Anonymous.

Disulfiram is today prescribed in lower doses than were used previously, usually 125 to 250 mg orally once a day. Its effects on the metabolism of alcohol may last for up to two weeks after ingestion. Consequently, if the patient wishes to drink after ingesting disulfiram, he or she must wait a significant period of time (allowing the person to reconsider the resumption of drinking) or risk suffering the quite uncomfortable effects that have been described. When disulfiram therapy is being initiated, the physician must educate the patient adequately concerning its use, including the need for awareness of hidden sources of alcohol, such as shaving lotion, perfume, certain vinegars, nonprescription liquid medications, mouthwash, and other nonbeverage substances that contain alcohol. While these contacts may be insignificant (as with perfume, for example), a mild disulfiram-alcohol reaction may occur, and an informed patient will be less frightened or more prepared to avoid it.

Once instituted, disulfiram therapy should generally continue for at least a year after initial establishment of sobriety. While some complications have been reported from long-term use of disulfiram, these appear to be infrequent and mild in comparison to the effects of ongoing active alcoholism.

Rehabilitative Model of Treatment

The medical descriptive model presented in the previous section is useful for the early diagnostic and detoxification phase in the treatment of alcoholism and drug abuse. The rehabilitative model utilizes a long-term, comprehensive program of education and therapy. Addiction is a chronic progressive illness that affects all areas of life. While specific diagnostic criteria may be employed for identification of the disorder, effective intervention requires a more *dynamic interactional approach* than that used in the medical model. This rehabilitative approach assumes an intimate knowledge of drinking and drug abuse behavior, not merely an ability to describe it. The approach also requires an in-depth understanding of the characterologic and defensive patterns typical of the substance-abusing personality. Without this more active and practical method, the clinician cannot put to effective use the diagnostic criteria described earlier in this chapter. Many diagnoses will be missed if the physician asks questions inexpertly and if the patient's denial is unchallenged. If a diagnosis is made under the medical model, treatment will be conceptualized only as a brief medical intervention for detoxification without long-term involvement in a recovery program. Such treatment usually results only in a revolving-door pattern of repeated relapse and increasing physical, psychological, and social destruction.

The rehabilitative model historically developed in the treatment of alcoholism. Over the past decade, however, it has been applied to the treatment of drug abuse and the very common mixed abuse disorders or cross-addictions involving both alcohol and drug abuse.

TREATMENT AND RECOVERY

An individual with an addictive illness (as is true for those with most other disorders) has the best chance of recovery if detection and intervention occur in the early stages of the disease process. To treat the illness effectively, a comprehensive program of education and psychological therapy is required.

Treatment should begin with the first contact the alcoholic has with people concerned with his or her illness, regardless of professional or nonprofessional role. In fact, anyone around the alcoholic has an opportunity to help. Because of ignorance of the disease, however, instead of being helped into treatment, alcoholics and drug addicts may rationalize their way out of seeking help with promises of doing better in the future. Many of the people who come in contact with active substance abusers misunderstand the situation and believe that if the abusers are helped to be more comfortable, their condition would improve. The truth is exactly opposite: only when alcoholics and addicts become uncomfortable with their disease will they seek or accept help to change.

There are many criteria the physician can use in diagnosing addictions. In substance abuse disorders, however, the ill person must *accept* the diagnosis if treatment is to be effective. The diagnostic process, then, must be one in which both the patient and the clinician come to understand the reality and seriousness of the disorder.

APPROACHES TO DIAGNOSING SUBSTANCE ABUSE

In their work, *The Patient with Alcoholism and Other Drug Problems,* Whitfield and Williams note that the physician can use three approaches to diagnose alcoholism (these approaches apply to other drug abuse disorders as well): (1) direct questioning, or simply talking to the patient; (2) inductive reasoning; and (3) quantitative testing such as the Michigan Alcoholism Screening Test or tests of blood alcohol or drug levels. If, while the drinking history is being taken, the patient becomes angry or evasive, states that he stopped drinking altogether, or says he drinks more than three drinks a day, the interviewer should consider the diagnosis of an alcohol abuse disorder. If this patient has just been admitted to a hospital, or is in the physician's office or clinic, and does not freely admit to being alcoholic, the examiner can order any or all of the following studies: a blood alcohol level, urine toxicology, and a structured questionnaire (such as the Michigan Alcoholism Screening Test in the Appendix at the end of this chapter).

At the end of the evaluation, a decision must be made as to whether the patient is alcoholic (or, "has a problem with drinking") or has a drug abuse problem. This can be done by synthesizing all the collected data. The physician should conclude by answering the question, "Does drinking or drug use interfere with any part of the patient's life?" The patient should then be presented the evidence for the diagnosis as a means of increasing his or her acceptance of the problem.

Confrontation
The process of communicating the diagnosis and the substantiating evidence to the patient, or the *confrontation,* can be done in the same serious and objective manner that a physician would use to inform the patient of any other serious chronic disease. If a physician has just diagnosed diabetes or cancer, there would be little hesitation about informing the patient. Informing and educating patients about their chronic illnesses are basic responsibilities of the physician. The goal of intervening in this manner is to get the patient to accept help. It is reasonable, however, to introduce the subject gradually and to confront the patient gently.

The doctor should anticipate denial—perhaps even angry denial—in the attempt to inform the patient of his or her alcoholism or drug dependence. The term *alcoholic* or *drug dependent* will often sound to the patient like name-calling rather than a medical diagnosis. The physician should anticipate a rebuttal from the patient and must not be dismayed if the patient gets annoyed. Physicians must remember that ultimately the disorder is the patient's problem and responsibility.

One very helpful maneuver is to attempt to get the patient to be the one to apply the label. In this gentle confrontation, the physician may begin by asking the question mentioned before, "Have you ever wondered whether you might be an alcoholic (or drug dependent)?" It has been LeClair Bissell's experience, for example, that over 60 percent of alcoholic patients will respond affirmatively. Most will go on to say that while they have wondered, they have concluded that they were not alcoholics "because an alcoholic is...". Typically, they will give a definition of alcoholism that does not fit them or is incorrect, and they will often reflect the skid-row stereotype that associates the disorder with constant, daily drinking. ("An alcoholic is someone under the bridge with no job and no family," or, "An alcoholic is someone who can't live without a drink.") This misunderstanding provides the physician with an opportunity to provide an accurate definition of alcoholism, or drug abuse, which can then be used by the patient to recognize his or her own illness. In such a discussion, the doctor can use a modified version of the definitions used in this chapter (that is, a substance abuser is someone who has had health, job, or family problems related to the substance abuse and, in spite of this, continues to use the chemical). Then the attempt should be made to have the patient relate his or her present situation to that definition. Patients should be shown objective evidence (for example, liver function tests, x-ray films of esophageal varices, a blood alcohol level, urine toxicology findings, or the Michigan Alcoholism Screening Test score) as a way of showing them how their health has been affected by the abuse pattern.

What the physician says must be backed up with medical facts. It is also important to remain professional and under control of the anger that can often occur during the confrontation process. There can be enormous frustration over denial of the alcohol or drug problem by a very ill patient. The clinician must remember that addicted persons simply cannot envision living without drinking or taking medications; they may see this threat as a death sentence and flee from treatment. In this delicate discussion, the patient-physician relationship is a key consideration. In discussions such as these, clinical medicine is at its height. The physician must be supportive but persuasive, calm yet persistent, and his or her concern, supported by relevant facts, must be conveyed. In such discussions, it is essential that one always be completely honest with the patient. Idle threats or false statements should never be made or the clinician will lose credibility if challenged.

Many patients will not accept the label readily. They have used denial for years, and it usually takes considerable time before the diagnosis is truly accepted. The physician should not persist in using the term "alcoholic," "alcoholism," or "drug dependent" in the face of continued or growing rejection of that label by the patient. However, *one does not have to wait until the patient accepts the diagnosis before anything is done.* The term "drinking problem" or "drug problem" still identifies a situation for which some action is necessary. Some patients will agree to stop drinking or using drugs even though they are still verbally denying their problem. The action usually must be initiated by the doctor, whether it be labeled "confrontation," "education about the disease," or "intervention." As the National Council on Alcoholism has said, "The worst treatment...is no treatment."

Referral or Consultation

Physicians should examine their attitudes toward the substance abuser and determine whether their skills are sufficient to engage in a type of therapy that involves close, open, and honest contact with the patient. Some physicians may elect not to treat such patients, but refer them elsewhere for assistance. This decision, made after careful self-scrutiny, is commendable. It is much better to refer than to become involved with such patients in a negative and antitherapeutic manner.

The physician who elects not to treat these disorders is responsible, however, for the following tasks: (1) suspecting the diagnosis; (2) establishing the diagnosis, at least preliminarily; (3) confronting the patient; and (4) referring the patient for further treatment. A physician who feels uncomfortable, or who for some reason cannot take the step of presenting to the patient the evidence for the diagnosis, should find someone else who will. Although it is probably more easily done by the patient's primary care physician, a knowledgeable consultant can effectively confront the patient. However, it is still up to the original physician to bring in a consultant and explain to the patient the reasons for so doing.

Engaging the Patient in Treatment

After presenting the evidence for the diagnosis to the patient, it is essential that the physician immediately offer specific help. This step of engaging the patient in treatment follows directly from the preceding step of confrontation. The way the patient has been confronted will also greatly affect his or her willingness to accept further help. The physician may offer to treat the patient or refer the patient to other professionals. The doctor should become familiar with local professionals (including selected physicians who specialize in this field) and treatment facilities.

After being presented with the evidence for their diagnosis and listening to an offer of treatment, many patients will refuse assistance. They may not have accepted the fact that they have a substance abuse problem, or firmly believe that they can solve their problems on their own. Most patients who have never tried to stop drinking or taking drugs think it will be easy. Even those who have made honest attempts seem to believe that they can do it this time, no matter how many times they may have failed previously. Attempting to engage the patient in treatment is partially a matter of getting the patient to want external help. It has been shown that patients have a much easier time staying sober if they allow others to help them, while it is likely to be very difficult for them to do it alone. Simple education—an explanation that the chances of success are much greater if he or she is willing to accept help—may be beneficial.

The doctor should not feel discouraged and abandon hope of helping a patient who refuses to accept treatment. There are alternative plans of action that can be initiated. The physician may tell the patient, "Think about what we have discussed; I plan to talk with you again about this subject." The patient should be assured that the doctor will be available at any future time should he or she decide to accept the offered treatment. (It is helpful to make sure that the patient has the office address and phone number.) The physician may also propose that the patient read educational material, such as the classic, *I'll Quit Tomorrow* by Vernon E. Johnson. Another option is to advise the patient to attend a meeting of Alcoholics Anonymous (or Narcotics Anonymous) or speak to an individual member of that program. If the suggestion is made that this be done as an educational experience, often the patient will follow through. Whenever possible, after obtaining the patient's consent, the physician should discuss the substance abuse problem with family members and offer assistance to them. Educational literature may be helpful here also. If the family is responsive, the physician may recommend that together they approach the patient in a nonjudgmental, loving manner to present their specific concerns; this should be attempted at a time when the patient is not intoxicated (if such a time can be found). Those closest to the patient can sometimes get him or her to accept treatment when the doctor cannot. If the serious nature of the problem and the necessity for complete abstinence are emphasized, most patients will agree at least to try to stop using alcohol or drugs. The door is then open for the doctor to say, "If you are unable to do it on your own, I'll be speaking to you again about treatment the next time I see you."

During one of the many crises that inevitably will occur in the person's life, the steps outlined above may then come into play and facilitate the alcoholic's entry into treatment. The physician's perspective, then, must be long term.

Selection of a Treatment Setting

Selection of the proper treatment setting is quite important. The first decision is between outpatient and inpatient treatment (hospital or rehabilitation center). Outpatient treatment can only be successful for patients who begin with some acknowledgement of their need for help and willingness to accept specific sources of aid. These sources include frequent professional counseling sessions (individual and/or group), regular attendance at Alcoholics Anonymous or Narcotics Anonymous, contact with individuals in these programs, and possibly the use of disulfiram to support abstinence from alcohol.

Successful outpatient treatment also depends on the presence of relatively good physical health, the absence of severe withdrawal symptomatology and complicating major psychiatric disorders, and the availability of a supportive family and work setting. It is, of course, unlikely that all of these factors will be present for any single patient. If certain critical areas are negative (for example, if the patient is likely to experience severe withdrawal, has a hostile or undermining family environment, or displays a low motivation to accept help), an outpatient program is likely to fail, and a more structured institutional treatment is indicated. The referring physician must keep in mind the devastating consequences of treatment failure for the patient and direct him or her accordingly.

Inpatient Treatment

If the physician has determined that inpatient treatment is the best course of action, he or she should be familiar with the treatment goals. These goals should be simple, even though the treatment regimen used to accomplish these goals may be complex. The goals of a good treatment program are to help patients (1) see that alcohol or drug use was a major factor in the majority of their problems, (2) accept the illness (disease concept), (3) clarify problem areas in their lives, and (4) make a commitment to long-term treatment in community support programs (such as Alcoholics Anonymous or Narcotics Anonymous).

After detoxification is complete, patients should move into a highly structured program of group and individual therapy. It becomes clear in this phase of treatment that feelings and perceptions are distorted and that the defense system is firmly entrenched. These patients, at this point, will still be blaming others for their problems and minimizing the negative effects that drinking or drug use has had on their lives and the lives of those around them. Through the educational components of a program and group therapy sessions, the patients soon begin to realize that their behavior and substance abuse patterns are remarkably similar to those of others in the group. As the patients become comfortable in the group, they begin to share and relate to various group members. Some patients may continue to deny their problems, but the peer group and staff continually bring reality to bear by pointing out distortions in their statements. The patients can then begin to relax their defensive stance.

Continuing peer pressure, education about alcoholism and drug abuse, and professional guidance from staff soon allow patients to identify themselves as alcoholics or drug addicts. When this happens, they gain a true picture of their existence over the past several years and can begin to see that substance abuse either caused or contributed to every major problem in their lives. Ceasing to drink or use drugs, however, will not automatically eliminate the years of damage. The next phase of treatment, consequently, is very important.

Clarification of Problems

While it is true that stopping drinking or using drugs will eliminate some problems, abstinence alone is not enough. Patients soon begin to look at the emotional damage done by their past behavior. The scars caused by lack of communication and anger over years of lying and covering up will leave much to be worked out among family members. The patients then must look at what can be done to achieve a healthy family, work, and social life. When alcoholics or addicts truly accept their disease, they accept responsibility for their actions and behavior in the past and in the future. In doing so, a sense of accomplishment is achieved but at the same time many sad feelings or even depression develop. Much has been lost, and the realization hurts.

These new feelings are real. Distorted thoughts and feelings experienced earlier are clearing. The patients begin to like themselves again because for the first time in years they are making an effort to correct past wrongs by receiving treatment for the illness they have had for years. They become honest with themselves and with those around them. Trust develops for themselves, peers, and staff members. They begin to disclose things that, until now, they had been unable to discuss. Feelings are being dealt with more realistically, and they begin to ask what needs to be done in order to keep the process moving. Newly sober alcoholics are searching for answers.

Alternative solutions to the previous lifestyle must now be explored. Habit patterns must be broken, drinking situations (or those that lead to drug use) must be avoided (at least temporarily), and associated friends may also have to be avoided. The treatment staff will provide helpful advice and guidance of a practical type. The patients now begin to set new goals for themselves. The kinds of things they do for fun and relaxation take on an important meaning. How many Alcoholics Anonymous (or Narcotics Anonymous) meetings should they attend weekly? How can they use the steps of their program in their daily routines? How can they help get their family life back in order? How will they reestablish their productivity at work? These questions and others help individuals set up immediate long-term goals. This kind of life planning brings a new perspective and sense of exhilaration and accomplishment to recovering persons. They feel a sense of commitment. Inpatient treatment is completed and the patients move into the next phase of the continuum.

Aftercare

The patients have now established a commitment to recovery; however, equally important is a commitment to an aftercare program. The transition phase, in which they learn to function in the family, on the job, and in social situations, is a delicate period. Many persons relapse and drink or use drugs again during this period if they do not have the structure of an aftercare program. It should be remembered that what alcoholics (or addicts) are being asked to do in recovery is abnormal for them—a deviation from the years of alcohol-oriented behavior (or behavior influenced by drug use). They are asked not to drink or use drugs when this has been an important part of their lives for years. They are asked to deal with feelings openly, when for years they have stifled such feelings. Until the patients are comfortable doing these things, professional guidance in an aftercare program can make the difference between success and failure. Putting into practical use what is learned in treatment is not an easy task.

Aftercare groups provide continued support and guidance by professionals. This process allows patients to continue in a group of peers until new close friendships in Alcoholics Anonymous or Narcotics Anonymous are developed. Gradually, patients will become less dependent on the aftercare group and will become firmly established in the self-help program. In this program they will grow and continue to change for the remainder of their lives. Along with an aftercare group and Alcoholics Anonymous or Narcotics Anonymous, there are a number of adjunctive therapies, such as family therapy or assertiveness training, that may be used. Treatment providers must be prepared to use as many tools as necessary to help the patients establish a solid recovery.

Recovery

Throughout this transition period and for the rest of the patients' lives, the recovery process continues to take place. This process has many facets. Gradually, recovering alcoholics or addicts begin to understand themselves and their illness. They are eventually established on an identifiable path of recovery. Attitudinal and behavioral changes are essential to long-term recovery. Recovering patients must begin to understand and accept their illness and thus begin to deal with the guilt and shame. They must also accept responsibility for their behavior, both in the past and the future. The self-centered willfulness of addiction must be replaced by a readier acceptance of guidance by others who can provide help. Acceptance of available help, then, remains crucial for long-term recovery. By utilizing available support, recovering alcoholics gradually develop a deeper understanding of their own needs (as well as the needs of others they are close to), better communication patterns, and an ability to tolerate frustration and cope with stress.

The Family Illness

The disease did not develop in a vacuum—substance abuse disorders involve the entire family. In fact, family members have often suffered as much as or more than the alcoholic or addict. Family treatment, then, should be part of the total treatment plan. The family usually must go through changes parallel to those of the alcoholic or addict if complete health is to be established for all. A full discussion of this process is beyond the scope of this text, but more information is available through the suggested readings and material from Al-Anon, a distinct self-help organization of those whose lives are affected by someone who is alcoholic or cross-addicted. In brief, family members must be prepared to change their reaction patterns and eliminate habits that facilitate the patient's addictive illness. The new environment that will be created will help remove major roadblocks to the alcoholic or addicted family member's recovery. The family must understand that the recovering person spends most of his or her time in the family environment. It is this environment that must cease nurturing the disease process—or recovery is unlikely to occur.

CONCLUSION

Substance abuse disorders are widespread, chronic, and potentially fatal. Detailed knowledge of both the medical and the psychosocial aspects of these diseases is essential. Specific understanding of the physical effects and detoxification methods appropriate to each abusable substance is crucial to early treatment. This initial phase, however, must be followed by a second one, in which patients are directed to a rehabilitative program. In that program they become more aware of the nature of their disease and the long-term recovery process into which they must enter. Only by assisting the patients and their families to establish new patterns of thinking, feeling, and acting will the physician achieve the treatment goal of long-lasting recovery from substance abuse.

Case 1. S.G. is a 31-year-old plumber who was seen repeatedly by his family physicians for complaints of nighttime needlelike pains in his stomach and recurring severe headaches. Despite repeated questioning, S. denied any excessive drinking and was not confronted by his physician or family. In the meantime S. was in fact steadily increasing his daily alcohol consumption to much more than a fifth a day. He had begun to drink excessively at around the age of 22, not long after his discharge from the service. He enjoyed alcohol greatly and never worried about the amount. As his intake accelerated, S. began to experience the physical symptoms noted above. His sleep decreased drastically, and his appetite became erratic. He developed periods of amnesia lasting many hours. Home life deteriorated and violent arguments and even physical fights occurred. S. began hiding bottles of liquor at work and at home. His job performance declined and he was increasingly absent from work.

The patient withdrew progressively from all except hard-drinking friends. He neglected all responsibilities and became very irritable and jittery. These feelings were relieved by several drinks but always returned within hours. Although S. knew that he had lost control of his drinking, he feared admitting it to anyone. Finally his boss threatened S. with loss of work unless he got treatment. He admitted himself to a hospital, was detoxified, and began therapy with disulfiram. S. also began to attend Alcoholics Anonymous meetings. His wife became involved with Al-Anon to help understand her life with an alcoholic. He has now been sober for eight months.

Case 2. G.L., age 41, and his wife C.L., age 38, have been married for 15 years and have three children. G. is a successful attorney, and C. works as an interior designer. They have always been a very popular and socially active couple. When they married, G. drank three to five martinis a night. C. did not drink at all, but her father had been an alcoholic. As his career advanced, G. worked longer hours and experienced even greater pressure from his expanding responsibilities. Periodically G. would drink quite heavily at weekend parties and become totally intoxicated. Later, these binges became increasingly frequent and occurred during the week as well. C. also began drinking to feel more comfortable with G. Gradually both C. and G. became dependent on daily drinking, which started by early afternoon. Their relationship grew more and more empty as the bottle replaced other ways of communicating and relating.

The patient continued to work regularly, but the quality suffered. Colleagues began to talk about G.'s obvious alcoholic excesses, but

G. remained oblivous. C. was more aware and worried, but she was afraid to confront G. about what she now realized was a mutual problem. She even made excuses for G. when he was late to court or other appointments. This situation continued to worsen for years. Finally, on their way home from a party where they had been drinking heavily, G. and C. caused a severe automobile accident. The occupants of the other car were seriously injured, and G. was convicted of drunken driving. The shock of their irresponsibility and its consequences jarred both into some honest self-examination. G. and C. admitted they had lost control of their alcohol consumption and turned to a close friend for counsel. He surprised them by telling of his own drinking history and took them to an Alcoholics Anonymous meeting. There G. and C. began the long process of achieving sobriety and relearning how to live without alcohol.

Case 3. B.H. is a 42-year-old mother of three children who required hospital admission for treatment of barbiturate and codeine abuse and dependence. She had initially been prescribed a combination medication for treatment of persistent, severe, generalized headaches. B. found herself relieved not only of her headache symptoms, but also of anxiety and tension and a nagging sleep problem. She began to increase her dosage. Aware of her physician's caution about renewing her prescription, B. sought out several other doctors in sequence. She was thereby able to rotate her prescription renewals and thus hide her habit.

Eventually the drug dosage reached levels that impaired B.'s personality and ability to function at work and in the family. Alternating lethargy and irritability resulted in her husband threatening marital separation. At this point B. admitted her drug addiction, and appropriate treatment was sought.

Treatment included supervised detoxification followed by education about the illness of addiction, assertiveness training, family therapy, and supportive followup group therapy.

APPENDIX
The Michigan Alcoholism Screening Test

Directions: If a statement says something true about you, put a check in the nearby space under *yes*. If a statement says something not true about you, put a check in the nearby space under *no*. Please answer all the questions.

	yes	no
1. Do you feel you are a normal drinker?	_____	_____
2. Have you ever awakened the morning after some drinking the night before and found that you could not remember a part of that evening?	_____	_____
3. Does your spouse (or parents) ever worry or complain about your drinking?	_____	_____
4. Can you stop drinking without a struggle after one or two drinks?	_____	_____
5. Do you ever feel bad about your drinking?	_____	_____
6. Do friends or relatives think you are a normal drinker?	_____	_____
7. Do you ever try to limit your drinking to certain times of the day or to certain places?	_____	_____
8. Are you always able to stop drinking when you want to?	_____	_____

9. Have you ever attended a meeting of Alcoholics Anonymous (A.A.)? _____ _____
10. Have you gotten into fights when drinking? _____ _____
11. Has drinking ever created problems with you and your spouse (or parents)? _____ _____
12. Has your spouse (or other family member) ever gone to anyone for help about your drinking? _____ _____
13. Have you ever lost friends or girlfriends or boyfriends because of your drinking? _____ _____
14. Have you ever gotten into trouble at work because of your drinking? _____ _____
15. Have you ever lost a job because of your drinking? _____ _____
16. Have you ever neglected your obligations, your family, or your work for two or more days in a row because you were drinking? _____ _____
17. Do you ever drink before noon? _____ _____
18. Have you ever been told you have liver trouble?
19. Have you ever had delirium tremens (DTs) or severe shaking, heard voices, or seen things that were not there after heavy drinking? _____ _____
20. Have you ever gone to anyone for help about your drinking? _____ _____
21. Have you ever been in a hospital because of your drinking? _____ _____
22. Have you ever been a patient in a psychiatric hospital or on a psychiatric ward of a general hospital where drinking was part of the problem? _____ _____
23. Have you ever been seen at a mental health clinic, or gone to a doctor, social worker, or clergyman for help with an emotional problem in which drinking played a part? _____ _____
24. Have you ever been arrested, even for a few hours, because of drunk behavior? _____ _____
25. Have you ever been arrested for drunk driving or driving after drinking? _____ _____

Scoring the Michigan Alcoholism Screening Test (Questionnaire)

Total possible score = 54 (most alcoholics score above 10 points)

    0–3 points = probably not alcoholic
    3–5 points = 81% diagnostic of alcoholism
    10 points or more = virtually 100% diagnostic of alcoholism

Scoring

Question No.	YES	NO	Question No.	YES	NO
1.	0	2	14.	2	0
2.	2	0	15.	2	0
3.	1	0	16.	2	0
4.	0	2	17.	1	0
5.	1	0	18.	2	0
6.	0	2	19.	5	0
7.	1	0	20.	5	0
8.	0	2	21.	5	0
9.	5	0	22.	2	0
10.	1	0	23.	2	0
11.	2	0	24.	2	0
12.	2	0	25.	2	0
13.	2	0			

References and Further Reading

Alcoholics Anonymous, 3rd ed., New York: Alcoholics Anonymous World Services, 1976.

Bell, R.G. *Critical Analysis of Problem Drinking.* Toronto: Donwood Institute.

Day by Day. Center City, Minn: Hazelden Foundation, 1974.

Dunner, D.L., Hensel, B.M., Fieve, R.R. Bipolar illness: factors in drinking behavior. *Am. J. Psychiatry* 136:583, 1979.

Gitlow, S. E. A pharmacological approach to alcoholism. *The A.A. Grapevine,* October 1968.

Goodwin, D.W. Alcoholism and heredity: a review and hypothesis. *Arch. Gen. Psychiatry* 36:57–61, 1979.

Goodwin, D.W. Genetic aspects of alcoholism. *Drug Therapy,* October 1982, pp. 57–66.

Goodwin, D.W., et al. Drinking problems in adopted and nonadopted sons of alcoholics. *Arch. Gen. Psychiatry* 31:164–169, 1974.

Heilman, R.O. Early recognition of alcoholism and other drug dependence. *Md. State Med. J.* 25(9):73–76, 1976.

Keller, M., McCormick, M. *A Dictionary of Words About Alcohol.* New Brunswick, N.J.: Rutgers Center of Alcohol Studies, 1968.

Living Sober. New York: Alcoholics Anonymous World Service, 1975.

Powell, B.J., et al. Prevalence of additional psychiatric symptoms among male alcoholics. *J. Clin. Psychiatry* 43:404–407, 1982.

Quitlein, F.M., et al. Phobic anxiety syndrome complicated by drug dependence and addiction. *Arch. Gen. Psychiatry* 27:159–162, 1972.

Rousaville, B.J., et al. Diagnosis and symptoms of depression in opiate addicts. *Arch. Gen. Psychiatry* 39:151–156, 1982.

Rousaville, B.J., et al. Heterogeneity of psychiatric diagnosis in treated opiate addicts. *Arch. Gen. Psychiatry* 39:161–166, 1982.

Schneidmule, A. *Basic Facts About Alcohol.* Baltimore: The Johns Hopkins Hospital Regional Training Program for Alcoholism Counselors.

Twelve Steps and Twelve Traditions. New York: Alcoholics Anonymous World Services, 1952–1953.

Twenty-Four Hours A Day. Center City, Minn.: Hazelden Foundation, 1975.

Wegscheider, S. *Another Chance: Hope and Health for the Alcoholic Family.* Palo Alto, Calif.: Science and Behavior Books, 1981.

Weissman, M.M., Meyers, I.K., Harding, P.S. Prevalence and psychiatric heterogeneity of alcoholism in a United States urban community. *J. Stud. Alcohol.* 41:672–681, 1980.

Whitfield, C.L., Williams, K., Liepman, M. *The Patient With Alcoholism and Other Drug Problems: Medical Aspects for Students, Residents, and Practicing Physicians.* Springfield, Ill.: Charles C Thomas, 1976.

6

Schizophrenic and Other Nonaffective Psychotic Disorders

C. GIBSON DUNN, M.D.

Schizophrenia has traditionally been described as one of the major functional psychotic disorders—that is, those severe mental disorders for which no organic etiology has been established. It was first recognized as a disease entity in the work of the Munich psychiatrist Emil Kraepelin in the 1890s. During that decade Kraepelin defined the two major groups of functional psychoses—dementia praecox and manic depression. As noted in Chapter 7, Kraepelin based his theoretical formulations on prolonged observation of psychiatric patients, relying heavily on differences in course and outcome for separating new nosologic entities. *Dementia praecox* was a term applied by Kraepelin to a severe disorder of presumably endogenous etiology, progressing to final deterioration in a great majority of cases; this mental deterioration took place despite a relative preservation of intellectual and memory functions. Kraepelin contended that dementia praecox was fundamentally characterized by a disruption of the coordination of functions. Most intensely affected were judgment, emotional impulses, volition, and initiative. Emotions were dulled and flattened, and thought processes disordered. Logical associations and contact with reality were frequently disrupted. Suggestibility and stereotypical behavior were noted. Delusions and hallucinations were often present, although not considered essential diagnostic features. Kraepelin stressed the loss of multiple mental functions, especially those contributing to active and successful function in the real world. His emphasis on the poor outcome of dementia praecox is particularly important.

In 1911, Eugen Bleuler of Zurich sought to extend Kraepelin's work. He published his studies under the title *Dementia Praecox or the Group of Schizophrenias*. Bleuler then derived the current term *schizophrenia,* which eventually replaced *dementia praecox.* Bleuler argued that the fundamental disorder in dementia praecox was a "split of mental processes." Thus, the term *schizo-phrenia* (split mind) was descriptive. The four main functions that he contended were impaired—associations, affectivity, ambivalence, and autism—came to be referred to as Bleuler's four A's.

Bleuler's work had far-reaching effects. Psychiatrists became increasingly interested in the psychological processes of the person with schizophrenia and less concerned with defining diagnostic criteria for the diagnosis. Bleuler's concept of illness was also quite broad, encouraging inclusion rather than exclusion of patients under this diagnostic entity. For these and other reasons, the diagnosis of schizophrenia was applied to increasing numbers of severely disturbed patients.

The introduction of lithium therapy in the late 1960s, led to a revival of interest in distinguishing among the various psychotic disorders. It became important not to misapply the diagnosis of schizophrenia, or a lithium-responsive manic depressive patient might go unrecognized. In the *Diagnostic and Statistical Manual of Mental Disorders,* Third Edition (DSM-III), the diagnostic criteria for schizophrenia are more specific and reflect this new emphasis on greater precision in applying the label *schizophrenia.*

Two new categories have been established in the DSM-III for those psychoses that are not affective but do not meet the criteria for schizophrenia. These entities, *schizophreniform psychosis* and *brief reactive psychosis,* are described later in this chapter.

Another category of psychosis, *paranoid disorder,* has long been recognized, although its relationship to the other nosologic entities has been debated. A residual category of *atypical psychotic disorder* includes cases that do not meet the criteria for any other psychotic disorder.

Schizophrenic Disorders, Schizophreniform Disorder, and Brief Reactive Psychosis

SIGNS AND SYMPTOMS

Schizophrenia, the most common of the schizophrenic disorders, has traditionally been called a *thought disorder,* reflecting the prominence of disturbance in the thinking processes. In fact, however, schizophrenia involves disorders in many more areas of mental functioning than thought processes alone. There is a pervasive and generalized breakdown in multiple areas of mental operations and functional abilities. Symptoms of schizophrenia often begin with increasing anxiety and fear, related perhaps to the pending dissolution of adaptive cognitive operations. Thinking may become tangential and associations loosened. Goal orientation may be impaired so that the person appears to be thinking or speaking past the point of thought. Total fragmentation of thought structure, including creation of meaningless neologisms, may occur. The following excerpt from a clinical interview illustrates the thinking disorder in schizophrenia. The patient was a 34-year-old hospitalized male (W_____ P_____) in the early states of recovery from acute psychotic decompensation:

Patient	To get down to a parallel level I will have to illustrate.
Interviewer	Talking parallel seems to confuse things, let's talk about the reasons for your feelings.
Patient	I don't know why I can't talk to you. Have you got a pen or a pencil?
Interviewer	What do you think? I guess there is some reason why you can't talk to me. It seems I make you uncomfortable.
Patient	You want to know what is happening for real....
Interviewer	Is that wrong?
Patient	No.
Interviewer	Is that something to be hidden? It sounds like you don't want other people to know what is happening inside of Willie Patterson. (Pause; patient borrows pencil and paper and writes.)
Patient (reading his work)	It is the time of day when everything is great and everybody is ok.... Then a little later on in the day you might start being a little bit more selective about your associates. When you do that, the associates that you have selected not including their jealousies are aroused; they might start to do things and say things they don't particularly care for you leaving them out of the big conversation. I don't consider myself big enough to have a big conversation. As far as I know I am one of the poorest patients in here. I mean financially I have about $30.00 or so in the checking account. That goes to show you that you can have charisma and people will want to talk to you.
Interviewer	Before you started writing, you asked if I want to know what's for "real."
Patient	That's for real.
Interviewer	It sounds like you're saying you feel like I want to know but you just don't feel comfortable about talking about it.
Patient	Maybe that's it. I don't know.

The patients may develop a loss of ability to assess the world. Unrealistic judgments and delusions of various types may occur. The most frequently observed delusions involve those of a paranoid nature of external control by real or unreal sources. Religious delusions may be present. Some patients also develop hallucinatory perceptions of hearing voices, and at times visual and even olfactory experiences may occur. These hallucinations are often felt to be absolutely real. Patients may also lose their sense of trust in those around them and withdraw from many routine activities. Then the illness progresses to a generalized breakdown in interpersonal and social functioning. Judgment becomes extremely impaired, and motivation to carry expected activities diminishes and disappears. This may be reflected in a decline in school or work performance. Unfortunately these patients may show a profound lack of awareness of the illness and may be quite indifferent to their own condition or to the concerns of others. In fact, they may have bizarre interpretations of the normal actions of others.

In this illness, mood and affect may also be disturbed. Along with anxiety and fear, significant anger or depression can develop during the acute decompensation. Expressed emotion may be inappropriate to the subject being discussed, or may be generally blunted. Along with the blunting, there may be a loss of interpersonal relatedness, which has been termed the *praecox feeling*.

It is also important to emphasize the functions that are maintained rather than impaired. Although concentration may be significantly diminished, memory remains intact. Intellectual abilities such as mathematical calculations and fund of knowledge are preserved. The ability to perform complex mental or behavioral operations is also retained when the person can adequately attend to the task.

In summary, then, the signs and symptoms of schizophrenia are characterized by pervasive breakdown in mental and behavioral functioning in multiple areas, with thought processes, initiative, and goal-oriented behavior most seriously impaired.

EPIDEMIOLOGY

As far as can be determined, schizphrenia occurs in cultures throughout the world. Its basic nature and prevalence appear to be remarkably consistent except for a few isolated, inbred cultural groups. While estimates of prevalence rates have varied according to the diagnostic criteria applied, an average prevalence of approximately one percent of the total population appears to be reasonably accurate. Distribution by sex is approximately equal; this is in marked contrast to the anxiety disorders, affective disorders, and substance abuse disorders. The social class distribution is skewed toward increased prevalence in lower socioeconomic groups. Despite earlier theorizing that the stresses of lower-class existence cause schizophrenia, it is now generally accepted that downward social drift caused by the dysfunction of schizophrenia leads to an accumulation of impaired individuals in the lower socioeconomic groups.

Onset, Course, and Prognosis
Most typically, the onset of schizophrenia occurs during adolescent and young adult years. While childhood schizophrenia is a recognized disorder, the illness is less frequent in this earlier period, and the precise relationship of the childhood illness to the disorder here being discussed remains clouded. Schizophrenia, especially in the paranoid form, may have an onset through the fourth decade of life. With advancing age, however, the diagnostician should maintain a higher index of suspicion for the psychotic presentation of an affective disorder. Onset after the age of 40 is likely to be indicative of a paranoid or affective disorder, as discussed elsewhere.

The nature and rate of onset of schizophrenia varies greatly. There may be a connection between the nature of onset and the course and prognosis of the disorder. Two broad patterns of schizophrenia have been described and given various labels. "Nuclear," "core," "process," and "poor prognosis" schizophrenia describe one category, while the other has been characterized as "acute," "reactive," and "good prognosis" schizophrenia. As the labels themselves imply, process or poor prognosis schizophrenia is a disorder characterized by insidious, gradual onset associated with profound interpersonal withdrawal and quiet though pervasive psychotic symptomatology. The course of this type of schizophrenia tends to be chronic and relatively unremitting, with poor functional outcome. Many of these patients have poor response to currently available neuroleptic medication. Acute or good prognosis schizophrenia is considered an illness of more rapid onset; florid symptomatology often follows a stressful precipitating event, and good response to neuroleptic medication, a high rate of remission, and generally more favorable outcome are found. Poor prognosis schizophrenia has been linked with a strong family history of the same illness, a schizoid or isolative type of premorbid personality, and a general paucity of interpersonal relationships. Acute schizophrenia has been associated with a history of affective illness in the family, associated depressive symptomatology, relatively normal premorbid personality, and much more frequent involvement in normal social relationships.

The wide discrepancy between these two categories of schizophrenia has been so striking that one must raise the question as to whether the illnesses in fact belong to the same category at all. As noted later in the discussion of differential diagnosis, many of the so-called acute schizophrenias may in face be atypical presentations of severe mania. The DSM-III criteria orient the diagnosis of schizophrenia to reflect the process of the illness by requiring that symptoms have lasted at least six months before the diagnosis can be applied.

Patients with schizophrenia often report its onset around events involving separation from family and intimate supportive persons. It has not been demonstrated, however, that these life events are in and of themselves precipitating factors in the initial illness episode. For example, schizophrenia frequently occurs in 18-year-old individuals; some may be going off to college, and some may be remaining at home. It could be argued that a life transition occurs at this age regardless of physical separation from the family, and that separation from loved ones may not be the trigger for illness. Thus, the long-term course and prognosis of a person with schizophrenia can be extremely variable, and expectations must take into account this range of variability. For the group of persons with "core" (i.e., especially severe) schizophrenia, the long-term prognosis is at best guarded; a minority of these will go on to consistently satisfactory functioning, but the majority will experience a life punctuated with periods of recurrence and probably repeated hospitalizations. At the other extreme, a small number will be poorly functional and severely impaired.

It is quite important to emphasize that outcome is not a homogeneous phenomenon. Three useful categories of outcome are based on continuing symptomatology, social function, and employment. Individuals may do well in one or two areas while doing considerably less well in the third. Strauss and Carpenter (1972) have found that the ability to form social relationships is the most significant predictor of outcome. There is only a partial intercorrelation of outcome measures. Treatment of each individual requires assessment of all three areas.

Complications

Several complications of schizophrenia require special mention. While there is frequent fear about potential for violence by schizophrenic patients, there is little evidence to show significantly increased violence by persons with this diagnosis. Occasionally paranoid psychotic patients may make major headlines by acting on their delusions and hallucinations, thus increasing public awareness and fear. While violence against others is uncommon, there is a definitely increased risk of suicide. This appears to be a result of the symptoms of fear and depressed mood combined with greater impulsivity. In addition, underachievement and relative occupational and social failure are frequent complications. There may be some increase in abuse of alcohol and drugs as well in people with schizophrenia.

ETIOLOGY

Schizophrenia remains a disorder of unknown etiology or etiologies. At the time of Kraepelin's description of dementia praecox, the illness was assumed to be of physical origin. This has generally continued to be accepted by most researchers throughout the world. For several decades, especially in America, a more intense search for possible psychogenic causes was undertaken. For some years the nature-versus-nurture debate was quite intense, and some clinicians still seem to be caught up in this rather sterile argument. Part of the intensity has come from a mistaken assumption that etiology must determine the nature of treatment. In fact, there are numerous biologically based illnesses (for example, diabetes mellitus and chronic renal failure) that require close attention to psychological and social factors in their treatment. At present, it is generally assumed that major biologic factors contribute to the onset of schizophrenic disorders but that the illnesses are multi-determined, with many forms having environmental contributions. It is useful to divide etiologic hypotheses into psychosocial theories and biologic theories, although it should be remembered that such division is simplistic and artificial.

Psychosocial Theories

The psychogenic and psychosocial theories of schizophrenia received their greatest impetus from the work of Freud and his followers and from Adolph Meyer and those whom he influenced in America. These schools have emphasized the enduring impact of emotional experiences early in life; attention had been focused mainly on contact between mother and infant but more recently has included the interaction within the entire dynamic family network. The theories themselves have generally been based on experience in therapeutic work. The most prominent theorists in this era—Harry Stack Sullivan and Frieda Fromm Reichmann, followed by Federn, Searles, Mahler, and Fairbairn—have emphasized the development in early life of severe ego disturbances resulting from disruption of the fundamental mother-child relationship. Basic ego functions, beginning with the distinction between self and other, fail to develop in the normal progression. This disruption of early *object relationships* results in distortion in all future contact with reality and interpersonal relationships. These theories, of course, do not rule out the existence of biologic factors, and many of these researchers have assumed the presence of a constitutional factor that influences the abnormal ego development.

Somewhat later investigators (most prominently Theodore Lidz, Steven Fleck, and Alice Cornelison at the Yale Psychiatric Institute) focused attention on interpersonal relationships in the families. Lidz and associates (1965) assumed the ongoing presence of pervasive deficiencies and distorting influences on the parents and families of their schizophrenic patients. They identified specific deficiencies of parental nurturance that led to the patients' difficulties in achieving individual autonomy—that is, independence and responsibility for the self. In addition, the family failed in the social role of directing the child's growth and development in the prevailing society. Finally, these families were inadequate at transmitting communication and other basic instrumental techniques of the surrounding culture of the child who eventually became schizophrenic. Thus, deprived of the satisfaction of basic needs, fundamental ego boundaries, an adequate sense of direction, and adequate interpersonal techniques to manipulate symbolic communication (language), the patient met the demands of growth, development, and individuation by retreat into a psychotic state.

While Lidz and his associates emphasized the multiple causes of family inadequacies, the abnormal patterns of marital schism and marital skew were frequently observed in the parents of schizophrenics. In *marital schism,* spouses were found to be in very divergent paths, often related to excessive individual needs. Such parents were unable to work together in a complementary or reciprocal fashion. Separation was a constant threat, and communication was used to coerce or defy the partner or to mask the seriousness of the situation. In families characterized by *marital skew,* there was serious psychopathology in which one marital partner dominated the home. In all of such families studied, the partner who was extremely dependent or masochistic was paired with a strong and protecting figure. Dependency or masochistic needs caused the weaker member to go along with any emotional distortions of the dominant parental partner. In all cases, the psychopathology of the dominant spouse created an abnormal family environment in which the basic needs of the eventually schizophrenic child could not be met. In these families, the child became an object of competition between the parents, with the intergenerational boundaries between parent and child violated in the struggle to retain the child's love and loyalty. This placed enormous stress on the child, who had to choose between the parents, resulting in anxiety and threatened loss.

Investigators Wynne and Singer found further that the disturbed communication and distortion of thinking within the family resulted in disturbance in the focusing of attention and blurring of meaning during the child's formative years. These distortions theoretically predisposed the child to the development of a schizophrenic thought disorder during later critical life periods. Thus, it was argued that disturbed interpersonal relationships caused disordered cognitive processes. A fundamental aspect of this pathology was a lack of differentiation of self from the environment and a fluidity of ego boundaries; consequently, later interpersonal relationships could not be established in the normal maturational sequence. The child had to remain a child of his or her parents rather than becoming an autonomous individual with a separate identity.

Gregory Bateson found on a specific aspect of the parent-child relationship believed to be of psychotogenic significance—the *double bind,* in which an overt direct communication was contradicted by a nonverbal covert message. The child consequently was caught in a serious emotional conflict of incompatible expectations, resulting in feelings of helplessness, anger, and fear. Alanen found that fear and aggression characterized early relationships between mother and child; the mother was particularly disturbed at the time of the birth and infancy of the eventually schizophrenic patient. Hartman emphasized that severe conflicts over uncontrolled aggression interfered with the development of autonomous ego functions and disrupted perception and logical thought processes.

Social and environmental factors have also been suggested as the etiologic factors in schizophrenia. In Redlich and Hollingshead's study of New Haven, schizophrenics were found to be clustered in the lower social groups, in which environmental stresses were more marked and social supports less available. It is now generally believed that this accumulation of individuals with schizophrenia in the lowest social classes results from intergenerational downward drift caused by the inability of impaired individuals to maintain their level in society. Some theorists have suggested that schizophrenic psychosis is increased among immigrants, because the stress of cross-cultural change leads to a psychotic breakdown. These studies have been inconsistent with regard to rate of psychosis and the question of whether the migratory pattern led to the selection of particularly predisposed individuals.

Biologic Theories

The biologic hypotheses of schizophrenia are even more diverse than the psychosocial theories. At this time none of these hypotheses is considered in any way definitive.

Genetic Inheritance. One of the most heavily studied areas has been that of a possible genetically inherited contribution to schizophrenia. The best-known work has been by

Gottesman and Shields (1973) from Great Britain and Kety and associates (1971) from the United States, but many other studies have been conducted. There appears to be a strong case for genetic contribution to many though by no means all cases of schizophrenia; the hereditary predisposition remains even when environment has been completely eliminated for all but a few weeks of life. According to various studies, the risk that relatives of schizophrenics will develop the disorder becomes greater as the degree of genetic relatedness increases. The sibling of a schizophrenic patient has approximately a 15 percent risk of becoming schizophrenic at some time; the risk in the general population is approximately 1 percent. This 15 percent risk seems to apply to most first-degree relatives, including the child of one schizophrenic and one nonschizophrenic parent. The Dizygotic twin of a schizophrenic patient likewise has genetic risk equal only to that of any other sibling. Monozygotic twins, however, have a concordance rate for schizophrenia of about 50 to 60 percent even when they are raised apart from birth. Similarly, the child of two schizophrenic parents has approximately a 40 percent risk of becoming schizophrenic.

Given that these studies have been carried out repeatedly and with large populations, the evidence is quite convincing that a genetic component probably contributes to some cases of schizophrenia. The mode of transmission, however, has not been determined, and both single gene and polygenic models have been proposed. In addition, it is unclear as to what might be transmitted genetically—that is, what fundamental diathesis is inherited. It should also be noted that in approximately 50 percent of schizophrenic patients, there is no identifiable genetic contribution. In these cases, as in the discordant monozygotic twin pairs, there is presumably an environmental or other biologic factor that has predominant influence.

Neurotransmitters and Endogenous Psychotogenic Substances. An area of biologic research that has received great attention involves neurotransmitters and endogenous psychotogenic substances. Most prominent within this research has been work on dopamine and the *dopamine hypothesis.* Investigators became quite interested in the role of the neurotransmitter dopamine in schizophrenia following the introduction of chlorpromazine in the early 1950s. It was discovered that chlorpromazine and all subsequently discovered neuroleptic medications had an extremely high affinity for binding to the postsynaptic dopamine receptor. This binding served to block the action of dopamine on the receptor site. The dopamine hypothesis states essentially that schizophrenia results from a functional overactivity of the neurotransmitter dopamine. At various times studies have indicated an excess of dopamine and increased receptor sensitivity present in the central nervous systems of schizophrenics. Interest in dopamine grew with the finding that many dopaminergic pathways are in close proximity to the limbic system and thereby might have profound effects on mood and cognitive processes. In addition, compounds like L-dopa, cocaine, and amphetamine, which increase the activity of dopamine, all tend to exacerbate schizophrenic psychoses.

The role of dopamine was explored in the work of Wise and Stein, who presented evidence showing that the enzyme dopamine-beta-hydroxylase is deficient in the brains of schizophrenic patients. This enzymatic deficiency theoretically would lead to the overproduction of 6-hydroxydopamine, which is toxic to noradrenergic neurons in the hypothalamic reward-and-punishment system. Damage to these neurons might contribute significantly to the major negative symptoms of schizophrenia, such as loss of goal-directed thinking and behavior, interpersonal withdrawal, and lack of initiative. At various times, also, there have been reports of excessive levels of dopamine or excessive dopaminergic receptor sensitivity in schizophrenics. Unfortunately, none of these observations has been consistently supported by well-designed studies.

Related to the dopamine hypothesis has been work on the inhibitory neurotransmitter gamma-aminobutyric acid (GABA), which is thought to inhibit dopamine activity. It would follow that an underactivity of GABA might result in a functional overactivity of dopamine.

Early schizophrenia research also focused on the possibility that some internal autotoxins might produce the psychosis of schizophrenia. Since it was known that exogenous hallucinogens such as lysergic acid diethylamide (LSD) and mescaline could produce a psychotic state, researchers hoped to identify an endogenously produced compound that was fundamental to the etiology of schizophrenia. Agents of interest have included transmethylated norepinephrine, dimethoxyphenylethylamine, bufotenin, and dimethyltryptamine.

Endorphins are a more recent area of research in the etiology of schizophrenia. The hypothesis that excessive endorphin activity might be schizophrenogenic receives some support from initial observations that the opiate antagonist naloxone may possess antipsychotic activity. There is also a suggestion that beta-endorphin might have actively antipsychotic properties itself.

In two recent hypotheses involving prostaglandins and monoamine oxidase, it has been postulated that deficiencies of these compounds might exist in schizophrenics. Monoamine oxidase deficiencies have, in fact, been observed in paranoid subgroups of the schizophrenic populations, and the platelets of some schizophrenics have been found to be deficient in their production of prostaglandin E_1 when stimulated by adenosine diphosphate. As with other hypotheses, the reliability and validity of these observations are as yet uncertain.

Gross Brain Abnormalities. Reports show an increased rate of abnormal electroencephalograms in psychotic patients, including those diagnosed as schizophrenic. Recent work by Weinburger and associates has employed computerized tomography to examine the brains of schizophrenic patients. They have identified a subgroup of schizophrenics with significant ventricular enlargement and cortical atrophy. While the import of this finding remains to be demonstrated, it is possible that there is a sizeable group of schizophrenic patients in whom this abnormality may have an etiologic role.

Viral Etiology. It has been observed in one group of schizophrenics that there is a clustering of births toward the late winter and spring. This has led to the hypothesis that a viral etiology might exist in some forms of schizophrenia. In such cases, the virus is presumably of a slow or latent type that is expressed long after birth. Related immunologic abnormalities in certain schizophrenic patients have been cited to support this hypothesis.

In summary, it can be said that the genetic and dopaminergic hypotheses for the etiology of schizophrenia have received the greatest investigation and support to date. In neither case, however, are the data sufficient to account for the disorders being investigated, and there has been no demonstrated association between genetic and biochemical findings. It is assumed that schizophrenia encompasses multiple disorders with multiple etiologies, and individual cases may reflect an interaction of several causal factors. A particularly interesting synthesis of observations has been made by T.J. Crow, who argues that a distinction should be made between positive and negative symptoms, which reflect two distinct disorders. Positive symptoms reflect the disorder characterized by an excess of dopaminergic transmission; this acutely psychotic state is responsive to current neuroleptic medication with a reversible outcome. Negative symptoms correlate with the chronic form of schizophrenia, which does not respond well to medication. In this disorder, there may be an illness resembling encephalitis, with resulting cell loss and structural changes in the brain such as those decribed by Weinburger and associates. This synthesis of observations in this area is still theoretical.

DIFFERENTIAL DIAGNOSIS

Schizophrenia must be differentiated from both functional and organically based psychotic states. Among functional psychoses, primary affective disorders may present the greatest challenge in differential diagnosis. Occasionally paranoid forms of psychotic depression can pose diagnostic difficulties. More commonly, severe forms of manic psychosis can appear extremely similar to, or indistinguishable from, acute schizophrenic psychoses. In these cases a heavier reliance must be placed on the patient's history and on the family history. The existence of affective disorders in relatives may be of major help in the differential diagnostic process. Among the anxiety disorders, severe obsessional states may reach levels so intense and so bizarre as to pose diagnostic difficulties. Finally, diagnostic difficulties may occur in certain severe personality disorders, including the paranoid, schizotypal, and borderline personality states. These disorders may be particularly difficult to distinguish from schizophrenia when the degree of functional impairment is marked. Again, strict reliance on the diagnostic criteria for schizophrenia, and a longitudinal history may be of major assistance.

Many organic psychotic disorders can appear quite similar or identical to schizophrenic disorders. Drug intoxications, especially with amphetamines and phencyclidine, may induce most of the schizophrenic symptoms. Amphetamine psychoses can sometimes be indistinguishable from paranoid schizophrenia. A careful history of drug use combined with laboratory data may be of assistance in the diagnostic process. Cocaine abuse may also create an agitated paranoid psychotic state. Alcoholic hallucinosis may cause diagnostic difficulties; in this disorder heavy alcohol abuse can create a paranoid psychosis with auditory hallucinations. While the disorder usually resolves within days to weeks, a few individuals may progress to a more chronic illness. These chronic illnesses may in fact occur in individuals who are predisposed to schizophrenia or who have already developed schizophrenia, since they decompensate simultaneously with the chemical insult. Therapeutically prescribed corticosteroids are known to induce psychotic disorders of several forms, including paranoid agitated states that appear similar to schizophrenia. This problem may actually occur in individuals already predisposed toward this type of psychotic disorder. Specific medical illnesses affecting the central nervous system are known to create schizophreniform psychotic disorders; among these are systemic lupus erythematosus, acute intermittent porphyria, and Wilson's disease. In addition, a paranoid schizophreniform psychosis can occur in association with temporal lobe epilepsy. Diagnosis of these disorders relies on comprehensive medical evaluation for each illness. In all cases, it is crucial to avoid premature closure of the diagnostic process. Overconfidence in the available data can result in the misdiagnosis of a serious and treatable disorder.

DIAGNOSTIC CRITERIA

There are no known pathognomonic symptoms or signs of schizophrenia or the schizophreniform psychoses. The diagnosis, therefore, must be established by the combined data of the individual's history, comprehensive mental status examination, and family history. The DSM-III diagnostic criteria for schizophrenic disorder, which are listed in Table 6-1, emphasize what has been referred to as *positive schizophrenia*—that is, active disorders of thought and perceptual processes. Emphasis is placed on a specific type of auditory hallucinations, including hallucinations of a voice commenting on the patient's actions or two or more voices addressing each other. This type of hallucination may eventually prove to be specific to schizophrenia; however, at this time, such hallucinations must be combined with other symptomatology to establish a diagnosis.

Table 6-1. Diagnostic Criteria for a Schizophrenic Disorder

A. At least one of the following during a phase of the illness:
  1. bizarre delusions (content is patently absurd and has *no* possible basis in fact), such as delusions of being controlled, thought broadcasting, thought insertion, or thought withdrawal
  2. somatic, grandiose, religious, nihilistic, or other delusions without persecutory or jealous content
  3. delusions with persecutory or jealous content if accompanied by hallucinations of any type
  4. auditory hallucinations in which either a voice keeps up a running commentary on the individual's behavior or thoughts, or two or more voices converse with each other
  5. auditory hallucinations on several occasions with content of more than one or two words, having no apparent relation to depression or elation
  6. incoherence, marked loosening of associations, markedly illogical thinking, or marked poverty of content of speech if associated with at least one of the following:
      a. blunted, flat, or inappropriate affect
      b. delusions or hallucinations
      c. catatonic or other grossly disorganized behavior
B. Deterioration from a previous level of functioning in such areas as work, social relations, and self-care.
C. Duration: Continuous signs of the illness for at least six months at some time during the person's life, with some signs of the illness at present. The six-month period must include an active phase during which there were symptoms from A, with or without a prodromal or residual phase.

Reproduced with permission from *Diagnostic and Statistical Manual of Mental Disorders,* 3rd ed. Washington, D.C.: American Psychiatric Association, 1980, pp. 188–189.

Table 6-2. Prodromal or Residual Symptoms of Schizophrenia

1. Social isolation or withdrawal
2. Marked impairment in role functioning as wage-earner, student, or homemaker
3. Markedly peculiar behavior (e.g., collecting garbage, talking to self in public, or hoarding food)
4. Marked impairment in personal hygiene and grooming
5. Blunted, flat, or inappropriate affect
6. Digressive, vague overelaborate, circumstantial, or metaphorical speech
7. Odd or bizarre ideation, or magical thinking, e.g., superstitiousness, clairvoyance, telepathy, "sixth sense," "others can feel my feelings," overvalued ideas, ideas of reference
8. Unusual perceptual experiences, e.g., recurrent illusions, sensing the presence of a force or person not actually present

Reproduced with permission from DSM-III, p. 189.

When all of the symptoms are evidence during the acute phase of illness, the diagnosis of schizophrenia may be reasonably straightforward. During the prodromal or residual phase of schizophrenia, when florid psychotic symptoms may not be evident, however, the diagnosis may rest more on the presence of *negative* symptoms combined with the eliciting of previous positive symptoms. The prodromal and residual symptoms of schizophrenia, which are listed in Table 6-2, may require considerably greater observation and interpretation. Such negative symptoms are quite important but are also more open to misinterpretation and blurring with other diagnostic categories. Nonetheless, as most investigators have noted, the residual negative symptoms may in fact be of major significance in the long-term outcome of patients with schizophrenia.

Basic Subtypes of Schizophrenia

Since the work of Kraepelin, schizophrenia has been divided into several subtypes. The generally accepted subtypes have varied from country to country and period to period. Kraepelin emphasized hebephrenic, catatonic, and paranoid subtypes, and later added simple schizophrenia. In the current diagnostic nomenclature, the subtypes include disorganized, catatonic, paranoid, and undifferentiated. *Disorganized schizophrenia* (previously termed *hebephrenic*) has the distinguishing symptom of marked incoherence of thought and language, absence of organized delusions, and inappropriate affect. *Catatonic schizophrenia* has as its diagnostic symptoms disorders of psychomotor activity, either withdrawn or excited. In withdrawn catatonia, the patient may be negativistic, rigid, or even stuporous. Catatonic excitement, on the other hand, is characterized by frantic and purposeless motor activity; there may be a classic posturing with an unusual muscle tone known as "waxy flexibility." In *paranoid schizophrenia,* there are characteristic delusions of a persecutory, jealous, or grandiose type. It is important to remember that excited catatonia and paranoid schizophrenia are most open to diagnostic confusion with extreme mania. *Undifferentiated schizophrenia* is diagnosed when the patient's symptoms meet the full diagnostic criteria for a schizophrenic disorder without the characteristics of any particular subtype.

Residual schizophrenia refers to a schizophrenic disorder without the marked positive symptoms described earlier but with continuing evidence of typical negative symptoms. If these symptoms resolve, the disorder is considered to be in remission.

Special mention should be made of *schizoaffective schizophrenia,* which is listed in DSM-III without specific diagnostic criteria. Although schizophrenia has always been defined as a disorder that primarily affects thought processes, there have been persistent observations of patients presenting not only with classic schizophrenic symptoms, but also with marked mood disturbance. The term *acute schizoaffective psychosis* was coined by Kasanin in the 1930s to describe this group of patients. In the United States, these disorders have generally been linked with the schizophrenic disorders. This categorization, however, has repeatedly been questioned, especially since lithium carbonate has led to the successful treatment of many supposedly schizoaffective schizophrenia patients. Many of these individuals are in fact experiencing variants of manic-depressive (or bipolar) affective illness and are probably not schizophrenic. These patients frequently have strong family histories for affective illnesses rather than schizophrenia. According to the DSM-III usage, the diagnosis of schizoaffective disorder should be applied to cases in which the clinician is unable to resolve the differential diagnosis between affective disorder and schizophrenia or schizophreniform disorder. From a practical point of view, when the diagnostic question is unresolved, the patient should be presumed to have an affective disorder and be treated accordingly.

New Categories

Two new categories of psychotic disorders have been added in DSM-III. One has been included to reduce the tendency to reach a premature diagnosis of schizophrenia, and the other category recognizes the existence of a reactive psychotic disorder that does not seem to be one of the schizophrenic or affective disorders.

Schizophreniform disorder is the category that pertains to patients whose symptoms meet the diagnostic criteria for schizophrenia but whose illness has lasted more than two weeks and less than six months (the time necessary for the diagnosis of schizophrenia). A practicing clinician will encounter many patients who are probably schizophrenic but who have not yet manifested the illness for a full six months. In such cases, the diagnosis should be schizophreniform disorder, which is later changed to schizophrenia if symptoms persist.

Brief reactive psychosis is a psychotic disorder of rapid onset in close relation to a psychologically stressful life event. The illness must last less than two weeks and be followed by full recovery to the premorbid level of function. There may be delusions, hallucinations, and loosening of associations, but there is also prominent emotional turmoil involving labile mood and affect. The patient may appear just as ill as an individual with schizophrenia or schizophreniform disorder, although affect tends to be better preserved. There may be preexisting psychopathology predisposing to development of this disorder, but this may involve some type of significant personality disorder. A disorder previously known as *hysterical psychosis* may have been a variant of this new diagnostic category. The onset tends to be in adolescence and young adulthood. Further information on epidemiology and long-term outcome of this disorder is available.

TREATMENT OF SCHIZOPHRENIA

The treatment of schizophrenia and other psychotic disorders remains one of the most complex and challenging of medical tasks. While it is generally recognized that current therapies are imperfect, remarkable progress has been made in reducing the severity of the illness during the acute phase and in helping the patient remain in the community with improved levels of function.

Acute Phase

For the purpose of treatment, schizophrenia can be divided into acute, early recovery, and residual phases. The acute phase of schizophrenic psychosis is characterized by the most florid of psychotic symptoms. In order to treat a person experiencing such symptoms, one should try to understand the patient's experience of the acute psychosis. The works of Bowers (1974) and Donlon and Blacker (1973) elucidate the psychotic experience. Patients initially cited feelings of conflict and the sense of being at an impasse, with the fundamental emotions of anxiety and intense dread. It should be emphasized that this anxiety is so pervasive that the continuity of life itself seems threatened. There may be feelings of excitement or loss of control, as well as fluctuations in mood. Patients may attempt to respond to the feeling of being out of control with an exaggeration of typical defense mechanisms. When these mechanisms eventually fail, an experience of heightened awareness follows in which sensory input is extremely intense and immediate. The patient may report a dissolution of barriers to sensations from both internal and external sources. A sense of urgency and anticipation may develop. The need for sleep decreases, and thoughts and perceptions may race. There may be feelings of horror at the primitive nature of these experiences. At this point, interpretation of stimuli may become individualistic (autistic), and otherwise disconnected or unrelated events will take on acutely personal meaning. Such interpretations by the patient will have much greater reality than input from treating clinicians. Thought, feeling, and perception mesh in an increasingly confusing fashion. Finally even the basic sense of self, generally considered fundamental, begins to fragment and dissolve. This sense of self is overwhelmed in the flood of psychotic experience, which is extremely frightening and painful. Once the dissolution has progressed, the patient may begin to construct delusions from the detached and free-floating sensory and experiential stimuli. The individual will seek to construct a comprehensible meaning out of the otherwise meaningless chaos that has been described.

The patient's experience of acute psychosis is a sense of being out of control. Thus, the initial phase of treatment must emphasize a highly structured environment, with provision of reality input (i.e., reality-based communication) and the active use of antipsychotic medication; all of these elements help the patient reestablish control. Treatment of this phase of schizophrenia is generally conducted in an appropriate hospital setting. While cooperation of the patient should be sought and is often forthcoming, the clinician, in conjunction with responsible family members, must take the initiative to direct the patients to a safe, secure environment. Whether or not these patients are capable of reaching this decision in their psychotic state, they will definitely benefit from guidance. Staff members should work to help patients maintain as much contact with reality as possible, gently correcting hallucinatory and delusional interpretations of the surrounding world.

In conjunction with the structured secure hospital environment, an active use of neuroleptic medication is strongly indicated during the acute phase. (The use of these medications is discussed in Chapter 21.) Each clinician must become familiar with a limited number of neuroleptic drugs so that he or she can feel confident in their use. For markedly agitated patients, haloperidol and chlorpromazine are most frequently prescribed. Once the patient's physical status has been evaluated, relatively rapid titration of medication is possible. Much higher blood levels of medication are obtained through intramuscular injection, which can be given every 30 to 60 minutes until adequate sedation or symptom control is achieved. Control of environmental sensory input may facilitate the positive effects of medication. The use of a quiet seclusion room can be markedly effective in reducing acute psychotic symptoms with a lower total dosage of medication. Employment of such a treatment technique, however, requires a highly skilled and dedicated staff who will pay careful attention to the patient's evolving condition.

If the total dosage of neuroleptic medication is being rapidly increased, careful monitoring of vital signs is essential. The combined anticholinergic effects of neuroleptic and antiparkinsonian medication can produce a severe tachycardia. Neuroleptics alone (primarily the aliphatic and piperidine phenothiazines) can produce a marked orthostatic hypotensive reaction. After initial titration of neuroleptic medication, a daily dosage can be determined by adding together the doses given in the previous 24 hours. Eventually this can be given on a once-daily basis, usually at bedtime, but during the early agitated phase, three or four daily divided doses may provide some additional sedation. With this method, the most prominent acute symptoms can be brought under control quickly—often in less than a day and usually in several days. Severely disturbed patients may remain in this acute phase for as long as several weeks, especially if there is some intolerance to the side effects of neuroleptic medication.

Recovery Phase

During the recovery phase, a more active psychological and social treatment program should be added to the environmental control and pharmacologic therapy. Clear expectations of contact with reality and appropriate behavior should always be set. Ambiguity is extremely frightening and stressful for the patient who was recently in a psychotic state. Gradually the patient should be reintroduced to increasing levels of interpersonal contact and expectations. While individual therapeutic sessions may be conducted, reality-oriented group therapy and activity programs are especially effective. Structured tasks, such as occupational and recreational sessions, are more easily tolerated than unstructured interpersonal contacts. There should also be careful assessment of the environment to which the patient is likely to return. This environment should be evaluated for the expectations, conflict, and support that the patient will encounter. The individual should also be assessed for the strength of coping resources that he or she will be able to muster to meet these demands. If, as is commonly the case, there is a significant discrepancy, it is the clinician's responsibility to address this discrepancy with both the patient and the responsible family.

Disposition planning should begin to prepare the patient and the receiving environment for the patient's eventual transition back to more independent function outside of the hospital. Careful preparation is critical since separation from the hospital is likely to prove stressful for the patient in this relatively early phase of reintegration.

The duration of hospitalization can vary widely depending on the individual patient, the particular hospital, and the available outside resources. There is evidence to suggest that prolonged hospitalization offers little if any benefit to most schizophrenic patients and may in fact be a negative factor. Extended absence from the community can lead to major functional regression and the development of institutional dependence.

A marked depressive syndrome may occur in the early recovery phase. This disorder, which has been termed *post-psychotic depression,* is found in a significant percentage of patients; it is characterized by lethargy, withdrawal, and depressive mood of varying intensity. The syndrome has been variously interpreted as (1) reflecting a grief reaction to the loss of health and identity during the acute psychosis; (2) a biochemically induced manifestation of the primary illness; (3) an unwanted effect of neuroleptic medication; or (4) in selective cases, the depressive phase of a misdiagnosed bipolar affective disorder. Even if the last category is eliminated the syndrome is still observed, and it appears to be a common aspect of schizophrenic illness. Treatment of the depression varies in its effectiveness. Psychological support and encouragement are generally necessary, but antidepressant medication has been of minimal value unless there is a clearly depressed mood accompanying the lethargy and withdrawal. Nonetheless, while the patient is being treated with a neuroleptic medication, the addition of an antidepressant is reasonable and acceptable therapeutic approach. For particularly severe and resistant cases, a course of electroconvulsive therapy may be warranted.

Residual Phase

Within weeks to several months following the initial psychotic experience, the patient usually enters the residual phase of schizophrenia. Some patients will eventually achieve complete remission, but most will continue to experience at least some residual symptoms punctuated by acute exacerbations of the illness. It is during this phase of the illness that most patients must be maintained in the community at varying levels of function. Undoubtedly, this is the most challenging task for the clinician. Although there are some patients who obtain minimal or no benefit from neuroleptic medication, the vast majority appear to require prolonged medication maintenance. The dosage may be reduced to approximately one-fourth to one-third of the level that was required during the acute illness. Continuation of neuroleptic medication appears to reduce the relapse rate by at least 50 percent, and probably by much more. Duration of treatment must be determined on clinical observation. After the first episode of schizophrenic psychosis, rough guidelines suggest that medication should be continued for six months to a year at a gradually decreasing dosage. After a second episode, medication should be continued for one to two years, and permanent maintenance should be considered following a third or subsequent episode.

Medication treatment fails most commonly because an inadequate dosage was prescribed or the patient did not comply with the prescribed dosage. In all areas of medicine, patients may be reluctant to cooperate with maintenance medication (including antihypertensive, antitubercular, and psychotropic agents). In addition, the paranoia that is often associated with schizophrenia makes these patients feel threatened by the presence of an exogenous substance in their bodies. Extensive patient and family education can assist in overcoming some of this problem, and a good doctor-patient relationship is invaluable. The clinician must conscientiously monitor the patient's ongoing tolerance of the medication. Some studies have discovered that undetected but aggravating side effects, particularly subtle akathisias, induce numerous patients to discontinue medication.

In addition to medication, however, an active psychosocial therapeutic regimen is essential. As described earlier in the chapter, outcome in schizophrenia is only partially related to symptomatic control; the outcome is also determined by interpersonal and occupational function. The negative symptoms of schizophrenia—that is, interpersonal avoidance, social withdrawal, and lack of initiative—have major effects on the patient's function in the community. Encouragement and even pressure to remain involved in society and work may be required. Special educational and vocational counseling and guidance may be invaluable. The patient should be evaluated for individual or group therapy (or both) in order to develop adequate self-esteem, confidence, and social skills. While there is little evidence to suggest that depth-oriented psychotherapy can resolve the fundamental aspects of schizophrenia, the individual doctor-patient relationship can assist the patient in growth and development. The relationship may provide the organizing point of an otherwise disorganized existence, and it can improve the patient's compliance with medication schedules.

In ongoing, long-term work with schizophrenic patients, special attention should be paid to anticipated life changes. These patients are markedly vulnerable to change, especially when it involves separation from family and other significant sources of emotional support. Symptomatic and functional decompensation most often occur around such events. Advance discussion, planning, and preparation can assist in easing through these critical periods. Concern over life change, however, should not be interpreted as permission or encouragement for the patient to become passive, apathetic, and uninvolved. The clinician and family should continue to provide positive and clear expectations, and goals must be individualized. Only by evaluating a patient's progress toward such mutually defined goals can the clinician assess the quality and effectiveness of the treatment program. If the patient is not progressing satisfactorily, there may be a need for a more active and structured therapeutic environment, such as a residential school or day hospitalization program. Active revision of the treatment plan may be essential to support a patient's continued function.

Role of the Family
In all phases of treatment, special emphasis should be placed on the role of the family. Family therapy was long the most neglected aspect of management of schizophrenia. This neglect is especially surprising since family involvement is obviously critical to the care of patients with many illnesses—particularly of those with schizophrenia, which involves issues of separation, individuation, autonomy, competence, and identity. When an individual becomes ill with schizophrenia, the entire family is affected. Certainly the acute phase of the illness is terrifying and devastating to most parents. They feel guilty about their possible responsibility for the disorder, and they fear that siblings may develop the illness later. The skilled clinician will involve the family from the beginning of treatment. He will help them understand that the illness is treatable, despite the bizarre initial symptoms. The family can be of great assistance in preparing the patient and the home for patient's discharge from the hospital. The family must support the patient's ongoing treatment regimen and help identify early signs of decompensation or regression. Particularly in cases of paranoid schizophrenia, the family may be the clinician's chief source of reliable information concerning the patient's function. The family can also be crucial in assisting the patient's development of new adaptive skills and in defining appropriate goals. Finally, family participation is vital in dealing with the regressive tendencies of the residual phase of schizophrenia. Families who are too willing to accept the patient's impairment can undercut even the best of therapeutic programs.

Brown and colleagues (1972) performed an especially dramatic and important study of the family's impact on outcome of schizophrenia. This study demonstrated that the index of emotion expressed by a key relative of the patient at the time of admission proved to be the single best predictor of symptomatic relapse in the nine months after discharge from hospital. The index of expressed emotion has three components: (1) the number of critical comments made by the relative when talking about the patient and his illness, (2) hostility, and (3) marked emotional overinvolvement. Schizophrenic patients who are exposed to an environment of highly negative emotion for the majority of waking hours are nearly four times as likely to relapse as patients from a home with low-expressed emotion. The clinician, then, should not hesitate to insist on family participation in the treatment process.

Clearly, treatment of the schizophrenic patient must be conceptualized on a long-term basis. For the majority of patients, the clinician will be encountering chronic illness, but levels of function vary widely. An aggressive use of all available community and treatment resources may be essential. The clinician's role is that of coordinator of multiple resources rather than that of sole care-giver.

TREATMENT OF SCHIZOPHRENIFORM DISORDER AND BRIEF REACTIVE PSYCHOSIS

The treatment of schizophreniform disorder is essentially identical to that for schizophrenia. The symptoms resolve more rapidly, however, and duration of neuroleptic therapy may be much briefer. The patient should still be seen at least on an intermittent basis to monitor continuing recovery.

Brief reactive psychoses will require even shorter periods of treatment. Medication can usually be discontinued within several weeks of onset without a requirement for maintenance. There may be a greater need for and ability to utilize insight-oriented psychotherapy for resolution of predisposing maladaptive personality traits and defenses.

Both of these disorders generally have favorable outcomes, and evidence indicates that prolonged neuroleptic therapy offers little benefit.

UNPROVED TREATMENTS FOR SCHIZOPHRENIA

Schizophrenic illnesses are frequently severe, and patients and families are especially vulnerable to exaggerated claims for efficacy of new therapies. Fringe treatments, however, tend to worsen rather than improve the situation in the long run. Among the unproved treatments currently being promoted are nicotinic acid therapy, other megavitamin therapies, special diets, trace element analysis, and hemodialysis. To date, documented controlled studies do not support the efficacy of these treatments. It is the responsibility of each informed clinician to hear the pain that drives people to such therapies and to provide hope without supporting the use of unsubstantiated treatment.

Paranoid Disorders

The paranoid disorders are recognized as a discrete group of psychotic conditions characterized by delusions of persecution or jealousy. The onset is later than that observed in schizophrenia and generally occurs during and after the fifth decade of life. The personality structure is better preserved than in schizophrenia, with daily functioning remaining largely intact. However, interpersonal and social relationships are generally significantly disrupted by the excessive sensitivity, resentment, anger, and jealousy characteristic of persons with this illness. Often the delusions may focus on the spouse or another single individual and can be utterly unshakable. The affected person may become reclusive and be considered the neighborhood eccentric; his or her nature becomes argumentative and litigious, and social ostracism frequently follows.

DIAGNOSTIC CRITERIA

The diagnostic criteria for paranoid disorder are listed in Table 6-3. In determining this diagnosis, it is essential to rule out the following: (1) a preexisting paranoid schizophrenic illness that has gone unrecognized; (2) a primary affective disorder, either depressive or bipolar; and (3) an organic delusional disorder which could have any of several causes. Paranoid disorders have a course distinct from that of both affective disorders and organic disorders. Subtypes of paranoid disorder include acute paranoid disorder (less than six months' duration), paranoia (six months' duration or longer), and shared paranoid disorder (an illness involving a shared delusional system with another intimately involved individual).

Table 6-3. Diagnostic Criteria for Paranoid Disorder

A. Persistent persecutory delusions or delusional jealousy.
B. Emotion and behavior appropriate to the content of the delusional system.
C. Duration of the illness of at least one week.
D None of the symptoms under criterion A of schizophrenia [see p. 96]. . . .
E. No prominent hallucinations.
F. Not due to full depressive or manic syndrome of organic mental disorder.

Reproduced with permission from DSM-III, p. 196.

COURSE AND PROGNOSIS

The course in paranoid disorders tends to evolve toward a chronic state. Deterioration of the personality and function are usually limited. Extreme social isolation and decline in level of self-care and social responsiveness may result. Job performance may deteriorate drastically because of the hostility associated with the paranoia.

DIFFERENTIAL DIAGNOSIS

The differential diagnosis of a paranoid disorder includes all of those disorders considered under the differential diagnosis of schizophrenia. Distinguishing a paranoid disorder from either paranoid schizophrenia or paranoid personality disorder can be difficult and may require observation over time.

TREATMENT

Treatment of paranoid disorders can be extremely difficult because the disorder itself induces a general resistance to cooperative endeavor. Often the affected individual comes to treatment only under marked duress from family members or as a result of court procedures. When brought to therapy, the patient will minimize or deny the existence of any difficulty, projecting all responsibility on those about whom the patient already had paranoid ideas; in addition these ideas can develop as a result of the pressure to seek and obtain treatment. While the effort should be made, success is rarely achieved in persuading the individual to accept treatment while still in the severe paranoid state. Neuroleptic medication tends to be a necessary part of treatment, although benefit may be gradual and incomplete. Dosage must reach an adequate antipsychotic level but may not need to be as high as that for severely agitated patients with psychotic illness. Once some degree of remission has been attained, the patient may become more compliant and accepting of treatment. Nonetheless, close monitoring and continued insistence on following recommended treatment are necessary. Injectable depot preparations of antipsychotic medication may be of practical benefit in long-term treatment. If the degree of remission is unsatisfactory, a reconsideration of the diagnosis may be warranted. In such cases a trial of lithium carbonate, antidepressant medication, or electroconvulsive therapy should be considered.

Case 1. G.H. is an 18-year-old high school graduate. He has always been a quiet, reserved boy who has a few acquaintances but no close friends, and he has never dated. His school work was satisfactory until age 17, when his grades declined to failing. The teachers were the first to notice his increasing distractibility and preoccupation in class. Over about eight months G. became increasingly withdrawn at school and at home. His parents noticed that G. was more and more irritable, asking only to be left alone and shouting angrily when questioned about whether anything was bothering him. He spent larger amounts of time alone in his room, eventually not coming out for days on end. His self-care deteriorated, with infrequent baths and careless dress. Although G. had talked to himself for months, one day he started to act as if he had an invisible companion with him. He argued aloud with no one present and became very upset with the voices he was apparently hearing. He looked frightened and exhausted, not having slept for days. Finally, G. barricaded his room, explaining that he was not going to let ''them'' get him. After repeated efforts at persuasion, his family and their doctor forcibly brought G. to the hospital, where he was admitted for psychiatric care. Eight weeks of treatment, including medications and individual and group psychotherapy, resulted in enough improvement that G. returned to school on a reduced schedule and completed his senior year. Plans for attending college were postponed.

Case 2. L.S. is a 23-year-old secretary who lives with her husband and three-year-old child. Her early life was fairly typical, although she was never an especially sociable person. She married after knowing her husband six months, and the relationship has gone well. Because of work demands, the family was forced to move across the country, away from L.'s parents and friends. Two months after the move, her behavior began to change rapidly, and she appeared increasingly anxious, fearful, and agitated. Her usually predictable and efficient performance at work and at home became erratic. She often failed to show up for work or suddenly left the office, and she began to neglect her child and husband. Finally L. would go out at all hours, talking to strangers in a confused and hard-to-understand way. Because of this change, along with a refusal to eat and a 10-pound weight loss, L. was taken to see her doctor, who referred her to a psychiatrist. Rapid hospitalization, treatment with medication, and discussion of the stress caused by moving away from supportive persons aided L. in regaining control of herself within three weeks. After extensive talks together, L. and her husband decided to return to their original home town, where L. has done well for the last two years. Outpatient contact on a monthly basis has continued. Medication was reduced gradually over the first year and then stopped.

References and Further Reading

Baldessarini, R.J. Schizophrenia. *N. Engl. J. Med.* 955–988, 1977.

Bleuler, E. *Dementia Praecox or the Group of Schizophrenias.* 1911. Reprint. New York: International Universities Press, 1950.

Bowers, M., Jr. *Retreat from Sanity: The Structure of Emerging Psychosis.* New York: Human Sciences Press, 1974.

Brown, G.W., et al. Influence of family life in the course of schizophrenic disorders: a replication. *Br. J. Psychiatry* 121:241–258, 1972.

Carpenter, W.T., and Strauss, J.S. Are there pathognomonic symptoms in schizophrenia? *Arch. Gen. Psychiatry* 28:847–852, 1973.

Donlon, J.T., Blacker, K.H. Stages of schizophrenic decompensation and reintegration. *J. Nerv. Ment. Dis.* 157:200–249, 1973.

Freedman, D.X. (Ed.). *Biology of the Major Psychosis.* New York: Raven Press, 1975.

Gottesman, I.I., and Shields, J. Genetic theorizing and schizophrenia. *Br. J. Psychiatry* 122:15–30, 1973.

Kety, S.M., et al. Mental illness in the biological and adoptive relatives of schizophrenics. *Am. J. Psychiatry* 128:302–306, 1971.

Kind, H. The psychogenesis of schizophrenia: a review of the literature. *Br. J. Psychiatry* 112:333–349, 166.

Klein, D., Rosen, B. Premorbid asocial adjustment and response to phenothiazine treatment among schizophrenic inpatients. *Arch. Gen. Psychiatry* 29:480–485, 1973.

Kraepelin, E. *Lectures on Clinical Psychiatry.* 1904. Reprint. New York: Hafner, 1968.

Langfeldt, G. *Schizophreniform States.* Copenhagen: Munksgaard, 1939.

Lidz, T. *The Origin and Treatment of Schizophrenia.* New York: Basic Books, 1973.

Lidz, T., Fleck, S., Cornelison, A.R. *Schizophrenia and the Family.* New York: International Universities Press, 1965.

MacKay, A.V.P., Crow, T.J. Positive and negative schizophrenic symptoms and the role of dopamine. Parts 1 and 2. *Br. J. Psychiatry* 137:379–386, 1980.

May, P.R.A. Rational treatment for an irrational disorder: what does the schizophrenic patient need? *Am. J. Psychiatry* 133:1008–1011, 1976.

McCable, M.S. Reactive psychosis and schizophrenia with good prognosis. *Arch. Gen. Psychiatry* 33:571–576, 1976.

Pope, H.G., et al. Schizoaffective disorder: an invalid diagnosis? A comparison of schizoaffective disorder, schizophrenia and affective disorder. *Am. J. Psychiatry* 137:921–927, 1980.

Schneider, K. *Clinical Psychopathology.* New York: Grune & Stratton, 1959.

Slater, E., Beard, A., Glithero, E. The schizophrenia-like psychosis of epilepsy. *Br. J. Psychiatry* 109:95–150, 1963.

Snyder, S.H., et al. Drugs, neurotransmitters and schizophrenia. *Science.* 184:1243–1253, 1974.

Stein, L., Wise, C.D. Possible etiology of schizophrenia: progressive damage to the noradrenergic reward system by 6-hydroxydopamine. *Science* 171:1032–1036, 19.

Strauss, J.S., Carpenter, W.T. The prediction of outcome in schizophrenia. *Arch. Gen. Psychiatry* 27:793–746, 1972.

Weinberger, D.R., et al. Lateral cerebral ventricular enlargement in chronic schizophrenia. *Arch. Gen. Psychiatry* 36:735–739, 1979.

Weinberger, D.R., et al. Structural abnormalities in the cerebral cortex of chronic schizophrenic patients. *Arch. Gen. Psychiatry* 36:935–939, 1979.

Affective Disorders I: Bipolar Disorder (Manic-Depressive Illness)

C. GIBSON DUNN, M.D.

This chapter and Chapter 8 cover the psychiatric disorders known as *affective disorders*. In these illnesses, the central feature is a disturbance of mood, which is often accompanied by an abnormality in expressed emotion, or *affect*. The disturbance may take the form of hypomania or mania in one direction or depression of varying intensity in the other. When mania of any intensity is present, the pathologic process is considered to be *bipolar*; however, depression without a history of mania is diagnosed as a *unipolar* affective disorder. Affective disorders may be *primary* in that they develop without any preexisting psychiatric illness, or *secondary* when the affective disorder occurs following the diagnosis of a preexisting illness. This chapter will consider the nature and treatment of bipolar affective disorder, previously called manic-depressive illness.

At approximately the same time that hysteria was being explored by Freud in Vienna, manic-depressive illness was being defined as a new, distinct psychosis by Emil Kraepelin in Heidelberg. Beginning with his *Compendium* and culminating in the fifth edition of his *Textbook* in 1896, Kraepelin led the field of psychiatry into a new era based on observation and description of individual patients suffering from a broad array of psychiatric symptoms. Kraepelin attempted to correlate prominent presenting symptoms with outcomes over many years of follow-up; he combined this method with an emphasis on the medical disease model, which required that diagnosis be connected with etiology. Through these approaches, Kraepelin was able to delineate the known organically based major psychiatric disorders such as chemical intoxications, cretinism, and general paresis. From remaining large numbers of disorders, Kraepelin was able to define two distinct, functional psychotic illnesses, dementia praecox and manic depression. Dementia praecox has since come to be known as *schizophrenia* while manic-depressive illness, in the *Diagnostic and Statistical Manual of Mental Disorders,* Third Edition (DSM-III) and this textbook, is called *bipolar affective disorder.* Kraepelin's great contribution was his ability to distinguish between these two major psychotic disorders and to connect the different presenting clinical features with his observation of generally distinct courses and outcomes. Kraepelin did this work long before there was any meaningful treatment for either disorder. The matching of distinct therapies to these two psychotic illnesses has confirmed Kraepelin's observation that the disorders are, in fact, separate and probably of different origin.

Despite having been recognized for more than 75 years, manic-depressive disorders continue to be among the most misdiagnosed psychiatric illnesses of our time. Properly diagnosed, manic-depressive illnesses can now be successfully managed in almost all cases. If untreated, however, these disorders can be catastrophic for the persons affected and for their families. An ability to recognize and diagnose bipolar affective disorders is a fundamental and critical part of psychiatric expertise.

Signs and Symptoms of a Manic Episode

There are two broad symptom patterns characteristic of the manic phase: an elated, euphoric, grandiose type and a more irritable, hostile, or paranoid type. There is usually a mixture of these two patterns in the individual patient, but in some cases these symptoms may be seen in fairly isolated form. The signs and symptoms of mania vary so greatly in intensity that it may be difficult to recognize them as belonging to the same disorder. The milder forms of manic symptoms are termed *hypomania*, reflecting the lower level of intensity. Carlson and Goodwin (1973), at the National Institute of Mental Health, have provided what is perhaps the best broad description of the manic episode. The authors chose to divide their observations of manic symptoms into three phases based on a predominant mood. In stage 1, euphoria was the predominant underlying mood; in stage 2, this altered toward irritability and anger; stage 3 is characterized by overwhelming anxiety and panic. The onset of a manic episode can vary widely in rate from hours to many days.

In the inital phase, according to Carlson and Goodwin, mania is characterized by increased psychomotor activity (rapid thought and speech) and increased physical activity. The mood can be quite labile, but the patient tends to be elated; however, irritability and frustration result when his or her demands are not met. Thought processes tend to be expansive, grandiose, and excessively confident. In this stage, thought processes are usually coherent but at times are tangential. Increased interests and activity occur in many areas, including sex, religion, spending money, smoking, telephone use, and letter writing. Insight is variable, although some patients continue to be aware of the altered state of their mental functioning and are able to exercise some self-control.

In stage 2, the authors found that patients demonstrate further increase in the pressure of speech and psychomotor activity, while mood tends toward increasing dysphoria and depression, often accompanied by open hostility and anger. Behavior can be quite threatening and even explosive. Thought processes further deteriorate into rapid shifting from one subject to another—known as *flight of ideas*—and increasingly disorganized cognition. Frank delusions of a grandiose or paranoid nature are also found in this stage.

The final stage is perhaps the most difficult aspect of mania for the clinician to recognize and treat. In Carlson and Goodwin's description, late (stage 3) mania is characterized by desperation, panic, and extreme dysphoria, often accompanied by frenzied and bizarre physical activity. Hallucinations, delusions, and disorientation to time and place are observed. In addition, the extreme sleep deprivation accompanying the excessive overall activation can further aggravate the clinical picture towards a more disorganized and bizarre presentation. During this stage, the misdiagnosis of schizophrenia is often made; the diagnosis of mania can be quite difficult to establish from the acute symptom pattern alone.

These brief descriptions contain the most prominent signs and symptoms of mania. It is important to appreciate that far more than mood is altered during manic episodes. To be sure, the expansive, euphoric, irritable, or paranoid mood changes must be present. Nonetheless, in addition, there is a clear change in thought and behavioral patterns. Classic changes include grandiosity, as previously noted, which may present merely as extreme overconfidence or unrealistic self-judgment, but which may also take the form of grandiose religious or historical beliefs that can distract the examiner from recognizing the existence of the primary disorder. High energy, driven behavior or increased acitivity is also very characteristic of the psychomotor change and may include excessive spending of money, sexual activity, telephone calling, talking, and writing.

Certain other features may be indicative of a manic episode. One patient may display excessive or inappropriate humor, speak in an excessively loud voice while being difficult to interrupt, or demonstrate extreme distractibility with accordingly poor concentration. Sleep is invariably decreased, and a change in sleep pattern in the direction of less total sleep time is often one of the first indicators of the onset of a manic period.

For the reasons that have been discussed, the recognition of a manic episode may require considerably more exploration than just a mental status examination. While the mental status features may be fairly clear-cut, a longitudinal history of behavior, usually obtained from collateral sources, may give a much more accurate and informative picture.

Perhaps the most complicated aspect of bipolar affective disorder is the *mixed state*, in which symptoms of both depression and mania are present at the same time, or in which they alternate with each other every few days. The mixed state also includes the primarily manic episode in which symptoms of depression are evident for a period of at least several days.

The examiner may fail to appreciate the significance and extent of the depression due to the patient's pressure of speech and the overwhelming nature of the irritability and grandiosity. During this time, while looking and feeling depressed, the patient may be markedly activated, agitated, pressured, and unable to establish self-control. This state can be especially dangerous for the patient in terms of suicide risk because of the potentially severe depressive symptoms with the accompanying pressured activation. As many as one-third of patients with bipolar affective disorder will experience this type of mixed state.

Epidemiology

For many years the prevalence of primary affective disorders was recorded by including in the same category patients with mania and those with only depressive episodes. This categorization reflected Kraepelin's initial view that severe depressions are merely the depressive phase of manic-depressive illness. Once the current class of unipolar depressions is eliminated, the prevalence of bipolar affective disorders is approximately 0.5 percent, with estimates varying from slightly below this to approximately 1.0 percent of the total population. The age of onset can vary greatly, but typically occurs somewhere between the adolescent years and age 30; it may also occur in childhood (before puberty) and in middle age or beyond. Various researchers have attempted to make much of the distinction between mania that develops early and that of later onset (*early* indicates onset before age 30, and *late* indicates onset after age 30). Higher genetic loading is found in patients with bipolar disorders of early onset than in those with illnesses of later onset. This finding, however, has not been uniformly upheld and is open to question. Response to treatment and outcome has not been consistently correlated with age of onset.

It is also quite apparent that initial episodes of mania may occur in the middle-age period or later. In older patients, the first manic episode may occur many years following what had been considered to be an isolated single episode or even several depressive episodes without any suspicion of a bipolar potential. In a significant number of cases, researchers have found that the onset of mania correlates with the existence of some serious cerebral organic disorder other than dementia. While the incidence of primary affective disorders in women is approximately twice that in men, the sex differential for bipolar affective disorder appears to be considerably smaller. In the elderly population, however, women appear to experience mania more often than men, although the differential is still small.

Classification and Diagnostic Criteria

As noted at the beginning of the chapter, the term *bipolar affective disorder* is employed when there is evidence of a past or current manic episode. It is not necessary that a depressive episode has occurred to establish the diagnosis of bipolar disorder. The diagnosis of bipolar disorder can be among the easiest or among the most difficult of psychiatric diagnoses to substantiate. If a patient presents in the midst of a classic and well-developed manic episode, the diagnosis is easy to establish. Quite often, however, a patient who in fact suffers from a bipolar disorder may present in a fashion that makes the diagnosis more obscure. Specifically, the patient may be experiencing a manic episode with few of the typical features evident. Also, the patient may present with a depressive disorder while the occurrence of a manic or hypomanic period has been at some time in the past. Alternatively, a patient may present for some other reason between major mood swings, but with related symptoms or impairment that would best be managed if the bipolar disorder is diagnosed. Each of these less-than-straightforward clinical situations requires expertise in the variants of bipolar affective disorder. A comprehensive knowledge of the presentation and evaluation of bipolar disorders is essential.

The diagnostic criteria for a manic episode are presented in Table 7-1. Since the affective disorders are called *mood disorders,* attention can easily be directed to the mood component of the bipolar disorder. In a manic phase, the mood may be elated, euphoric, expansive, or irritable. Some change in mood is essential to establish the diagnosis, but there are many cases in which a dysphoric component (that is, something experienced as unpleasant) may be quite prominent while to some degree obscuring the overall elevation or irritability of mood. There may also be a significant intermingling of depression with the elevated mood. In any case, the mood change should persist for at least one week to establish this diagnosis firmly.

The quality of pressure in thought, speech, and activity is at least as important as the mood alteration. This pressure may take a psychic form primarily, with racing thoughts, flight of ideas, and constant talkativeness, or it may assume a more high-energy or physical form in which the patient becomes overinvolved in numerous activities or becomes extraordinarily productive and creative; it is possible that both forms may be present. Impairment in concentration and continuity of thought occurs with the classic alteration of flight of ideas, in which the patient may skip from thought to thought with inadequate connections or pauses between. Sleep is almost always significantly disturbed and its amount diminished. At times patients may demonstrate sleeplessness or hyperactivity for days on end.

When these symptoms are present, the diagnosis is quickly established. Unfortunately, stage 3 mania (as noted previously) may be considerably more bizarre, with prominent delusions and hallucinations. Anxiety, which may be of panic proportions, is often quite incapacitating. In its most severe stage, symptoms of psychotic mania may be virtually indistinguishable from those of schizophrenic psychosis. In this situation, attention must be given to the nature of onset of the current episode (that is, rapid rather than insidious) and

Table 7-1. Diagnostic Criteria for a Manic Episode

A. One or more distinct periods with a predominantly elevated, expansive, or irritable mood. The elevated or irritable mood must be a prominent part of the illness and relatively persistent, althought it may alternate or intermingle with depressive mood.

B. Duration of at least one week (or any duration if hospitalization is necessary), during which, for most of the time, at least three of the following symptoms have persisted (four if the mood is only irritable) and have been present to a significant degree:
   1. increase in activity (either socially, at work, or sexually) or physical restlessness
   2. more talkative than usual or pressure to keep talking
   3. flight of ideas or subjective experience that thoughts are racing
   4. inflated self-esteem (grandiosity, which may be delusional)
   5. decreased need for sleep
   6. distractibility, i.e., attention is too easily drawn to unimportant or irrelevant external stimuli
   7. excessive involvement in activities that have a high potential for painful consequences which is not recognized, e.g., buying sprees, sexual indiscretions, foolish business investments, reckless driving

C. Neither of the following dominate the clinical picture when an affective syndrome (i.e., criteria A and B above) is not present, that is, before it developed or after it has remitted:
   1. preoccupation with a mood-incongruent delusion or hallucination...
   2. bizarre behavior

Reproduced with permission from *Diagnostic and Statistical Manual of Mental Disorders,* 3rd ed. Washington, D.C.: American Psychiatric Association, 1980, pp. 208–209.

to the possible existence of more typical elevation of mood and manic symptomatology earlier in the clinical course. Progression of symptoms may occur gradually or rapidly, and careful history taking from collateral sources may be necessary. In addition, a careful history of the patient and his or her family may establish a previous pattern suggestive of an affective disorder or a genetic loading in this direction. The diagnosis is more readily established when the delusions and hallucinations are mood congruent—that is, the delusions are of a grandiose or elated nature consistent with a primary mood disorder. At other times, however, the delusions may be quite paranoid and difficult to distinguish in a single evaluation. In such a case, obtaining to a personal family history is essential.

If a patient presents with a depressive episode (the features of which are described in the Chapter 8), there is no way to establish the diagnosis of bipolar disorder from evaluation of the depressive episode alone. In such a case, the search for a previous manic episode must be carried out and a family history taken in order to evaluate possible genetic contributions for bipolar disorder.

Finally, it is important to emphasize that a patient may present with a complaint that is not directly attributable to a clear-cut mood swing. Typical examples include problems with alcoholism or anxiety, as well as marital difficulties that may be related to minor mood swings or simply occur in someone with previous difficulties with bipolar mood disorder. It is important to evaluate the possibility of a bipolar disorder in every patient seen since only by taking a careful personal and family history can one gain the necessary information to rule out a bipolar disorder.

It is important to understand how to ask the questions to establish the diagnosis of bipolar affective disorder. Often when interviewing a patient, the physician assumes the patient knows what the physician is thinking and tends to ask overly vague or general questions that the patient feels incapable of answering.

This is especially true in mood disorders. When asking about an elevated mood, for example, one needs to specify to the patient that one is talking about a mood well beyond normal or one that appears out of proportion to any environmental stimuli and is sustained for a period of a week or more. In addition, one should be specific in seeking the other diagnostic features including changes in sleep patterns, sexual activity, spending of money, interpersonal contact and output of energy. Often patients will not recall an alteration in mood, but may remember a period when sleep was greatly decreased and they felt excessively stimulated and even overwhelmed with energy. This may sometimes be remembered with great fondness, but often will be seen as something unusual and uncomfortable. Many patients will concur that they have experienced these symptoms, and it is only with repeated questioning around the areas of persistence of changes and degree of change from baseline that the history can be delineated accurately.

This procedure is emphasized because establishing a correct diagnosis of bipolar affective disorder can truly alter the course of a person's life for the better. At the same time, this diagnosis strongly suggests a long-term or even lifelong commitment to maintenance treatment with lithium carbonate. This is a serious matter that will cost the patient time, money, effort, and some risk of complications and should not be undertaken lightly.

Differential Diagnosis

If it presents in a classic pattern, a manic episode is easy to distinguish from other diagnoses. In its psychotic stage, however, mania may closely mimic paranoid schizophrenia. Numerous retrospective studies have been carried out reevaluating patients diagnosed as paranoid schizophrenic. A sizable percentage of patients, often a majority, are found to have been experiencing a manic disorder with psychotic features rather than a schizophrenic psychosis. Features favoring the diagnosis of mania over schizophrenia include: (1) rapid onset, (2) psychotic features that are mood congruent, (3) any previous mood disorders, including depression; and (4) a family history of affective disorder especially bipolar disorder. A later onset of psychotic disorder (beyond the middle twenties) also favors a diagnosis of an affective disorder. Good premorbid adjustment, while sometimes found in schizophrenia, is far more typical of mania than of schizophrenia. Finally, even in a paranoid manic patient, there is more of a tendency toward people-seeking behavior than is seen in the paranoid schizophrenic. While this differential point should not be overemphasized, it occurs repeatedly in severely paranoid manic patients and is worth noting.

If a patient has had a previous episode similar to the current one, the degree of recovery is a significant evaluative point since patients with bipolar affective disorder tend to experience better return of function than do schizophrenic patients. It is also important to appreciate that numerous adolescent psychotic illnesses are now believed to be bipolar illnesses. Catatonic features, once considered strongly diagnostic for schizophrenia, are now understood to occur frequently in mania.

The differentiation of bipolar disorders from schizoaffective disorder can be extraordinarily difficult. This latter diagnosis has been applied to a broad array of clinical situations, but most accurately it pertains only to patients who demonstrate symptoms consistent with diagnoses of both schizophrenia and bipolar affective disorder. It should only be employed if inadequate or incomplete results occur with every effort to treat the patient for bipolar affective disorder and if schizophrenic features persist.

The differential diagnosis of bipolar disorder versus unipolar affective disorder can also present problems. Specific patients include those with one or two depressive episodes and a family history of bipolar disorder; in these patients, symptoms of such severe agitation should raise the question as to whether the current depressive episode is part of a larger bipolar illness. This question cannot be established from a single clinical presentation, but the examiner should try to clarify the diagnosis by seeking evidence of a previous manic of hypomanic episode. Perris, in his important work distinguishing between unipolar and bipolar affective disorders, found that if a patient had experienced three consecutive depressive episodes without a manic episode, the chances were only 1 in 6 (17 percent) that the patient would experience a manic episode in the future. If there had been four depressive episodes, the chances that a manic episode would occur dropped to less than 5 percent. As will be discussed later, it is important to distinguish between unipolar and bipolar disorders in treating depression because of the effect of antidepressants on a latent bipolar disorder.

The final differential diagnostic point to consider is that of drug intoxications or drug-induced psychoses. Amphetamines, other sympathomimetic drugs (such as cocaine), marijuana, and steroid drugs can induce psychosis indistinguishable from mania. Often it can be difficult to determine whether these drugs have merely precipitated latent tendencies or have in fact induced a psychotic state by the drug effect alone. Generally speaking, amphetamines and cocaine can produce a psychosis through drug effect alone, while the other medications or drugs tend to precipitate an endogenous tendency toward bipolar disorder.

Special note should be given to the problem of precipitating a manic episode by antidepressant medication. Every practicing psychiatrist has treated a patient who presents with a depression, begins to recover, but then becomes hypomanic or floridly manic under the effects of catecholamine-active agents. In these cases it appears that the medication has truly precipitated a latent bipolar disorder. Often the manic episode must then be treated independently, although some milder forms may subside with the removal of the antidepressant. This is an embarrassing and inelegant way to obtain evidence for the diagnosis of bipolar affective disorder, and a careful family history may save a great deal of pain for both the patient and the physician.

Secondary mania caused by medical disorders is relatively uncommon but not rare. As mentioned, exogenous steroid medication can precipitate or generate a manic episode; the same result can occur under conditions of endogenous excess of steroids, including Cushing's disease and hyperadrenalism. In addition, secondary mania, especially in older patients and particularly in older men, is known to result from direct physical insults to the central nervous system. Reported cases include head trauma, tumors, and cerebral vascular accidents, and the condition may occur in patients with no previous history of bipolar disorder or with a history of only a single depressive episode. In these cases treatment of more than just the primary medical disorder may be necessary, and it would follow the same lines as for other manic episodes.

Course, Complications, and Prognosis

The natural history of bipolar affective disorders is extremely variable. The age of onset can vary from childhood to old age. Most literature designates the thirties as the typical age of onset for this disorder. In more recent years, however, with greater attention being paid to the early diagnosis of bipolar affective disorders, it is clear that onset may be considerably earlier in many cases than previously recognized. Onset in adolescents is now known to be quite common, and many cases previously diagnosed as schizophrenic episodes have, in fact, been manic episodes. In addition initial manic episodes may occur after the age of 60. As a general rule, however, bipolar affective disorders peak in onset in the third and fourth decades of life, with the frequency of initial episodes trailing off in both directions from that age period.

It appears that most initial episodes are of the hypomanic or manic type, but it is also quite common for initial episodes to be of a depressive nature. With each successive depressive episode not accompanied by mania, the likelihood of developing a bipolar disorder decreases.

Individual hypomanic or manic episodes can also greatly differ in length. Episodes are known typically to last from days to months or longer. Very rapid cycling on a 24- to 48-hour basis are known, but these are infrequent occurrences. There is no way of determining the probable duration of a single episode during an initial illness. Previous manic episodes may provide a rough guide as to what might be expected, but this is at best approximate.

The period between recurrent manic or depressive episodes is equally variable. A significant percentage of individuals will experience only one manic or depressive episode in the course of their lives. Estimates for this percentage vary from 5 to 50 percent, depending on whether the studies were performed before or after the introduction of lithium therapy. The family history may provide some assistance in this area if other family members have experienced a single episode or recurrent affective disorders.

For persons experiencing recurrent manic, or manic and depressive episodes, the natural history is one of episodes that are increasingly frequent and severe, although briefer. A patient cannot be left with the impression that he or she will simply outgrow a primary affective disorder. This natural history also strongly reinforces the importance of prophylactic treatment once the recurrent pattern has become established. Individuaals with bipolar disorders usually have function that is normal or nearly normal between episodes; however, many do develop a subchronic or chronic course and continue to experience troubling impairment of function in many areas unless adequately treated.

The complications of bipolar affective disorder can be quite severe. On the most basic level, the mood instability associated with this disorder may cause severe disruption of function in family, social, and business affairs. Although the premorbid personalities of those with bipolar affective disorders have not been found to be particularly disturbed, there is no doubt that recurrent mood swings of even a mild nature distort intimate relationships. Mild mood elevations, for example, can lead a person to be extremely narcissistic, demanding, and difficult, causing great pain in a marriage or in rearing children. Every clinician who has treated manic depressive patients will have observed the rage of the patient's family over this narcissistic quality. In addition, mood elevations can affect judgment so greatly that the affected person becomes involved in actions and behaviors that he or she would have avoided otherwise. Grave damage to personal reputation or financial standing can ensue. It is common, for example, to see a person suffering from manic-depressive illness who has lost enormous sums of money or destroyed a business that he or she had worked many years to create; this results from the impaired judgment and impulse control of a hypomanic illness. Alcohol abuse and dependence also appear to be a significant complication of bipolar affective disorder. Although the percentage is unclear, it is a pervasive impression that bipolar patients consume more alcohol or become dependent on it more frequently than is true in the population at large. The reasons for this have been debated at length, but one possible explanation is that alcohol is used as self-medication for mood elevation or depression.

Special emphasis must be placed on the risk of *suicide,* the most serious complication of manic-depressive illness. Persons with bipolar disorder have an enormously increased rate of suicide as compared with other psychiatric patients or the population at large. It has been estimated that up to 15 percent of the deaths of bipolar patients result from suicide. This is a staggering statistic, over 1,000 times the rate in the general population, and it must constantly be remembered when one is responsible for treating a person with this disorder. This risk for suicide seems to exist not only in the depressive phase, but also in the mixed phase, when symptoms of depression coexist with the marked activation and pressure of the manic episode.

Etiology

The data indicate that bipolar affective disorder has a biologic etiology. The most commonly accepted hypothesis is that the central nervous system is affected by a disturbance in catecholamine metabolism. A relative noradrenergic overactivity is thought to contribute to the occurrence of a manic illness. Attention has also been focused, however, on abnormalities of dopamine, serotonin, and acetylcholine activity in facilitating or contributing to the manic illness. This hypothesis receives some general support from the established observations of drugs that affect these neurotransmitters; these drugs—antidepressants, amphetamine, and cocaine—are capable of triggering hypomanic or manic mood swings.

The more fundamental cause of this abnormality in neurotransmission is still being investigated. There is no doubt that a genetic contribution exists in many bipolar disorders. Research has suggested that this genetic contribution may be more significant for persons experiencing the onset of bipolar disorder before age 30 than for those with later onset. For the early-onset group, there is a well-established familial contribution to the illness, as determined from family histories and twin studies. It is quite common, on taking a careful history, to be able to trace the presence of a bipolar affective disorder through multiple generations. In first-degree relatives of an index case, the morbidity risk for bipolar disorders is approximately 15 percent. If both parents of an individual suffer from bipolar disorders, the risk increases greatly. The concordance rate for monozygotic twins is approximately 75 percent, while that for dizygotic twins is the same as the risk for first-degree relatives. The mode of genetic transmission has been investigated at length but is still uncertain. Considerable evidence suggests an X-linkage of bipolar disorder, but father-son transmission is known to occur. It may be that a subtype of this illness is X-linked, while other cases are transmitted in a different genetic pattern or occur without any genetic contribution.

In some cases, as noted previously, specific toxic or medical factors may contribute to a secondary manic disorder. Studies that explored the possible psychological basis of bipolar disorder have been unconvincing and are no longer considered particularly significant in understanding the fundamental causes. Nonetheless, it is apparent that psychological factors may play a major role in precipitating some mood swings. Psychologically stressful events, particularly ones involving emotional loss or threatened loss, can induce the onset of a manic episode, which then becomes autonomous in its course, once initiated. Years ago the observation of this association between emotional events and the onset of mania led to a psychological theory that manic-depressive illness is a "flight from depression." Indeed, mania may be viewed in this light, but such a defensive function does not appear to be a primary determining cause for the existence of the illness.

Treatment

Treatment of the patient suffering from bipolar disorder can be extremely challenging but also very rewarding. Treatment, of course, cannot be initiated until the diagnosis is established. Comprehensive and careful evaluation of the individual patient's mental status and assessment of his or her history and that of the family are critical to formulating the correct treatment plan. Once a diagnosis of a manic episode is established, the treatment of choice is lithium carbonate. Only special circumstances can justify not initiating lithium therapy for the treatment of manic disorder.

In order for treatment to begin, however, the affected person must come to or be brought to a physician. If a patient is experiencing a manic episode, this may be easier said than done. Many persons during a manic episode deny the existence or significance of their illness; other patients enjoy the elation, deny the destructive aspects, and do not wish treatment. When an individual is profoundly depressed or grandiosely elated, the reluctance to seek help can be extremely difficult to overcome. Obviously the best situation is for the person to bring himself or herself to treatment. This should not be considered the only path, however. As mentioned earlier, the consequences of an untreated bipolar illness can be devastating or fatal. If it is evident that someone is suffering from a manic episode but is resistant to treatment, a family member or friend who cares about that person must take over. Often this will require the advice and guidance of the physician. The assertion of control can provoke angry, even abusive responses, but such responses are further proof of impaired judgment. Only by outside influence will the disastrous consequences of the mood swing be reduced and eventually stopped. The physician can anticipate that most of these disturbed persons will eventually be grateful for this care and protection.

Once a person with a bipolar disorder is brought to a physician, a psychiatric referral should follow immediately; this referral may be to the doctor's office or to a hospital, depending on the severity of symptoms. Psychiatric hospitalization is indicated if (1) the patient is so symptomatic that close observation and care are needed; (2) a significant suicide risk exists; (3) the patient poses a danger to his or her own emotional, physical, social, or financial well-being because of poor judgment or impaired impulse control; (4) attempts at outpatient treatment have proved inadequate or unsuccessful; or (5) coexisting medical illness makes psychiatric treatment more difficult or excessively risky.

Hospitalization can be voluntary or involuntary. Involuntary commitment should occur when the impairment is so great that the patient is unable to assess the illness realistically. The physician must remain aware of the consequences if treatment is not obtained promptly and must take the responsibility for ensuring that the patient receive correct treatment.

When the proper conditions for treatment have been arranged, either in the office or the hospital, the responsible physician should inform the patient thoroughly as to the treatment process that will be followed. In bipolar disorders, even more than in other illnesses, a cooperative and informed patient is invaluable. A person with this condition seems particularly sensitive to issues of control and feelings of inadequacy related to the illness. Careful patient education and establishment of a collaborative approach will go far to overcome these potential complications to treatment.

USE OF LITHIUM AND OTHER MEDICATIONS

It is essential that the responsible physician be fully informed and confident about the use of lithium carbonate. (Chapter 21 discusses the use of lithium in greater detail.) The patient with a bipolar disorder will respond positively to such confidence and expertise; any uncertainty or anxiety can be perceived and may lead to discontinuance of medication at a premature or inappropriate time. Some patients may also decide to stop lithium treatment because they enjoy the mildly or moderately intense mood elevations of their illness. In addition, there are many annoying and at times frightening side effects or toxic effects from the use of lithium, and patients may often overreact to these transient problems. It is the rare patient who cannot tolerate lithium treatment, buy many ambivalent or reluctant patients need clear explanation and some persuasion to appreciate the importance of lithium therapy in altering the potentially disastrous course of their illness. The support and encouragement of a knowledgeable physician may be critical in giving manic patients the ability to cope with their problems.

Special mention should be made of recent research suggesting that carbamazepine (Tegretol) may be useful either instead of or in addition to lithium in bipolar disorders.

If the patient continues to be ambivalent or recalcitrant about treatment, the physician should feel impelled to involve concerned family members, who may be much more aware of the consequences of the manic episode than is the patient. Taking a passive role with such a manic patient is both inadequate and irresponsible. Often it is the physician who must engage the entire social system to support appropriate treatment for the patient.

Other medications in addition to lithium carbonate may be necessary in the early treatment of a severe manic episode. Any of the antipsychotic medications may be used during periods of extreme pressure, agitation, mood elevation, and sleeplessness. Generally, chlorpromazine and haloperidol have been most frequently employed in combination with lithium treatment. There has been concern about the combined effects of haloperidol and lithium carbonate treatment. Usually this combination can be used safely as long as the serum lithium level is carefully monitored and haloperidol dosage is tapered rapidly as the lithium level approaches the therapeutic range. The combination of neuroleptic medication and lithium carbonate appears to have some troublesome side effects, including increased severity of extrapyramidal symptoms and some increase in organic brain toxicity; these effects may be caused by increased intracellular concentration of one or both of the medications. Again, the primary means of protecting against this is careful monitoring of the serum lithium level and rapid tapering of the neuroleptic dosage.

It is not uncommon that a manic episode will be followed by a depressive episode, either directly or after only a brief euthymic period. In such cases, it may be necessary to add an antidepressant, which is generally given in addition to the ongoing lithium therapy; the dosage is carefully monitored and adjusted based on an assessment of the patient's mood state. Because an antidepressant can stimulate a manic period despite an adequate serum lithium level, the antidepressants tend to be given in lower dosage and for a more limited period than in the unipolar depressive disorder. In order to obtain initial response to the antidepressant, however, one may need to use the higher dosage range.

The duration of therapy with lithium carbonate following an initial episode can be difficult to determine. As noted previously, some persons may experience only one manic episode in the course of their lives. In such a case, it would obviously be unwise and unnecessary to maintain the individual on lithium permanently. At this time there is no clear-cut standard of practice for duration of lithium treatment in such instances, and it is impossible to identify these persons with much confidence. Maintenance of treatment for at least a year following the episode, however, appears reasonable and appropriate; discontinuance should occur only after full discussion of the risks with the patient and his or her family if at all possible. The physician should work with the patient and the family to identify early warning signs of mania so that treatment can be resumed as soon as possible if a manic episode begins.

If, as is usually the case, the person comes to treatment only after two or more major mood swings, the general recommendation is for life-long maintenance on lithium carbonate. While there appear to be some risks of thyroid and renal complications from lithium treatment, these risks can be minimized through careful monitoring of organ function. In addition, any risk and difficulty of treatment must be weighed against the very serious nature of bipolar disorders. It is essential to remember that this is a potentially fatal illness and that the risk from the illness is high. With treatment, however, it is apparent that manic and depressive episodes will occur less frequently, and any episodes that do occur will be less severe. Work by Dunner, Murphy, Stallone, and Fieve confirm this outcome pattern with the observation that patients who experience manic episodes are hospitalized much less frequently if they are receiving lithium therapy than if they are not.

PHYSICIAN-PATIENT RELATIONSHIP

It is apparent that the physician's relationship with the patient who has a bipolar affective disorder will be an ongoing one. The patient will experience life crises and periods of mood instability and may undergo one or more hospitalizations. It is now apparent that the frequency and intensity of mood swings, even on medication treatment, can be affected by the nature of the physician-patient relationship. This supportive and therapeutic relationship not only helps the patient improve the quality of his or her life, but can also have a direct and significant impact on the course of the disorder. The more open, direct and collaborative the nature of this relationship, the more successful will be the patient's outcome. Issues of self-esteem, independence, success, and dependency should be expected and sought. Many patients will desire only psychopharmacologic treatment, which may be all that is needed or all that can be accepted. If this is the case, the physician will have to work from this point, always making clear to the patient that they can discuss and attempt to deal with these other matters if they arise. Other patients are more motivated to understand the emotional factors involved in their illness, either contributing to the mood instability or associated with it. The frequency of therapeutic involvement is determined by many events, but a surprisingly large amount of psychotherapeutic work can occur with even infrequent visits over many years.

Finally it should be emphasized that treatment should extend whenever possible to involve the patient's family. The family has always been affected by the patient's illness. Marital and parent-child relationships can be severely distorted by guilt, anger, and fear. The physician should give the family an opportunity to identify and ventilate these concerns, attempt to provide more realistic understanding of the nature of the illness, and seek some resolution for the maladaptive behavior patterns that may have become established prior to treatment. In addition, the family may be critical in bringing the patient to treatment at times of relapse. An established working relationship between the physician and the family may be the major tie to health during such crises.

It should be apparent that treatment of the person suffering from bipolar affective disorder is general medical practice in its purest form. Expertise in the biologic, psychological, and social spheres is called on repeatedly in treating such persons, and only by a combination of these areas of knowledge will treatment prove successful.

Case 1. R.W. is a 41-year-old man who was brought to the hospital by his family because of his strange behavior. Over the past week, the patient had become increasingly energetic and active. He had not slept for several nights and seemed to talk constantly. Alcohol consumption had increased drastically and R.'s sexual preoccupation had become extreme. Over the last 24 hours, R.'s family had become aware that he was arranging many strange business deals and committing himself to enormous expenditures that he could not meet. When R. called the state's governor to propose a new way of financing the annual budget, the family decided something had to be done.

This patient had a past history of two hospitalizations, one for severe depression at age 25, and one for similar uncontrolled hyperactivity at 34. During the depression, R. had become acutely alcoholic and suicidal. His mother had a history of mood swings, and one uncle and one cousin had been hospitalized for depression.

He resisted hospitalization but was committed by the court. His diagnosis was bipolar affective illness, manic phase. Treatment included close supervision in the hospital, lithium carbonate, and high doses of an antipsychotic tranquilizer. The hospital course was initially quite stormy, but the problems subsided rapidly over the first two weeks, The total time in the hospital was five weeks, and an excellent treatment outcome and full return of function were noted.

Case 2. N.T. is a 38-year-old female attorney who was brought to a psychiatrist's office after causing a major disruption at work. Colleagues had noticed her increasing irritability over the last three weeks, but her work output had increased significantly. Although appearing fatigued and lately confused, N. had written many complete briefs over a short period of time. She had become more demanding and critical of those around her. For about a week she had become more guarded, accusing others of stealing her superlative ideas. When the firm's senior partner finally confronted N. regarding her behavior, she became incensed and began throwing objects around her office.

This patient had been hospitalized once before at age 18 for an acute psychosis that was diagnosed as schizophrenia. After that N. experienced a prolonged period of depression before full recovery. She returned to college and went on to study law. A very outgoing woman, N. married at 26 and had two children. She experienced several other periods of depression, lasting one to three months, of overly energetic, irritable expansiveness not requiring hospitalization. Her family had learned simply to "bear with mother" during such times.

On this last hospitalization, the correct diagnosis of bipolar affective disorder, manic type, was made and treatment with lithium carbonate was started, with good results.

Case 3. S.B., a 45-year-old woman married to a physician, was brought to hospital for treatment of severe manic agitation. The patient had experienced her first manic episode eight years previously. The diagnosis was established without problem at that time and the patient treated appropriately with lithium carbonate.

During the ensuing years, however, the patient had frequently complained of side effects that she attributed to lithium. These included a mild tremor of her fingers, a feeling of being slowed down, and facial and chest ache. After the occurrence of each side effect, the patient would discontinue her medication, stating she felt that it was being forced on her by her husband and his colleagues. Intermittently during the periods after she discontinued the medication, the patient would again become manic, causing great distress to her family and havoc in her social environment. The patient had been rehospitalized on six separate occasions, each time signing out of the hospital prematurely and eventually discontinuing her medication without her psychiatrist's approval.

During the current episode, S. had signed out of the hospital after 10 days and returned home. There she was so agitated, pressured, hostile, and violent that the family combined to bring her to the hospital against her will. Although her attorney had previously been quick to help her sign out of the hospital, he had apparently become sufficiently informed about the nature of S.'s illness that he refused to do so during this episode.

On admission, S. was angry, pressured, grandiose, and rather paranoid. She stated that she believed that this entire treatment was simply a conspiracy to control her for her husband's betterment and that she knew that all medical personnel were in a conspiracy against her. She threatened to sue the admitting psychiatrist and the hospital. The patient was extremely abusive to nursing staff and refused to take any medication. After being allowed to remain off medication for a day and a half, the patient became increasingly bizarre and agitated, eventually requiring environmental control through seclusion. At this point, treatment with lithium carbonate and intramuscular injections of chlorpromazine was begun. Over a period of three weeks, S. achieved a therapeutic serum lithium level and deescalated greatly in her mood and behavior. As the patient improved symptomatically, great attention was given to individual, group, and family psychotherapy sessions. The individual and group sessions focused on the patient's resistance to treatment, her underlying fears of being too dependent on her husband (combined with the fear that she might lose him), concerns over her aging, and general fear of experiencing a depressive mood. All sessions continually reestablished the connection between the patient's mood changes and the chaos of the patient's life. A further connection was made between lithium treatment and avoidance of such life disruption in the future. Family therapy sessions allowed the patient, once under adequate control, a forum to verbalize her individual and marital conflicts, while the husband was able to confront the patient with his reactions to her manic behavior.

By the time the patient was ready for discharge, she had made considerable headway in understanding the nature of her illness, its treatment, and the necessary follow-up to avoid continuation of the obviously worsening pattern. To date, the patient has continued on her lithium carbonate while maintaining therapy with her outpatient psychiatrist, both on an individual basis and jointly with her husband. Manic or depressive mood swings have not recurred.

References and Further Reading

Abrams, R., et al. Manic depressive illness and paranoid schizophrenia. *Arch. Gen. Psychiatry* 31:640–642, 1974.

Ambelas, A. Psychologically stressful events in the precipitation of mania. *Br. J. Psychiatry* 135:15–21, 1979.

Browden, C.L., Saraba, F. Diagnosing manic depressive illness in adolescents. *Compr. Psychiatry* 21:263–269, 1980.

Bunney, W.E., et al. The "switch process" in manic depressive illness. *Arch. Gen. Psychiatry* 27:295–302, 1972.

Carlson, G.A., Goodwin, F.K. The stages of mania. *Arch. Gen. Psychiatry* 28:221–228, 1973.

Cohen, M. B., et al. An intensive study of twelve cases of manic depressive psychosis. *Psychiatry* 17:103–127, 1954.

Garvey, M. J., Tuason, V.B. Mania misdiagnosed as schizophrenia. *J. Clin. Psychiatry* 41:75–78, 1980.

Himmelhoch, J.M., et al. Incidence and significance of mixed affective states in a bipolar population. *Arch. Gen. Psychiatry* 33:1062–1066, 1976.

Kotin, J., Goodwin, F.K. Depression during mania: clinical observations and theoretical implications. *Am. J. Psychiatry* 129:679–686, 1972.

Kraepelin, E. *Lectures on Clinical Psychiatry.* 1904. Reprint. New York: Hafner, 1968.

Krauthummer, C., Klerman, G.L. Secondary mania. *Arch. Gen. Psychiatry* 35:1333–1339, 1978.

Lipkin, K.M., et al. The many faces of mania. *Arch. Gen. Psychiatry* 27:262–267, 1970.

Ollerenshaw, D.P. The classification of the functional psychoses. *Br. J. Psychiatry* 122:517–530, 1973.

Reich, T., Winokur. G. Post-partum psychoses in patients with manic depressive disease. *J. Nerv. Ment. Dis.* 151:60–68.

Rifkin, A., et al. Lithium carbonate in emotionally unstable character disorder. *Arch. Gen. Psychiatry* 27.519, 1972.

Shulman, K., Post, F. Bipolar affective disorder in old age. *Br. J. Psychiatry* 136:26–32, 1980.

Taylor, M., Abrams, R. The phenomenology of mania. *Arch. Gen. Psychiatry* 29:520–522, 1973.

Taylor, M.A., et al. Manic depressive illness and acute schizophrenia: a clinical, family history, and treatment-response study. *Am. J. Psychiatry* 131:678–682, 1974.

Affective Disorders II: Depressive Disorders
C. GIBSON DUNN, M.D.

A sad or depressed mood, a frequent occurrence in normal life, is familiar to everyone. It is generally considered normal to experience sadness after a negative event occurs, when the reaction seems approximately proportional to the seriousness of the event. Such reactive sadness is tolerable and transient. Since the beginning of recorded time, however, mood states have occurred in which the depression has been experienced as unbearable, out of proportion to precipitating events, or of excessive duration. Early descriptions of what would now be considered a clinical depressive disorder were provided by Greek physicians, who termed it *melancholia* (from the etiologic theory that the disorder results from an excess of black bile). Much of subsequent dramatic literature also concerned itself with the experience of severe depression and the search for some meaning in suffering. Recent researchers, novelists, journalists, and others, sharing this interest of earlier physicians and writers, have become extremely concerned with the problems of depression. Current psychiatric investigation is probably more attentive to this group of illnesses than to any other. Depressive disorders, when grouped with manic-depressive illness, constitute probably the most frequently diagnosed psychiatric illnesses presenting in physicians' offices. The associated morbidity and even mortality are enormous. For these and other reasons, therefore, it is especially important for the practicing medical clinician to be thoroughly familiar with the manifestations, diagnostic criteria, complications, and treatment of the depressive illness.

Signs and Symptoms of Depression

Depressive disorders are often described as disorders of mood (meaning internal emotional state) or affect (manifest or expressed emotion). Depression and manic depression are often joined under the heading of *affective disorders*. In either case, the most prominent signs and symptoms of depression are those of emotions rather than thought processes. With rare exceptions, a depressive disorder will be characterized by a mood that the patient will describe as sad, blue, depressed, gloomy, or negative. The technical term *dysphoria* is also applied to this mood. Several other symptoms are frequently associated with this depressed mood. There may be the feeling of lack of pleasure or an inability to enjoy normally pleasurable pursuits. This condition, which is termed *anhedonia,* is considered by many to be a critical symptom of major depression. There may be associated feelings of helplessness and hopelessness. Interest in routine activities may be decreased, and sexual desire may be blunted or absent. There is a general loss of initiative, and lack of energy or lethargy may be especially evident. Frequent and easy tearfulness is often reported. The patient may express a general pessimism toward the future. Anxiety may be prominent, although it is not invariably present. With these symptoms and signs, it should not be surprising to learn that depressed persons often withdraw from their normal family, social, occupational, or school activities and display a tendency toward isolation. The person's view of himself or herself is generally adversely affected; feelings of worthlessness or guilt may be expressed. Depressed individuals frequently feel easily overwhelmed and may be irritable when pressed to participate in or contribute to their surrounding environment.

There may be obvious changes in what are called *neurovegetative signs*—that is, sleep, appetite, gastrointestinal function, as well as the previously mentioned energy and sexual activity. Sleep may be either increased or decreased in depression. A decrease in sleep may occur in one or more patterns, including difficulty falling asleep, awakening in the middle of the night (waking up restlessly during the night and having difficulty returning to sleep), or early morning awakening (waking up considerably earlier than the appointed time, without return to sleep). When total sleep time is increased, the increase may be very striking—some people report 12 or more hours of sleep per 24-hour period. Even if total sleep time is not greatly changed, there may be reports of inefficient sleep with persistent fatigue. Appetite, like sleep, may be increased or decreased, although in diagnosable clinical depressions decreased appetite is most frequent. In profound depressions, there may be annoying and persistent constipation. If anxiety is a prominent symptom, however, diarrhea is sometimes the complaint.

These alterations in the rate of functioning of both mental and physical processes are called *psychomotor changes*. When the basic functions of thinking and moving are slowed, *psychomotor retardation* is present, while the term *Psychomotor agitation* is applied when thought processes are pressured and there is physical agitation. Such changes can be profound and extreme. Retardation may progress to actual stupor. Agitation may result in constant pacing, hand wringing, or even clawing at parts of the body until bleeding occurs.

One of the most serious symptoms of depression is suicidality (this is discussed at greater length in Chapter 18). Suicidal symptoms may begin with a wish to be relieved from the suffering of depression by death. It may process to include self-induced, life-threatening, or life-ending acts. For every completed suicide, there are many attempted acts of self-destruction; and for every actual attempt, there are many thoughts and impulses contained solely within the patient's mind.

Along with these signs and symptoms of depression, there may be a specific change in affect that has been characterized as *blunting* or *flattening*; these terms describe a generalized decrease in the range and intensity of expressed emotion. While not specific to depression, blunting or flattening is a frequent concomitant of a depressive disorder.

Although depression has already been defined as a disorder of mood and affect, thought processes are significantly altered in most clinical depressions. Thought content tends to be gloomy, negative, and pessimistic. There may be preoccupation with past or present or anticipated loss, guilt, or death. In depression with psychotic features, such preoccupations may become delusional and involve a partial or complete break from reality. Themes in delusions are considered *mood congruent* when they deal with a depressive subject, such as those listed previously: inadequacy, destruction, or deserved punishment. The patient may experience related hallucinatory phenomena, most commonly auditory but also possibly visual or olfactory. Once again, these are generally mood congruent. In addition to the content of specifically psychotic changes, cognitive processes are more generally altered in a depressive disorder. There is often a marked impairment in concentration and attention span, which may be experienced and even observed as a disorder of memory. This impairment can be so severe that the clinician might make a misdiagnosis of a dementing illness in older depressed patients. Such depressed individuals also have difficulty organizing and categorizing new information presented to them. The flow of thought may become quite circumstantial or even tangential.

While often not listed among formal diagnostic criteria, somatic preoccupations and even specific bodily symptoms may be among the most prominent of depressive symptoms. Such a pattern appears to be especially common in older patients who are already experiencing more physical illness and appear to be sensitized in this direction. Somatic symptoms may involve any organ system. Complaints of joint pain, headache, and gastrointestinal disturbance seem to be the most common. Certainly, complaints of changes in sexual function may be a manifestation of an unrecognized depressive disorder.

Epidemiology

Depression has classically been considered a disorder of adult life. It is now appreciated, however, that depressive disorders can begin at virtually any age from childhood onward. The frequency of depression definitely increases with increasing age, and the rate continues to climb through the productive years and into the senium. This increase with age is especially important to appreciate in order to avoid the misdiagnosing depressive disorders in elderly patients. To illustrate, it might be noted that more than 50 percent of hospitalized patients aged 60 to 70 have affective disorders; the proportion is only slightly less in those aged 70 to 80. Suicide rates increase accordingly, although they tend to level off somewhat earlier than the rate for all affective disorders. The diagnosis of depression is made approximately twice as often in women as in men. This differential appears to reflect the actual frequency of the disorders rather than a diagnostic bias. Approximately 1 in 5 females and 1 in 10 males will experience a major depressive episode at some point during their lives. Except for isolated inbred populations, ethnicity or race does not appear to be a significant factor. Depressive disorders do tend to cluster in families, and both genetic and environmental factors are probably involved (this is covered further in the discussion of etiology).

Course, Complications, and Prognosis

In considering the course of depressive disorders, investigators have often raised the question as to whether a specific premorbid and possibly predisposing personality pattern might exist. The literature in this area, as reviewed by Chodoff (1972), is extremely imprecise and difficult to compare. There has been a general opinion that an obsessive, worrying personality antedates the development of mid-life agitated involutional depression more often than chance alone would allow. At most this appears to be a subgroup of all depressive disorders. When unipolar depressives are compared with bipolar depressives, there is again a rather poorly substantiated opinion that more abnormalities exist in the premorbid personalities of unipolar patients. Historically it has been argued that bipolar depressives more often have premorbid personalities with low-intensity mood swings in evidence before the major illness is manifested; more recent data suggest that their premorbid and intermorbid personality structures may be relatively normal when compared with unipolar patients. Chodoff notes that certain investigators have identified the presence of a more oral-dependent personality structure in the bipolar patients than found by other authors.

In conclusion, however, it must be stated that there is no well-established connection between a specific premorbid personality structure or adaptation and the later development of a depressive illness. Furthermore, whatever premorbid personality patterns may be identified, there is the question as to whether these attributes are causal or whether they are incidental to or results of the depression. Virtually every practicing clinician has seen patients with significant depressive illnesses who have problematic personality disorders; however, the traits of introversion, dependency, worrying, and unassertiveness have been particularly noted.

Depressive illness can definitely be precipitated by life events. In persons of either sex or any class, it is apparent that stressful life events, especially those of a negative nature or those that involve emotional losses from real or psychological events, can induce the onset of a major depressive disorder. The risk for onset of depressive illness may be increased fivefold or more for the six months following such stressful events. Critical early life events of a similar nature—that is, loss of significant supportive figure such as parents or other caretakers—may also increase not only the risk for depression, but also its subsequent severity.

Once a depressive episode has begun, the course of that episode and of subsequent episodes may be extremely variable. The duration of a single depressive episode may range from weeks to years. There is a demonstrated increased risk for symptomatic relapse if antidepressant therapy is stopped during the eight-month period after the onset of symptoms. Weissman and associates (1979) followed 150 women with depressive disorders for one year of maintenance treatment for depression. Approximately 30 percent of the patients remained in complete remission; 12 percent remained chronically symptomatic and 60 percent experienced recurrence of symptoms. In a study by Murphy and co-workers (1974), the five-year follow-up found that 16 percent were chronically ill throughout the follow-up period, 24 percent had no recurrence, and the remaining 60 percent had from one to nine recurrences of depression. Recurrent episodes varied in symptomatic duration from two weeks to one year. Winokur and Morrison found that long-term outcome varied widely depending on the parent's sex and the age at the onset of the depressive episode. Men who were older at the onset of the episode were more likely to have recurrences, and the subsequent episodes were more frequent than was true for women with early onset. Chronicity was more common in the early onset women, however. The overall probability of having only a single episode of a major depression is approximately 50 percent. The other half of those who experience an initial episode appear likely to have one or more recurrences. It is evident, therefore, that a significant minority of patients with depression will develop a fairly chronic impairment of some degree, although this can vary from mild to severe. Total disability from depression is quite uncommon, but it does exist. For most patients, however, either considerable or total recovery is to be expected.

The most severe complication of depression is suicide. In the population at large, up to 1 in 6 patients (12 per 100,000 population) with a primary affective disorder may complete suicide. This is an enormous risk when compared with that of the population at large, and it emphasizes the importance of accurate diagnosis and aggressive, complete treatment. In addition to suicide, however, there may be significant long-term interference with interpersonal and occupational function and even an increased risk for death from other causes. It is known that a major depression is accompanied by increased sympathetic activity with concomitant increases in heart rate and blood pressure. These effects may produce an increased long-term risk for the development of atherosclerotic cardiovascular disease.

There has also been much discussion about alternative manifestations and complications of depression, including alcohol and drug abuse, sociopathy, and hysteria. Winokur has emphasized the concept of a *depressive spectrum disorder* as one subtype of depression in which these other illnesses may be alternative manifestations of the depressive disease. At present, however, such theories remain unproved. The relationship between depression and alcoholism, in particular, is complicated and unclear.

The postpartum period is a time of particular risk for the development of major depressive symptoms. It is generally recognized that mild depressive symptoms, often referred to as "maternity blues," are a nearly ubiquitous concomitant of the post-delivery stage. Such symptoms usually develop two or three days after delivery and persist for up to one to two weeks. In a minority of women, however, there appears to be a risk for the development of a major depressive disorder. It is uncertain whether this risk is increased significantly beyond the risk that would pertain to women of the same age who have not just given birth. While the data are unclear, it does appear that at least some women, especially those with bipolar affective disorders, are at increased risk for the development of a serious mood disorder in this period. This risk may be the result of either the significant postpartum endocrine shifts or the major emotional stress of the responsibility for the constant demands of a newborn infant. It is likely as always that a combination of biologic, environmental, and psychological factors are involved.

Classification and Diagnostic Criteria

Historically there have been numerous classifications of depressive illnesses. These taxonomies have generally attempted to distinguish between milder, transient disorders and those that are more severe and require medical intervention. Depressive disorders in the former category have been variously labeled "reactive," "exogenous," and "neurotic." The more severe disorders have been described as "endogenous," "melancholic," "autonomous," and "psychotic." Reactive, exogenous, and neurotic depressions have been associated with milder impairment, relatively normal neurovegetative signs (that is, no serious changes in sleep, appetite, or libido), inconsistency in depressed mood, and lack of diurnal variation. Autonomous, endogenous, and psychotic depressions characteristically are more intense and unrelieved, with abnormal neurovegetative signs and positive diurnal variation (worsening in the morning). The neurovegetative changes include loss of appetite, energy, sex drive, and sleep. The sleep disturbance typically is one involving awakening in the middle of the night and early in the morning. There may be marked psychomotor changes such as agitation or retardation. Hallucinations or delusions may be present and may especially focus on themes of guilt, worthlessness, bodily dysfunction, or death.

There are obvious limitations in the classifications that have just been described. Most evident is the blurring of levels of severity with theories of etiology. For example, the term *neurotic* implies a disorder resulting from an internal psychological conflict. When contrasted with the term *psychotic,* it suggests a mild illness without hallucinations or delusions. And while an *exogenous* depression might occur as a result of an environmental precipitating event, it might also possess many of the features supposedly typical of an endogenous disorder. Repeated research efforts to make a definitive distinction between these dichotomies have failed to validate the previous categories. This inconsistency was so prominent that it led Donald Klein (1974) to coin the term *endogenomorphic* for the depressions that follow an environmental precipitating stress but include abnormal neurovegetative signs, especially anhedonia (loss of the ability to experience pleasure).

More recent classifications of affective or mood disorders have emphasized observable descriptive features in an effort to achieve greater validity and reliability. These classifications include distinctions between the bipolar and unipolar disorders and between primary and secondary disorders. A *bipolar* depression is a depressive disorder that follows a manic or hypomanic illness, whatever the intervening period. A *unipolar depressive disorder* is one in which only depressive episodes occur. The term *primary depressive disorder* indicates that no other diagnosable psychiatric illness has preceded the depression. *Secondary depressions* follow some other nonaffective psychiatric illness.

While these terms are only descriptive, there has been a general tendency to equate a primary affective disorder or depression with the older concept of endogenous depression. Many clinicians have further assumed that primary disorders involve a need for pharmacologic or other somatic intervention. It is now increasingly appreciated that the category of *primary depressive disorder* is excessively global and obscures clinically important distinctions. While the categories and criteria of the *Diagnostic and Statistical Manual of Mental Disorders,* Third Edition (DSM-III) are utilized in this text, it is important to note their limitations. As yet, there is no direct, firm linkage between a category and any specific clinical management. Clusters of symptoms, such as Klein's (1974) endogenomorphic features or the DSM-III subcategory of melancholia, more strongly suggest the need for somatic treatments, either pharmacologic or electroconvulsive. Carrol's pioneering work with the dexamethasone suppression test has also produced a new marker for somatic treatment (see Chapter 3). Other promising techniques now being evaluated include sleep electroencephalographic studies and investigations of the effects of thyrotropin-releasing hormone on thyroid-stimulating hormone.

For the practicing clinician, however, the DSM-III criteria for depressive disorders provide the current standards for diagnosis. The main disorder is labeled *major depressive disorder,* and the diagnostic criteria for it are listed in Table 8-1. As is evident, these criteria emphasize associated neurovegetative changes. The disorder may be accompanied by psychotic features, which may be either consistent with the depressed mood or mood incongruent. Psychotic features include delusions or hallucinations and are considered mood congruent when the themes are inadequacy, guilt, disease, nihilism, or deserved punishment. In the most extreme form, depressive stupor may occur. As a further subcategory, the patient can have depression *with melancholia* in which case at least three of the following must occur (from DSM-III, p. 215):

1. Distinct quality of depressed mood, i.e., the depressed mood is perceived as distinctly different from the kind of feeling experienced following the death of a loved one
2. The depression is regularly worse in the morning
3. Early morning awakening (at least two hours before usual time of awakening)
4. Marked psychomotor retardation or agitation
5. Significant anorexia or weight loss
6. Excessive or inappropriate guilt

A major depressive disorder must be distinguished from three other categories: uncomplicated bereavement, adjustment reaction with depressed mood, and dysthymic disorder. *Uncomplicated bereavement,* which is not considered a diagnosable clinical disorder, refers to depressive symptoms occurring in immediate reaction to the death of a loved one. This reaction may, however, evolve into a

Table 8-1. Diagnostic Criteria for Major Depressive Episode

A. Dysphoric mood or loss of interest or pleasure in all or almost all usual activities and pastimes. The dysphoric mood is characterized by symptoms such as the following: depressed, sad, blue, hopeless, low, down in the dumps, irritable. The mood disturbance must be prominent and relatively persistent, but not necessarily the most dominant symptom, and does not include momentary shifts from one dysphoric mood to another dysphoric mood, e.g., anxiety to depression to anger, such as are seen in states of acute psychotic turmoil. (For children under six, dysphoric mood may have to be inferred from a persistently sad facial expression.)

B. At least four of the following symptoms have each been present nearly every day for a period of at least two weeks (in children under six, at least three of the first four).
 1. poor appetite or significant weight loss (when not dieting) or increased appetite or significant weight gain (in children under six, consider failure to make expected weight gains)
 2. insomnia or hypersomnia
 3. psychomotor agitation or retardation (but not merely subjective feelings of restlessness or being slowed down) (in children under six, hypoactivity)
 4. loss of interest in pleasure in usual activities, or decrease in sexual drive not limited to a period when delusional or hallucinating (in children under six, signs of apathy)
 5. loss of energy; fatigue
 6. feelings of worthiness, self-reproach, or excessive or inappropriate guilt (either may be delusional)
 7. complaints or evidence of diminished ability to think or concentrate, such as slowed thinking, or indecisiveness not associated with marked loosening of associations or incoherence
 8. recurrent thoughts of death, suicidal ideation, wishes to be dead, or suicide attempt

C. Neither of the following dominate the clinical picture when an affective syndrome (i.e., criteria A and B above) is not present, that is, before it developed or after it has remitted:
 1. preoccupation with a mood-incongruent delusion or hallucination...
 2. bizarre behavior

Reproduced with permission from *Diagnostic and Statistical Manual of Mental Disorders*, 3rd ed. Washington, D.C.: American Psychiatric Association, 1980, pp. 213–214.

major depressive disorder. An *adjustment disorder with depressed mood* is considered to be present when symptoms of depression occur within three months of the onset of an environmental stressor and when those symptoms are considered to be in excess of the expectable reaction to the stressor. It is assumed that the depressive symptoms, which are not severe enough to meet the full criteria for major depressive disorder, will remit spontaneously on removal of the stressor. *Dysthymic disorder,* the DSM-III category most closely equivalent to the older concept of depressive neurosis, is a chronic disturbance of mood of at least two years duration unrelieved except for brief periods of days to weeks. The symptoms, however, should not be so severe as to justify the diagnosis of a major depressive episode. The onset is usually gradual, and there are no clear-cut precipitants. There should be no associated psychotic features.

Differential Diagnosis

The differential diagnosis of major depressive disorders must include consideration of a great number of both medical and psychiatric illnesses. Virtually any medical illness can manifest itself as a depressed mood. When lethargy and lack of interest are especially prominent complaints, it can be particularly difficult to feel confident that one has eliminated possible medical causes. The medical disorders that are most likely to create a depressive picture include disorders of thyroid function (especially hypothyroidism), parathyroid disorders, pituitary and adrenal malfunctions (Cushing's and Addison's diseases), connective tissue diseases, viral infections, hepatitis, infectious mononucleosis, hypoglycemia, diabetes mellitus, and occult malignancies (especially carcinoma of the pancreas). Exposure to industrial or other environmental toxic products, especially heavy metals or compounds containing petrochemicals or cholinesterases, can cause depression. Specific medications that can induce a depressive disorder include catecholamine-depleting agents such as reserpine and propranolol, systemic steroids, and nonsteroidal antiinflammatory drugs.

Significant depressive symptoms can be associated with virtually any psychiatric disorder. When making the diagnosis of a major depressive disorder, it is most important to seek out indications of previously unrecognized bipolar or cyclothymic disorder. Depression can also be associated with incipient schizophrenic disorders, even without meeting the criteria for a complete schizoaffective picture. Organic brain disorders are a particularly important area to consider. While depressed mood can occur with any of the organic brain syndromes, it is also quite easy to misdiagnose the presence of a dementia or to accept as permanent the degree of impairment present with a dementia when a depressive disorder may be making a major contribution to the impairment. It is simply impossible to determine to what degree depression may be aggravating or even creating a dementiform picture without undertaking an adequate therapeutic trial for treatment of the depression. Only a high index of suspicion will minimize the risk of consigning a patient to the ranks of the untreatable when there is in fact a readily treatable illness present.

The relationship of depression to the personality disorders has long been problematic. DSM-III has eased this difficulty somewhat by placing these diagnostic groupings on separate axes. It remains important, however, to recognize the presence of a personality disorder when considering the therapeutic approach to undertake. Depression may occur in association with any of the personality disorders. Depression may also be a frequent complication of severe anxiety disorders, particularly agoraphobia and obsessive-compulsive disorders. When diagnosable, the depressive disorder should be treated in its own right.

The psychiatric disorders most commonly associated with depression, however, are probably those of alcohol and substance abuse. Alcohol and many of the central nervous system depressant drugs appear to be able to generate major depressive symptoms. Withdrawal from these or from sympathomimetic agents, such as amphetamines or cocaine, can also produce a very severe depression. It is generally impossible to determine which of the disorders—

substance abuse or depression—is primary and which is secondary until the individual is totally free of the effects of the abused substance. It may require several weeks to observe the degree of spontaneous mood improvement before a diagnosis of depressive disorder can be established. This diagnosis has significant implications for treatment approach and should not be made precipitously without adequate time and the proper environment in which to observe the patient's course.

Etiology
As noted in the discussion of classification, the depressive disorders are a heterogeneous group of illnesses. This diversity extends not only to symptom clusters, severity, and course, but also to etiologic factors. In addition, a distinction can be made between the precipitating factors and the more fundamental predisposing conditions.

Precipitating factors are not necessarily present for all depressive disorders. Apparently spontaneous, unprovoked depressions definitely occur. In other cases, the link between any precipitating events (external or internal) may seem tenuous at best. Post hoc theorizing as to cause and effect is always open to doubt. This uncertainty seems especially true as the time gap between the purportedly triggering event and the onset of the illness increases. A large percentage of depressive disorders, however, do in fact seem to be precipitated by life events. These events may come in a series, and no one of them alone might have proved overwhelming but collectively they exceed the individual's strength for coping.

LOSS AND GRIEF
As has long been recognized, and more recently proved by Weissman's (1979) group, life events associated with the onset of depression are usually ones involving some type of loss. The loss may involve death, divorce, or separation from some possession, a job, or a life role. In addition, the loss may be almost solely of an internal origin, such as a perceived lost opportunity or hope. The final common pathway for all such traumatic experiences may be the loss of positive, sustaining input to the person's self concept—that is, loss of love, caring, praise, reassurance, and companionship. It must be acknowledged, however, that virtually everyone experiences such losses in the course of a lifetime.

Normally the individual response to such loss is with the experience of grief, which may involve many of the symptoms and signs of depression, including sadness, tearfulness, loss of appetite and interest, discouragement and even dispair, disturbed sleep, and irritability. In the vast majority of people, however, the grief reaction is time-limited and resolves without clinical intervention. Why, then, do some people differ in developing the illness that has been described previously as a depressive disorder? It now appears that a range of social, psychological, and biologic factors can be involved; the relative weighting of each is difficult to determine, and certainly varies among the different depressive disorders.

SOCIAL, PSYCHOLOGICAL, AND BIOLOGIC FACTORS
Little can be said for certain about social (environmental) factors in depressive disorders. Common experience suggests that traumatic losses are better tolerated when supportive persons and resources are immediately available. Women with disturbed marriages, for example, seem to be more likely to develop postpartum depression than are women with stable marriages. The rates of depression and suicide do not increase equally with age in every culture, which suggests an environmental factor. Such evidence is at best indirect but supportive of environmental input.

Individual psychological factors, of course, have long received attention. Freud noted that severe depression (melancholia) differed from normal mourning by the added presence of guilt and self-reproach. This observation led him to suggest that a clinical depression was the result when anger toward a lost object (person) was directed inward against the self; the lost person was thought to have been internalized, thereby becoming part of the self. When anger was directed toward the now unavailable person, it was essentially directed against the self, resulting in severe self-criticism, guilt, and depressed mood. Later (ego) psychologists suggested that depression resulted from the loss of positive input to the self.

Certain developmental experiences in personality constellation may also predispose to the occurrence of depression under the impact of negative life events. As noted previously in this chapter, the childhood loss of a parenting figure may sensitize a person in adulthood to later emotional losses of various types. Early life deprivation of caring and adequate emotional nurturing from any cause may create a similar diathesis. Aaron Beck (1979) has suggested such experiences may create a cognitive set of "depressogenic premises and schemata" that predispose the individual to interpret experiences in the world in a negative, pessimistic, and eventually depressing fashion.

Particular personality profiles also seem to be more commonly associated with depressive disorders. One type is rather passive, emotionally needy (dependent) and self-perceived as helpless. When struck by a negative life event, such people quickly collapse into a depressive state. Here Seligman's (1974) concept of depression as "learned helplessness" truly seems to apply. Another personality type often seen in association with depression is one that is demanding, critical, rather rigid, perfectionistic, and emotionally constricted. In these individuals, the punitive conscience does seem to be attacking the self-concept for failing to achieve some unrealizable life ideal.

But are these psychological factors sufficient to cause depression? Especially in the more severe depressive disorders, researchers have long suspected the existence of fundamental biologic factors. Kraepelin's concept of manic-depressive illness included patients with major depressions even when mania had not occurred. The merging of these disorders continued until the 1960s, when improved genetic studies in Scandinavia separated out some unipolar depressive disorders from manic-depressive illness. This separation, however, only strengthened the presumption of a biologic basis. Today it is clear that many depressive disorders have as their etiology some physiologic abnormality. Family and twin studies taken in their entirety are quite convincing in this direction. Once again, monozygotic twin concordance is much higher than that for dyzygotic twins and siblings.

Winokur (1972) has argued for the existence of two types of depressive illness: (1) depressive-spectrum disease, and (2) pure depressive disease. In the spectrum disorder, the prototype is a woman whose illness is of early onset and who has an excessive incidence of depression in female relatives and of alcoholism and sociopathy in male relatives. In the pure depressive disease, the typical proband is a male with the onset after age 40; both male and female relatives show equal amounts of depression and there is no increase in alcoholism or sociopathy. To date, however, the precise mode of genetic transmission has not been identified.

Over the last two decades, the greatest attention to biologic factors in depression has focused on the biogenic amine hypothesis of depression. According to this theory, depression results from alteration in the metabolism of centrally active biogenic amines. These amines function as neurotransmitters and include norepinephrine, serotonin, and dopamine. Earliest attention was drawn to alterations in norandrenergic activity induced by the drug reserpine. It was observed that this drug is capable of inducing a profoundly depressed state; its major physiologic effect is depletion of neuronal norepinephrine. Certain medications with antidepressant effects increase the availability of norepinephrine at the neuronal synapse. Subsequent research raised the possibility that deficiencies in serotonin metabolism might also be involved, while it is now suspected that abnormalities in dopamine activity may be significant in mania and delusional depressions.

Schildkraut and Maas have suggested that subgroups of depressive disorders might be identified with specific deficiencies in either norepinephrine or serotonin. If accurate, this hypothesis would have major implications for selection of particular antidepressant agents for the different subgroups (desipramine or imipramine for norepinephrine deficiency, and nortriptyline or amitriptyline for serotonin deficiency). In addition to biogenic amines, alterations in acetylcholine metabolism might be involved in affective disorders, according to some suggestions. Davis has used this theory in arguing that a depression may represent a disturbance in balance between central cholinergic and noradrenergic neurotransmitter activity. Depression would result from relative cholinergic dominance, while noradrenergic dominance would lead to mania.

Most recently, investigation has advanced into the neuroendocrine aspects of affective disorders. Hypothalamic-pituitary disinhibition has been identified in certain patients with major depressions. Whether this alteration is etiologic or secondary remains unclear.

Management and Treatment of Depression

As in all other psychiatric disorders, competent management and treatment of depressive disorders requires an initial careful diagnostic assessment to rule out other, more fundamental psychiatric or medical disorders. Once it has been established that a significant depressive disorder is present, the clinician must assess the degree of severity, and especially the risk of suicide. Evaluation of suicide risk is *always* a priority in managing a depression, given the greatly increased incidence in this patient population. Such an evaluation can be done in a nonthreatening fashion, without increasing the likelihood of suicidal. Assessment should further include the family psychiatric history, the family history of suicidality, and the patient's psychiatric history. The clinician should then proceed to assess the degree of impairment caused by the depression, including the presence or absence of neurovegetative changes and anhedonia.

SOMATIC THERAPY

Treatment per se remains empirical and may involve multiple modalities. An early and ongoing question in the management of a depression is, "Should the patient receive some somatic therapy?" Generally this therapy would involve an antidepressant medication, but electroconvulsive therapy (discussed in Chapter 22) might also be considered. Although there are no absolute indications for somatic intervention, the presence of neurovegetative changes (alterations in patterns of sleep, appetite, and sexual activity) is generally accepted as an indication for a trial of antidepressant medication. If there is serious doubt, it is preferable to observe the patient for at least a second session while assessing his or her response to interpersonal contact, ventilation, and support. If a decision is made to use an antidepressant, it is crucial to prescribe the drug correctly and to educate the patient about the appropriate expectations of benefit and side effects to increase the likelihood of compliance.

PSYCHOTHERAPY

Even if the clinician prescribes medication, psychotherapy generally has a major role in the treatment of depression. Individual, marital, and group therapy may be employed singly or in combination. The decision as to the type of therapy and probable length (brief versus long-term) may depend on the assessment of factors that contributed to the onset of the illness. If sudden, uncontrollable loss (for example, the death of a spouse) was the precipitant, the clinician may recommend only supportive individual sessions with encouragement of the normal grieving process and gradual resumption of a socially involved life pattern. On the other hand, the clinician may find more persistent maladaptive psychological or interpersonal patterns requiring longer and intensive psychotherapy. For example, a person with an overly rigid personality structure with a highly critical conscience and unrealistic ideals and standards may require intensive therapy to resolve the psychological factors predisposing to depression. Likewise, a passive-dependent individual, who is unable to assert himself or herself in painful interpersonal situations, may benefit from extended group therapy. Finally, marital therapy as well as individual or group sessions might be helpful to someone who is depressed over a conflictual marital situation and is experiencing excessive dependency needs and separation anxiety.

There has been considerable research to suggest that psychotherapy and pharmacotherapy act on different areas of depressive disorders. Medication may be most beneficial to acute symptoms while psychotherapeutic intervention may best alter maladaptive social and interpersonal personality patterns. There is also considerable evidence to suggest that these therapeutic techniques may be synergistic in their benefit, rather than in any way conflictual.

COGNITIVE THERAPY

An especially interesting recent area of study is that of cognitive therapy by Beck et al. (1979), Kovacs and Beck (1978), and others. Cognitive therapy, as described by Beck et al. (1979) is generally a short-term intervention focused on altering persistent thought processes that predispose to depression. These thought processes, presumably learned early in life, are generally of a negative, pessimistic nature and lead the individuals to assess their experience in the present and anticipated experience in the future in an unfavorable, unpleasant manner. By identifying these fundamental thought processes and instructing the patients in methods of altering these processes, the therapist helps them change their basic view of the world around them in a more positive direction. Preliminary data suggest that this therapeutic approach may be especially effective in depressive disorders.

HOSPITAL TREATMENT

The decision to hospitalize a patient can be difficult. Depressed patients may be especially resistant, given the associated negativism and hopelessness that accompany the illness. Specific indications for hospitalization include marked suicidality, gross impairment of daily function, failure of adequate outpatient therapy, the presence of a physical condition that makes use of essential antidepressant medication hazardous (leading to the need for frequent monitoring), and a lack of adequate external social supports to ensure sufficient time for outpatient therapy to become effective. In addition, hospitalization may be wise when there are indications for electroconvulsive therapy (see Chapter 22).

Case 1. L.B. is a 34-year-old separated mother of three children ages 4, 6, and 9. Eight months earlier, L. separated from her alcoholic husband of 14 years. The husband's drinking had worsened to the point that he lost his job and became increasingly abusive to L. and the children. After one especially violent argument, L. moved into her own apartment. Since then, L. attempted to work full time while applying for welfare and caring for her three children. Despite her exhausting schedule and financial pressures, L. began to date again and met a separated man whom she liked very much. She had become quite hopeful for this relationship, but it ended suddenly when the man decided to return to his estranged wife. After this event, L. became increasingly discouraged and depressed. Her energy decreased markedly, she began to awaken during the night, and her appetite fell off. When L. failed to appear for work on four consecutive days, L.'s supervisor stopped by her home after hours. There she found L. sitting alone, crying. The supervisor learned that L. felt the future was hopeless and no longer cared about living. The friend talked with L. for some time and persuaded her to go to her local mental health center the next day. She did this and began twice-weekly sessions of psychotherapy and some medication to help her sleep. Within two weeks, L. began to feel better and become more active. Her spirits brightened, and her routine normalized. Within six weeks, L. had begun dating again, this time with a more realistic attitude about meeting a man and what to expect from him.

Case 2. J.W. is a 50-year-old married man who was referred from his family doctor for "nerves." He presented as a very agitated, sad-looking man who stated that he was miserable. His trouble had begun eight months earlier, when he learned that his business partner had overcommitted their company to a large inventory purchase. This had put in jeopardy the business for which he had borrowed money by mortgaging his house. Furthermore, both this company and a family store were losing money. J. had become intensely worried by a fear of losing everything. He began to lie awake at night, tormented by feelings of doubt and hopelessness. J. was sure his career was at an end and felt ashamed when he saw friends and associates in his home town. Alcohol consumption went from one to four drinks a night in an effort to blot out the worries. In the meantime, J. tried to arrange a sale of the indebted business in order to relieve the pressure. When a likely prospect backed out, J. became more despondent and sought treatment.

He was hospitalized for depression at age 32 after a major physical illness had disrupted his plans for law school. Symptoms had been similar then, although more intense.

Treatment for the current episode involved supportive talking therapy, antidepressant medication, and encouragement to turn over more of the business to his colleagues in the short run. J.'s anxiety and sleeplessness improved, and his mood brightened partially. The stress of the still-unstable business seemed to prevent complete recovery at that time.

Case 3. F.N., a 53-year-old married mother of three adult children, was admitted to the hospital with a four-month history of intensifying depression. She had begun looking sad and tearful, according to her husband, the month before they moved into a new apartment. The couple had agreed that their old home was too big for them now that the children were grown. She had been much more concerned about the move, since the apartment took her away from her neighbors of 35 years. Soon after the move, F. began to sleep fitfully, and her appetite decreased steadily. Her activity level and responsiveness to family and friends declined greatly. In the last several weeks, F. had become almost totally housebound. She ate and drank little and became quite anxious. Two days before admission, F. began to say that God was punishing her for her past sins and that she deserved to die. She seemed to be hearing voices and responded aloud to them. On the day of admission, she suddenly tried to jump from the apartment window, explaining afterward that she would be doing the world a favor if she killed herself.

She was known to have experienced a major depression after a miscarriage at age 30, and had been hospitalized and treated successfully with electrotherapy.

Because of F.'s severe depression and determined suicidal intent, a decision was made to begin her on a course of unilateral electrotherapy two days after her admission. After three treatments, F. ceased her suicidal preoccupation and began to eat. Within eight treatments, she was back to her normal mood and thinking. Several therapy sessions involving both patient and husband were held, and ways that she could keep in touch with her old friends were discussed. Three weeks after admission, F. was discharged home on a moderate daily dose of an antidepressant.

References and Further Reading

Allen, M.G. Twin studies of affective illness. *Arch. Gen. Psychiatry* 33:1476–1478, 1976.

Avery, D., Lubrano, A. Depression treated with imipramine and ECT: the DeCarole's study reconsidered. *Am. J. Psychiatry* 136:559–562, 1979.

Baldessarini, R.J. An overview of the basis for amine hypotheses in affective illness. In R.J. Friedman and M.M. Katz (eds.), *The Psychobiology of Depression: Theory and Research*. Washington, D.C.: Winston, 1974, pp. 69–83.

Beck, A.T., et al. *Cognitive Therapy of Depression*. New York: Guilfield Press, 1979.

Chodoff, P. The depressive personality. *Arch. Gen. Psychiatry* 27:666–672, 1972.

Hill, D. Depression: disease, reaction or posture? *Am. J. Psychiatry* 125:445–457, 1968.

Klein, D.F. Endogenomorphic depression. *Arch. Gen. Psychiatry* 31:447–454, 1974.

Klerman, G.L., et al. Treatment of depression by drugs and psychotherapy. *Am. J. Psychiatry* 131:186–191, 1974.

Kovacs, M., and Beck, A.T. Maladaptive cognitive structures in depression. *Am. J. Psychiatry* 135:525–533, 1978.

Lloyd, C. Life events and depressive disorder reviewed. I. Events as predisposing factors. II. Events as precipitating factors. *Arch. Gen. Psychiatry* 37:529–548, 1980.

Murphy, G.E., et al. Variability of the clinical course of primary affective disorder. *Arch. Gen. Psychiatry* 30:757–761, 1974.

Nelson, J.C., Charney, D.S. The symptoms of major depressive illness. *Am. J. Psychiatry* 138:1–13, 1981.

Seligman, M.E.P. Depression and learned helplessness. In R.J. Friedman and M.M. Katz (eds.), *The Psychobiology of Depression: Contemporary Theory and Research*. Washington, D.C.: Winston, 1974.

Weissman, M.M. The psychological treatment of depression. *Arch. Gen. Psychiatry* 36:1261–1269, 1979.

Weissman, M.M., et al. The efficacy of drugs and psychotherapy in the treatment of acute depressive episodes. *Am. J. Psychiatry* 1365:555–558, 1979.

Winokur, G. Types of depressive illness. *Br. J. Psychiatry* 120:265–266, 1972.

Anxiety Disorders

C. GIBSON DUNN, M.D.

Anxiety, perhaps the most frequently experienced painful human emotion, is experienced by most people at some point during the course of an average day. For the majority, anxiety is a normal part of life and can actually serve a variety of useful functions. Specifically, anxiety can be a warning of danger (minor or major) from the outside world or from a person's internal emotional or physical state. In this context, anxiety is a normal adaptive and transient alerting response that is useful to the individual. For some people, however, anxiety becomes so intense and sustained that it interferes with comfort and function. When this pattern develops, the affected person is suffering from pathologic anxiety, either as a distinct disorder or as part of some other illness or situation.

Probably because of their prevalence, the anxiety states were among the first psychiatric disorders to become the subject of concerted research efforts. As early as 1871, anxiety conditions were described in two major articles that are still recognized today. J.M. Da Costa published his famous article, "The Irritable Heart," describing the syndrome that was later and more enduringly labeled *anxiety neurosis* by Sigmund Freud in 1894. In the same year Westphal defined *agoraphobia,* which has received increasing attention in recent years. Following these early efforts, however, there appears to have been a period of relative decline in interest, perhaps as a part of the general trend away from descriptive and biologic psychiatry. In the last 15 or 20 years, however, the delineation of the panic anxiety states and the identification of simple and effective pharmacologic and behavioral therapies have rekindled latent interest in these areas.

Anyone planning to practice clinical medicine in any specialty must be alert to the existence of anxiety symptoms and familiar with the recognition, diagnosis, and management of anxiety states. While the psychiatrist tends to have the most training in this area, far more anxiety disorders or anxiety complications of other medical or psychiatric disorders are seen by the general physician or nonpsychiatric specialist. To illustrate, it has been estimated that from 10 to 15 percent of patients consulting cardiologists are experiencing primary anxiety disorders. This chapter is intended to give practical help in the diagnosis and management of people with these disorders.

Anxiety Signs and Symptoms

The term *anxiety* is generally applied to a cluster of symptoms related to subjective experience of fear, the source of which is largely unrecognized by the individual or which is substantially out of proportion to an actual external threat. This subjective experience may or may not be recognized or labeled by the suffering individual as anxiety, but rather may be experienced as nervousness or tension. At other times, however, the emotional experience may be so extreme that intense fear, dread, or even terror is reported. This mental representation is usually accompanied by one or more of the somatic manifestations of anxiety, including (in rough order of reported frequency) palpitations (involving the awareness of heart beat or rapid heart beat), easy fatigability, shortness of breath, chest pain, tightness in the chest, headache or other muscular pain, paresthesias, shakiness, sweating, dry mouth, nausea, abdominal pains, diarrhea, blurring of vision, dizziness or vertigo, cold extremities, and urinary frequency or urgency.

As may be apparent, these symptoms involve multiple organ systems and are, by and large, symptoms of the generalized autonomic nervous system discharge that accompanies anxiety to varying degrees of intensity. In any given individual, the relative intensity of the subjective and somatic experiences of anxiety may vary, often resulting in the major emphasis being given to reports of physical discomfort and symptoms rather than to the more clearly emotional. It is very easy for a clinician, therefore, to find his or her attention directed primarily to a specific organ system while missing the underlying problem of anxiety.

The signs and symptoms of anxiety as described may occur in different patterns of varying duration and relationships to internal and external stimuli. These patterns are discussed in the sections on the primary anxiety states and differential diagnosis.

While the signs and symptoms of anxiety are easily recognizable when listed or identified as manifestations of autonomic hyperactivity, men and women in modern society tend to obscure the patterns by individual and social modification. Very often people with anxiety may present as worrying, irritable, or pressured personalities, which may obscure the more fundamental symptoms; the clinician may respond to these personality features without observing what is behind them. In order to recognize the key signs and symptoms, the clinician must attempt to dissect these aspects of personality into symptom patterns without losing sight of the whole individual suffering with them.

Epidemiology

Epidemiologic data on anxiety states are of somewhat limited value. Different diagnostic classifications have been used over the years, and often anxiety states have been lumped together in many of the studies done. Nonetheless, certain information is available that is of practical significance in diagnosing and treating anxiety disorders. In the general population, the prevalence of pathologic anxiety states has been estimated as being from 2 to 5 percent, with the rate being much higher among persons seeking medical treatment. Individuals with lesser although uncomfortable degrees of anxiety no doubt constitute a considerably larger portion of the population.

To a great degree, prevalence estimates depend on how the data have been gathered and what criteria of severity are applied to findings. In the study by Agras and colleagues (1969) on the epidemiology of phobias among the general population, the total prevalence of phobias was approximately 75 per 1,000 at a "mildly disabling level of intensity." When only severely disabling phobias were counted, however, the prevalence dropped to 2.2 per 1,000. It is apparent, therefore, that a great many people who might not be recognized as having a clinically diagnosable disorder nonetheless suffer significant morbidity. The same prevalence no doubt holds true for the anxiety states other than phobias.

The age of onset varies somewhat among the subtypes of anxiety states but the condition virtually always appears before the age of 40. Phobias can begin in childhood and through the twenties; simple phobias tend to begin in childhood, social phobias in late childhood or adolescence, and agoraphobia from the late teens through the twenties. Panic anxiety states may begin the late adolescence or early adult life, but they may also develop in those in their thirties. Generalized anxiety disorder also tends to have its onset from adolescence through the early thirties, although not usually after that period. Onset after the thirties should lead the clinician to consider whether the anxiety symptoms are secondary to some other disorder, often of a depressive type. Obsessive compulsive disorders tend to have the broadest range in the age of onset; they occur from childhood through the mature adult years. Generally, however, the practicing clinician should be suspicious of anxiety symptoms that are reported to have begun after the age of 35 regardless of the subtype.

The sex ratio of anxiety disorders varies somewhat with subtype; the general finding is that the condition has a higher incidence in women than in men. This predominance seems to be especially true for the phobic disorders. Obsessive compulsive disorder appears to be diagnosed with approximately equal frequency among men and women. Among patients referred for psychiatric treatment, there is some evidence that the sexual differential is reduced or eliminated, suggesting that the more severe forms of anxiety may be more equally distributed.

Cultural aspects are far more difficult to evaluate since there is a definite difference between the actual occurrence of anxiety disorders and the report of these same problems. Furthermore, the manifestations of anxiety appear to vary widely from culture to culture; certain ethnic groups tend to express anxiety or symptoms complicated by anxiety more openly and actively than is true of other groups. So far as is known, race is not a significant predictor of the prevalence of anxiety states.

Classification and Diagnostic Criteria for the Primary Anxiety States

Over the years, there have been many classifications of anxiety symptoms and disorders. A pragmatic and workable distinction utilized in the *Diagnostic and Statistical Manual of Mental Disorders,* Third Edition (DSM-III) and throughout this text is that between anxiety that is the predominant or *primary* clinical disturbance and anxiety that is accessory or *secondary* to some other presumably more fundamental disorder—either functional or organic. The following section considers secondary anxiety and the problem of distinguishing primary anxiety that presents with symptom patterns more suggestive of medical disorders. In discussing the primary anxiety states, the classification that will be most prominent and influential over the next decade is undoubtedly that presented in DSM-III. Table 9-1 presents the

Table 9-1. DSM-III Anxiety Disorders

Phobic disorders
   Agoraphobia with panic attacks
   Agoraphobia without panic attacks
   Social phobia
   Simple phobia
Panic disorder
Generalized anxiety disorder
Obsessive compulsive disorder
Posttraumatic stress disorder, acute, chronic, or delayed
Atypical anxiety disorder

diagnostic classes and the disorders within each class listed in order of decreasing comprehensiveness.

PHOBIC DISORDERS

The first of the anxiety disorders to be considered are the phobic disorders. An essential feature of any phobia, as noted in DSM-III, is "persistent avoidance behavior secondary to irrational fears of a specific object, activity, or situation." Without avoidance behavior or a strong urge to avoid the phobic stimulus, there is no pathologic phobia. Unlike persons suffering from psychotic disorders, the phobic individual on questioning will acowledge that his or her fear is unreasonable as measured by the actual threat posed by the dreaded object, activity, or situation. As noted in the discussion of epidemiology, mild phobias are extremely common throughout the general population while more severe phobias are much less common; however, they can be quite disabling when intense. Phobic disorders are subclassified into agoraphobia, social phobia, and simple phobia. Approximately 60 percent of clinically significant phobias are of the agoraphobic type, and this phobia is by far the most disabling of the common phobias.

Agoraphobia

The term *agoraphobia,* previously rarely heard but recently much more publicized, is derived from the Greek word for fear of a market place or place of assembly. It is, however, more correctly considered a fear of leaving a familiar setting such as the home or other secure environment. It appears to be a phobia since individuals afflicted with agoraphobia try to avoid going out and away from the familiar and thereby create the appearance of avoiding the destination of their journey. This kind of phobic individual, therefore, may complain of being frightened to go to the store or to a movie theater, but the more fundamental anxiety results from the fear of leaving home to any destination. Individuals suffering from agoraphobia are consequently constricted in their geographic mobility; alternatively, they may achieve the usual range of movement only with the assistance of a companion or at the emotional expense of considerable suffering. The degree of restriction can vary widely—at one end of the spectrum are those with a full range of movement (although they experience difficulty), while at the other end, the affected individuals are virtually confined to the home. This is a truly miserable state in its severe form and is clearly quite incapacitating. The DSM-III diagnostic criteria for agoraphobia are listed in Table 9-2.

It is very important to appreciate that agoraphobia has a close association with panic anxiety disorder. The occurrence of panic attacks (as described in the section dealing with that disorder) appears to be a major cause of the development of agoraphobia. In what is probably the great majority of severe cases of agoraphobia, panic anxiety attacks have been the chief factor in creating the phobic anxiety of leaving a secure setting. These are many patients, however, in which no history of clearcut panic attacks can be elicited; in these cases the diagnosis of agoraphobia without panic attacks is more correct. Much more commonly, however, recurrent panic attacks generate a severe anticipatory anxiety that an attack will occur, and that anxiety manifests itself thereafter as a phobic avoidance of traveling alone or of being in unfamiliar settings.

Social Phobia

Another category of phobic disorders, social phobia, has as its central feature the persistent excessive fear of situations in which the individual may be observed by others, leading to a compelling desire to avoid such situations. The phobic individual may also experience fear that he or she will behave in a manner that will be judged humiliating or embarrassing. As with all phobias, much anxiety develops as the affected person anticipates entering a situation exposed to public view (such as speaking before an audience or even eating or writing in public). Such phobias are more a cause of inconvenience than they are seriously incapacitating. Nonetheless, significant morbidity may result over time, and these phobias should not be dismissed lightly when brought to the attention of the clinician. The diagnostic criteria are presented in Table 9-3.

Simple Phobia

The third category of phobias, *simple phobia*, represents a condition that is usually quite specific and limited to one stimulus. It is characterized by persistent and irrational fear of an object or situation, except when that fear falls into the categories described by the diagnoses of agoraphobia or social phobia. To be diagnosed, the phobia must be of sufficient distress that it causes the individual significant discomfort and leads to a desire to avoid the phobic situation or object. The most common simple phobias found in the general population involve animals, followed by fears of specific places such as enclosed areas or heights. When exposed to the phobic stimuli, any or all of the

---

Table 9-2. Diagnostic Criteria for Agoraphobia

A. The individual has marked fear of and thus avoids being alone or in public places from which escape might be difficult or help not available in case of sudden incapacitation, e.g., crowds, tunnels, bridges, public transportation.
B. There is increasing constriction of normal activities until the fear or avoidance behavior dominate the individual's life.
C. Not due to [another psychiatric disorder]. . . .

Reproduced with permission from DSM-III, p. 227.

Table 9-3. Diagnostic Criteria for Social Phobia

A. A persistent, irrational fear of, and compelling desire to avoid, a situation in which the individual is exposed to possible scrutiny by others and fears that he or she may act in a way that will be humiliating or embarrassing.
B. Significant distress because of the disturbance and recognition by the individual that his or her fear is excessive or unreasonable.
C. Not due to another mental disorder. . . .

Reproduced with permission from DSM-III, p. 228.

symptoms characteristic of anxiety may be experienced or demonstrated. Table 9-4 lists the diagnostic criteria for simple phobia.

PANIC DISORDER

An especially crucial classification of anxiety disorders for the practicing physician to recognize is that of panic disorder. An episode of panic disorder, or a panic attack, involves the experience of extraordinarily severe anxiety symptoms, which are often reported by affected individuals as being totally terrifying. There may be a true sense of dread or fear of dying. The autonomic discharge associated with these attacks is extremely intense and may produce a fear of fainting, losing control, or dying. Along with generalized anxiety disorder, panic disorder is most often reported in terms of some specific physical discomfort or symptoms; thus there is a great likelihood that

Table 9-4. Diagnostic Criteria for Simple Phobia

A. A persistent, irrational fear of, and compelling desire to avoid, an object or a situation other than being alone or in public places away from home (agoraphobia), or of humiliation or embarrassment in certain social situations (social phobia). Phobic objects are often animals, and phobic situations frequently involve heights or closed spaces.
B. Significant distress from the disturbance and recognition by the individual that his or her fear is excessive or unreasonable.
C. Not due to another mental disorder. . . .

Reproduced with permission from DSM-III, pp. 229–230.

the patient will be wrongly diagnosed as having a primary medical disorder.

Along with the more frequently reported anxiety symptoms, individuals suffering panic disorder may report feelings of unreality and depersonalization, which may be reported as a sense of being "spaced out" or detached from oneself; they may describe a feeling that the mind is separated from the body and even observing it from afar. Panic attacks may occur at any time of the day or night and last from seconds to hours, although several minutes is a more typical period of time. The initial onset may occur with dramatic suddenness, and patients can often report their first attack with great precision after many years. These episodes are relatively discrete, although they may be followed by considerable anxiety that they will recur. Eventually, the anticipatory anxiety about another attack may merge with the panic attack to create a virtually constant state of agitation and anxiety. The unpredictability, suddenness, and intensity of the attacks further aggravate the problem and create great suffering and incapacitation; this discomfort also leads to agoraphobia, as already noted.

The diagnosis of panic disorder results largely from the work begun by Roth (1959) and Klein (1964); their work unfortunately continues to be largely unappreciated by the medical profession and the general population.

Recognition by the informed physician of a panic disorder is one of those rare occasions in which clinical acumen can actually save years of suffering and incapacitation. It is not uncommon in my experience to identify panic anxiety disorders that had been active but incorrectly diagnosed for more than a decade; some patients were diagnosed as having some medical disorder such as a cardiac illness or a disorder of the inner ear, while others were treated with prolonged psychotherapy for manifestations of some specific internal psychological conflict. The possible etiology and precipitating factors of this disorder are covered in the discussion of etiology. The diagnostic criteria are presented in Table 9-5.

Table 9-5. Diagnostic Criteria For Panic Disorder

A. At least three panic attacks within a three-week period in circumstances other than during marked physical exertion or in a life-threatening situation. The attacks are not precipitated only by exposure to a circumscribed phobic stimulus.
B. Panic attacks are manifested by discreet episodes of apprehension or fear, and at least four [of the previously described symptoms of anxiety] appear during each attack.
C. Not due to a physical disorder or another medical disorder.
D. The disorder is not associated with agoraphobia [in which case diagnosis of agoraphobia with panic attacks should be made].

Reproduced with permission from DSM-III, pp. 231–232.

GENERALIZED ANXIETY DISORDER

The category of generalized anxiety disorder represents the DSM–III view of the condition that was previously called *anxiety neurosis*. It is characterized by generalized anxiety symptoms of at least one month's duration without the characteristic symptoms of phobic disorders or obsessive compulsive disorder. This illness tends not to be as disabling as panic disorder, although the periods of anxiety may become quite intense in this disorder; some care must be given to differentiate it from panic disorder. If there is any doubt, it is preferable to assume the diagnosis of generalized anxiety disorder since its treatment tends to involve less intensive psychological and pharmacologic intervention. If the individual does not respond to the treatment as described later in this chapter, however, one should reconsider the possible existence of a panic anxiety disorder. The overall impairment in function in generalized anxiety disorder tends to be less severe than in agoraphobia or panic disorder, although at times anxiety symptoms may interfere significantly with day-to-day function. The diagnostic criteria for this are given in Table 9-6.

Obsessive Compulsive Disorder

Obsessive compulsive disorder was previously labeled obsessive compulsive neurosis. While the compulsive personality disorder (see Chapter 13) is a common psychiatric problem, a true obsessive compulsive disorder is seen much less frequently. Nonetheless, when fully developed, this is an extremely painful and disabling psychiatric illness and requires quite sophisticated management.

The essential features of obsessive compulsive disorder are recurrent *obsessions*—persistent ideas, thoughts, images, or impulses that the individual experiences as alien and uncomfortable. This awareness distinguishes an obsession from a delusion, in which the patient may fully accept the reality of the thought. Very often individuals attempt to resist the obsessional thought in order to avoid its anxiety-inducing or anxiety-associated experience. The most common obsessions include thoughts of violence, contamination, doubt, or loss. Sexual obsessions are also fairly common. Worry, especially in an intense form, may be conceptualized as a form of obsessional rumination; however, to be diagnosable, the worry must become fairly specific and repetitive.

Compulsions—repetitive and seemingly purposeful stereotyped acts—are essentially the behaviors resulting from obsessions. Thus, if an individual is obsessed with the thought of his or her hands being contaminated with dirt or bacteria, hand washing might result as a compulsion. People affected by compulsions experience themselves as, in fact, being compelled to undertake such actions in order to ward off the anxiety associated with their ruminations. While they may be able to resist acting on an obsession of mild intensity or to

Table 9-6. Diagnostic Criteria for Generalized Anxiety Disorder

A. Generalized, persistent anxiety is manifested by symptoms from three of the following four categories:
   1. motor tension
   2. autonomic hyperactivity
   3. apprehensive expectation
   4. vigilance and scanning
B. The anxious mood has been continued for at least one month.
C. Not due to another mental disorder.
D. At least 18 years of age.

Reproduced with permission from DSM-III, p. 233.

delay acting on a more intense obsession, eventually they relent and attempt to seek relief through the compulsion, only to find the anxiety resuming again once the compulsion is complete. In addition to hand washing, other common compulsions include checking, counting, touching, and straightening.

When first encountered by a nonpsychiatric physician, a person suffering from obsessive compulsive disorder can seem quite bizarre. The patient is equally amazed at what is happening to him or her and is usually quite ashamed of it. The responsible physician should not underestimate the pain and impairment that can result from this uncommon, but not rare, illness. The diagnostic criteria for obsessive compulsive disorder are presented in Table 9-7.

POSTTRAUMATIC STRESS DISORDER

While anxiety is not necessarily the main characteristic of posttraumatic stress disorder (acute, chronic, or delayed), anxiety is frequently a major symptomatic component. The essential feature of the disorder is the development of interfering symptoms after an emotionally traumatic event, which is usually outside the range of human experience. To justify this diagnosis the stress of the event must be considered of sufficient intensity to evoke significant symptoms of distress in most people. If anxiety symptoms predominate, these symptoms would be similar to those listed previously for anxiety. Depression or irritability may be more common than in other anxiety disorders. The diagnostic criteria for posttraumatic stress disorder are listed in Table 9-8.

The term *acute* is applied when the onset of symptoms occurs within six months of the trauma or when the total duration of the symptoms is less than six months. The term *chronic* is used when duration of symptoms is six months or more, and the term *delayed* is applied when the onset of symptoms occurs more than six months following the stress.

ATYPICAL ANXIETY DISORDER

The final category, atypical anxiety disorder, is a residual classification for any clinical picture in which anxiety predominates but the symptoms do not meet the diagnostic criteria of any of the disorders previously described.

Table 9-7. Diagnostic Criteria for Obsessive-Compulsive Disorder

A. Either obsessions or compulsions:
   Obsessions: Recurrent, persistent ideas, thoughts, images or images that are ego-dystonic. . . . Attempts are made to ignore or suppress [the thoughts that invade consciousness and are experienced as senseless or repugnant].
   Compulsions: The repetitive and seemingly purposeful behaviors that are performed according to certain rules or in a stereotyped fashion [usually in close association with an obsession. The behavior is designed to prevent some future event or situation]. The act is performed with a sense of subjective compulsion coupled with a desire to resist the compulsion (at least initially). The individual generally recognizes the senselessness of the behavior. . . and does not derive pleasure from carrying out the activity, although it provides a release of tension.
B. The obsessions or compulsions are a significant source of stress to the individual and interfere with social or role functioning.
C. Not due to another mental disorder.

Modified with permission from DSM-III, p. 235.

Table 9-8. Diagnostic Criteria for Posttraumatic Stress Disorder

A. Existence of a recognizable stressor that would evoke significant symptoms of distress in almost everyone.
B. Reexperiencing of the trauma as evidenced by at least one of the following:
   1. recurrent intrusive recollections of the event
   2. recurrent dreams of the event
   3. sudden acting or feeling as if traumatic event were reoccurring because of an association with an environment or ideational stimulus
C. Numbing of responsiveness to or reduced involvement with the external world. . . .
D. At least two of the following symptoms that were not present before the trauma:
   1. hyperalertness or exaggerated startle response
   2. sleep disturbance
   3. guilt about surviving . . .
   4. memory impairment or trouble concentrating
   5. avoidance of activities that arouse recollection of the traumatic events
   6. intensification of symptoms by exposure to events that symbolize or resemble the traumatic event

Reproduced with permission from DSM-III, p. 238.

Differential Diagnosis of Anxiety Symptoms
As noted earlier, a pragmatic distinction can be made between anxiety symptoms that represent a primary clinical disturbance and anxiety that is secondary to some other, more fundamental psychiatric or medical disorder.

OTHER PSYCHIATRIC DISORDERS
The preceding section discussed the diagnostic features of the primary anxiety disorders. Far more common is anxiety associated with a broad array of psychiatric and medical illnesses. Anxiety may accompany psychiatric disorders of various classifications and degrees of intensity. Anxiety frequently accompanies affective disorders, both depressive and bipolar. In either case, other diagnostic features should be present leading to a diagnosis of the more inclusive illness. Anxiety also is a major feature of the psychotic disorders and organic brain disorders. Efforts to treat the anxiety as a primary disorder when there is an underlying psychotic process will be unsuccessful. For the diagnostic features of the preceding groups, see the appropriate chapters in the text.

Anxiety accompanying personality disorders presents another type of differential diagnostic problem; however, under the DSM-III diagnostic system, anxiety disorders and personality disorders are recorded on different axes. This system allows the physician to attend to two aspects of an individual's functional impairment, but it can also pose a pragmatic problem as to which disorder might be considered more fundamental. For example, if a patient were found to be suffering from a borderline personality disorder (see Chapter 13), it would be essential to approach treatment differently than would be the case if major anxiety symptoms were present without this coexisting personality disorder. Medication selection, psychological therapy, and social management might vary considerably depending on whether or not the personality disorder coexisted with the anxiety symptoms.

Anxiety symptoms may also accompany organic brain disorders of various etiologies. Once again, treatment and management might be quite different in the patient with an organic brain disorder than in one with a primary or isolated anxiety disorder. In all of these cases, the practicing clinician must be familiar with the full range of psychiatric disorders as discussed in the text, with an awareness of the approach to treatment of each. Failure to make the concurrent or more primary diagnosis is likely to result in inadequate or unsuccessful efforts to treat the anxiety symptoms.

SUBSTANCE USE DISORDERS
Substance use disorders or their complications are frequent causes of anxiety symptoms and might be unappreciated as such by the physician. Anxiety symptoms may appear either in direct response to an abused chemical or as part of a relative or total abstinence syndrome. Sympathomimetic or stimulant medication, such as amphetamines, may generate severe anxiety symptoms. Withdrawal from central nervous system depressant chemicals—including alcohol, barbiturates, benzodiazepines, or hypnotics—usually causes major anxiety symptoms as part of the total picture. Only a careful history and high index of suspicion, as well as an active use of laboratory monitoring (such as urine toxicology), may reveal the diagnosis in patients who are less than candid with their physicians.

A rather special, although not uncommon, chemical cause of anxiety symptoms is *caffeinism*. Caffeine is present in a wide range of foods, beverages, and medications in common use, and many people are unaware of the total dosage being ingested from these various sources. The combined effects of several cups of coffee, cold tablets, and cola beverages may produce a syndrome that closely resembles an anxiety disorder but is clearly secondary to the excessive use of the chemical. Once again, a careful history may be the most useful tool in establishing this diagnosis.

In all of the examples of anxiety stemming from other disorders, while anxiety symptoms and even syndromes may be prominent, treatment must be based on the associated or underlying disorder. It is important to reemphasize that all anxiety is not the same, as will be described more fully in the section on management of the different primary disorders. Just as *fever* is no longer an adequate medical diagnosis, the word *anxiety* has become an inadequate description of a clinical phenomenon.

PHYSICAL AND MEDICAL DISORDERS

There are also numerous physical and specific medical disorders that may generate anxiety symptoms or symptoms that mimic anxiety. Again a high index of suspicion is essential if underlying disorders are not to be overlooked. A thorough medical evaluation should be part of any differential diagnostic process, including not only a routine physical examination but also laboratory evaluations. Medical illnesses that most commonly create anxiety symptoms include hyperthyroidism (either endogenous or exogenous), hyperadrenalism from tumors of the adrenal medulla or pituitary, pheochromocytoma, paroxysmal atrial tachycardia, and other arrhythmias. Certain medications, such as corticosteroids or the more stimulating antidepressants, can also generate anxiety symptoms.

A particularly troublesome question has been raised concerning the *mitral valve prolapse syndrome* (MVPS), which has been implicated as the cause of many symptoms similar to those in the primary anxiety disorders. Wooley (1956) contended that many so-called anxiety states are, in fact, secondary to MVPS. This syndrome is characterized by the prolapse of the mitral valve leaflet during the midsystolic phase and may create symptoms indistinguishable from those associated with severe anxiety attacks. More recent work has also complicated this question by finding the concurrent existence of both anxiety states and MVPS in probands and their family members. At times only a careful cardiac evaluation can establish this differential diagnosis adequately.

Functional hypoglycemia presents another difficult diagnostic problem. While there is no doubt that tumors of the pancreas, specifically insulinomas, can cause marked hypoglycemia and reactive sympathetic stimulation similar to anxiety, the prevalence and significance of functional hypoglycemia is quite unclear. In my experience, hypoglycemia is an uncommon cause of symptoms mimicking anxiety, and individuals who blame hypoglycemia, in fact, often have significant anxiety or personality disorders. There is a body of literature supporting this observation. Nonetheless, if there is a question, a glucose tolerance test is easy to obtain and relatively definitive in establishing a diagnosis.

Anxiety, of course, is also a common part of the human reaction to any serious medical illness. Since the anxiety is a reaction to the medical disorder, this anxiety is correctly considered secondary. It can, however, be of such intensity that it is a major aspect of the patient's overall management. In such a patient the diagnosis of acute stress reaction might be justified. Management of such disorders will be considered later.

The previous discussion has emphasized the importance of seeking an associated or underlying medical illness when evaluating anxiety symptoms. An equally important, or perhaps even more significant, problem occurs when the physician continues to search for medical illnesses in patients whose fundamental problem is an anxiety disorder. As delineated in the section on anxiety signs and symptoms, people with moderate or severe anxiety often seek medical treatment believing that the somatic manifestations of anxiety in fact represent a specific physical disorder. For example, approximately 10 percent of the patients in a typical cardiology practice have an anxiety disorder that will receive inappropriate and unsuccessful treatment if the anxiety problem is not recognized. This diagnostic challenge applies to all organ systems, and the clinician must accept it as an important one for his or her patients. Consequently, once reasonable medical evaluative procedures have been completed, the clinician must shift his or her attention to the diagnostic criteria for primary anxiety disorders; it is important to communicate the reliability and importance of the diagnosis to the patient. Only thorough familiarity with the diagnostic criteria for anxiety, as well as confidence in one's clinical experience, will enable the physician to succeed with this approach. To fail to do so, however, will expose the patient to a useless and even dangerous medical evaluation and prolongation of the fundamental problem (see Tables 9-9, 9-10).

Table 9-9. Medical Conditions Commonly Presenting with Anxiety Symptoms

1. Cardiovascular
    a. Angina pectoris
    b. Hyperdynamic beta-adrenergic circulatory state
    c. Mitral valve prolapse syndrome (systolic click murmur syndrome)
    d. Paroxysmal tachycardias
2. Drug related
    a. Caffeinism
    b. Stimulant abuse
    c. Withdrawal from central nervous system depressant drugs, including alcohol
3. Endocrine
    a. Hyperadrenalism, Cushing's disease
    b. Hyperthyroidism
    c. Hypoglycemia
4. Neoplastic, predominantly pheochromocytoma
5. Respiratory; chiefly hypoxia of various origins, most often chronic obstructive pulmonary disease
6. Seizure disorder, especially temporal lobe epilepsy

Table 9-10. Common Medical Misdiagnoses for Anxiety Disorder

Angina pectoris
Acute myocardial infarction
Hypoglycemia
Menière's disease
Menopausal syndrome
Migraine headaches
Thyroid disorders
Peptic ulcer

Complications, Course, and Prognosis

The most common complication of anxiety states is secondary depression, usually of a mild or moderate severity. If the depressive symptoms progress to the point of meeting the diagnostic criteria for depressive disorder, then this diagnosis supersedes the anxiety disorder. In the more severe anxiety disorders, especially panic disorder, there appears to be an increased risk that drug or alcohol abuse might develop, presumably because the patient is trying to modify the anxiety symptoms. Drugs in this disorder tend to be of the sedative or hypnotic type; they may have some initial antianxiety effect, but they prove inadequate in treating the basic disorder. This complication may also be present in intense generalized anxiety disorder, but not in the more isolated phobic disorders. Agoraphobia with panic anxiety disorder, of course, presents the same risk as the panic state itself. Sexual maladjustment can also result from prolonged anxiety symptoms.

While much has been written about the relationship personality type in those affected by anxiety and medical disorders such as peptic ulcer or cardiovascular disease, there is no convincing evidence that an anxiety disorder predisposes an individual to any medical illness. Not uncommonly, the physician finds that the anxiety is a manifestation of developing physical illness that has previously gone unrecognized.

The course, impairment, and prognosis vary significantly among patients with the different anxiety disorders. Within the phobic disorders, social and simple phobias tend to be of a chronic nature once present in adulthood, but they are rarely incapacitating. The course may worsen if the affected person is forced into the presence of the phobically avoided situation or stimulus, but this tends to remit once the provocative stimulus is removed. Agoraphobia can vary considerably in intensity and often has a waxing and waning course with periods of nearly total remission. Among cases identified as severe, follow-up studies have found that one-quarter were seriously impaired at the time of follow-up and another quarter had nearly or totally recovered. The remaining one-half experienced continued phobic anxiety symptoms of some degree, but were more functional than at the time of initial identification. Since most cases of agoraphobia are milder than those cited above, the course and resulting impairment tend to be milder.

Among patients with obsessive compulsive disorders, the milder cases appear to have a good prognosis, with 60 to 80 percent being asymptomatic or much improved. Individuals who were severely impaired at one time continue to have more impairment on an ongoing basis. The course of the disorder tends to be chronic, and symptoms of moderate or severe intensity wax and wane. Of patients who need to be hospitalized, approximately one-third are improved; two-thirds appear to be functioning as well as before hospital treatment. Total disability is a rare outcome of this disorder.

The data for outcome in generalized anxiety disorder must be taken from studies of the previously utilized disorder of anxiety neurosis. Those studies show that approximately one-half of the patients recover or improve greatly at long-term follow-up. Of the remaining 50 percent, symptoms persist in one-quarter, but only 1 in 10 persons is severely impaired as a result.

The anxiety disorders tend overall to have moderate to good outcomes but with intermittent exacerbations. Disability can vary widely but is rarely total. In patients whose anxiety is incapacitating, however, careful clinical attention can be crucial.

The complications, course, and outcome of posttraumatic stress disorders vary depending on the diagnostic subtype. Impairment may be transient; complete recovery may occur in acute reactions, while the chronic disorders by definition are significantly more incapacitating.

Etiology

As with most psychiatric disorders, the precise etiology of anxiety disorders is uncertain. There is a considerable body of evidence, however, that indicates a multifactorial determination of anxiety states. That is, there is evidence of contributions from the biologic, psychological, and environmental spheres, with the ratios varying among individuals. In the biologic sphere, there are considerable data supporting a genetic contribution to many anxiety disorders. There is a great overrepresentation of anxiety states in the children and the original families of probands with anxiety problems, as well as a much higher concordance rate for anxiety states between monozygotic twins and dizygotic twins. The greatest information has been gathered on anxiety neurosis and the panic anxiety states, both of which may have genetic contributions. There is also an overrepresentation of obsessional traits and conditions in the parents of obsessive compulsive patients. The precise inheritance pattern is unclear and must be considered undetermined at this time.

Physiologic differences in patients diagnosed with anxiety disorders have often been reported. Specifically, anxiety patients have been found to overrespond physiologically to standard exercise or stress tests and to respond to infusions of sodium lactate with symptoms indistinguishable from anxiety. This work has been challenged by other authors, and the exact significance remains uncertain. There is also evidence of increased forearm blood flow at rest, increased skin conductance in response to spontaneous fluctuations, and a decreased rate of habituation to stimulation.

More recent studies by Sweeney and associates have proposed that there is an abnormality of central nervous system metabolism of norepinephrine in patients with anxiety states; the locus ceruleus is identified as the primary area of dysfunction. This is an extremely promising area of research, but it is not yet completely explored.

In the interface between biology and psychology, it has been noted that anxiety patients often have had unusually intense reactions to separation in childhood. *Separation anxiety* appears to be a distinct form of anxiety, and panic anxiety has been interpreted as a recurrent form of separation anxiety. Whether this unusual separation anxiety is biologically or psychologically determined is also unclear, but it does appear to be an enduring trait of patients who develop panic disorder. Furthermore, this disorder is often precipitated by a specific type of event—that is, an actual or threatened loss of an important source of support. For example, recent death of a loved one, divorce, and forced geographic separation are overrepresented among the precipitating events in panic anxiety disorder.

Psychological theories of etiology or anxiety disorders have been greatly explored. A behavioral conditioning paradigm that has been suggested for certain phobias pairs the phobic stimulus with an anxiety-inducing stimulus. The anxiety is then transferred to what should be a neutral object or situation. Depth psychology (psychodynamic) studies have suggested that anxiety symptoms result from a conflict between an internal drive and an emotional prohibition against that drive. Specifically, internal impulses of a sexual, hostile, or aggressive nature may trigger repressive reactions within the individual's mind. When these repressive efforts of the person's psyche are only partially successful, anxiety may be a symptom resulting from the conflict between the drive and the prohibition. Presumably this conflict has been established in the individual's early emotional development as a result either of overly strong drives or of excessively strict standards communicated to the person by the parenting individuals. The specific anxiety disorder that develops depends on the age of the affected individual, the impulse which is repressed, and the nature of the prohibition.

Finally, it must be recognized that precipitating events are quite common before the onset of the anxiety disorders. As already noted, separations are particularly involved in the onset of panic disorder, but the loss of a supportive person may trigger any of the various disorders. Other precipitating events are usually of the type of a threatening nature involving some external demand that the individual change himself or herself. This is a broad definition of what is called *stress,* and particularly predisposed individuals may respond with increased and sustained anxiety symptoms. Sometimes the environmental event is one that triggers the internal impulses; the actual precipitant of symptoms is internal but has been set off by the external situation. It must be recognized, however, that the specific precipitating event is often only the last in a chain of events or situations and by itself might not have been adequate to cause the onset of the disorder. In this case, excessive attention to the particular event is unwarranted.

From the discussion above, it should be recognized that the etiology of anxiety disorders is probably multidetermined and interactional; all the major spheres contribute to individual function and adjustment. Correct management, therefore, must assess all three areas—biologic, psychological, and environmental—if the patient is to achieve the best outcome.

Treatment

As in the treatment of any medical disorder, the treatment of an anxiety state begins with the proper approach to the patient. The physician should first, of course, recognize the presence of the anxiety symptoms and appreciate how this anxiety affects the person seeking his or her aid. An anxious patient comes to a physician hoping for relief and seeking someone to give help, but considerable tentativeness and fear of accepting such help is experienced. This stance reflects the patient's feeling of being threatened and vulnerable. The initial approach to the doctor, in fact, may create more anxiety in the patient and make him or her feel worse during the first interview. The clinician, therefore, should proceed slowly and deliberately rather than firing off a series of questions before the patient has an opportunity to tell his or her own story. A restrained, steady professionalism is much more effective than either the cross-examination politely known as a review of systems or the bland reassurance that an anxious person cannot accept anyway. The physician is challenged in effect to establish a relationship of trust and confidence with the patient through his or her conduct rather than by the exertion of power.

An initial attentiveness and communication of interest is very important. The anxious person is often ashamed at having what he or she may recognize as unrealistic fears and consequently may be very sensitive to any slight or sense of rejection. The physician can then proceed to a gradual but thorough exploration of the symptoms, leading the patient to treatment as well as determining the duration and circumstances around the onset of the disorder. Through this process the physician can attempt to rule out other psychiatric or medical disorders that may be associated with the anxiety symptoms. A family history should be explored since this may help with the diagnostic process. The physician should also give careful attention to the possible presence of an alcohol or drug abuse problem, since this may influence the diagnosis or subsequent treatment. It is usually worthwhile to attempt to identify specific precipitating or contributing life events or environmental factors.

DIAGNOSIS AND FORMATION OF TREATMENT PLAN

Once evaluation is under way, the physician should try to conceptualize the relative contributions of biologic, psychological, and environmental factors to the anxiety disorder. The physician should also establish a preliminary diagnosis of the particular type of anxiety disorder identified.

When this stage is completed, a treatment plan can be formulated; the clinician and the patient discuss the therapeutic modalities available for each of the different etiologic factors involved. To begin with, one should never underestimate the value of a stable, supportive doctor-patient relationship. Society invests great power in the role of doctor, and the anxious patient will respond to this if the individual clinician does not interfere. The availability and reliability of the doctor are enormously reassuring and therapeutic, and his or her specific actions are less important than is being there in a predictable way. Planning brief but continuous visits may achieve great relief for the patient. During such visits the patient can be allowed to ventilate feelings about possible precipitating events or simply share his or her symptomatic distress.

If there are specific environmental factors contributing to the anxiety disorder, the physician may help the patient appreciate the significance of these factors and develop ways of avoiding or decreasing the external stress. Encouraging the patient to utilize supportive family members or other close friends or co-workers may be necessary and quite helpful. Some anxious persons are reluctant to acknowledge the significance of their symptoms and tend to push themselves into continuingly stressful situations. The patient should then be encouraged to see that avoidance or alleviation of these stresses is appropriate and therapeutic rather than weak or malingering.

MEDICATIONS

Medications are discussed more fully in Chapter 21, but mention of them will be made here. The benzodiazepines are the current medications of choice for generalized anxiety or mild anxiety symptoms associated with other psychiatric or medical disorders. Despite the current publicity about abuse of certain medications, the overall abuse potential of the benzodiazepines is low, and the vast majority of patients use these medications appropriately. In fact, anxious patients are usually quite reluctant to accept an appropriate medication and tend to undermedicate themselves. The anxiety itself tends to generate excessive fears of addiction, and an informed directiveness can be essential in obtaining adequate patient compliance with such treatment. For fairly mild symptoms of anxiety, intermittent use of the benzodiazepines may be sufficient. If symptoms are more intense and interfere with function, a regular dosage should be prescribed, usually for a week or more; it should be recognized that long-term maintenance medication may be necessary with some patients (long-term in this case may involve several months, although with many patients I have not found it necessary to give benzodiazepines for more than six to eight weeks). The responsible physician will monitor the patient's medication intake and thus avoid unrealistic fears of addiction and lessen the likelihood that the patient will become excessively dependent on the benzodiazepines.

For panic disorders, the benzodiazepines are totally inadequate. While a mild amount of symptomatic relief may be achieved, the basic panic attacks continue unaffected. Individuals with panic anxiety may, in fact, be vulnerable to excessive medication use in an attempt to avoid these devastating experiences.

Over the last 15 years, fortunately, it has been determined that several other medications are extremely effective for panic anxiety states (this treatment is discussed in Chapter 21). The treatment of choice is the tricyclic antidepressant imipramine, which appears to have a beta-adrenergic blocking effect that decreases or inhibits the panic anxiety. Unlike the treatment of depression, the treatment of panic anxiety may require much lower doses (as little as 10 mg orally) several times a day rather than larger doses once a day. Response to treatment may be more rapid in this anxiety disorder, although the more typical one- to two-week period may be necessary. Anxious patients also tend to respond to these medications with overstimulation more often than do depressed patients.

In some cases tricyclic antidepressants other than imipramine may prove effective, although changing to another medication is not usually necessary. Studies have also been done with the use of the monoamine oxidase inhibitor phenelzine (Nardil), and this medication appears to be at least as effective as imipramine. Currently it is a drug of second choice. There have also been studies carried out with the beta-blocking drug propranolol, which appears to block the somatic manifestations of anxiety but is less effective against the subjective fear.

With all of these drugs, once the panic attacks have been adequately controlled, significant residual anxiety (often of an anticipatory type) may persist. The use of a minor tranquilizer or low-dose neuroleptic medication may be necessary to assist with this anxiety. If an agoraphobic pattern has developed, the patient may need reassurance and directive therapy to return to the phobically avoided travel or other avoided situations.

A special situation exists with regard to medication use in alcoholic or previously drug-dependent individuals who are suffering from a serious anxiety disorder. If a patient is still drinking excessively or abusing drugs, it is inappropriate to prescribe any medication; the more fundamental disorder requires attention, which may involve hospitalization. If the patient has stopped abusing alcohol or drugs but is quite anxious, the conscientious physician will avoid prescribing an addictive medication because of the increased risk of drug dependence in such persons. Generally, the use of supportive groups or individuals, including the physician, is preferable to the use of any medication. If anxiety is so intense that the physician believes some medication is necessary, a nonaddictive drug, such as low-dose phenothiazine, appears to be safe and avoids the likelihood of recurrent physical dependence.

PSYCHOLOGICAL THERAPY

The indication for longer-term psychological therapy should be considered in patients with anxiety disorders. While a more complete discussion of psychological therapies is presented in Chapter 20, it should be recognized that these therapies can be quite effective for patients with anxiety disorders, especially when an individual psychological issue or response to an environment situation can be identified.

There are several specific types of psychological therapy that should be considered. Behavior therapy, such as systematic desensitization, is the treatment of choice for individual phobias. Progressive muscle relaxation can be most useful in any of the anxiety disorders, especially those in which muscle tension is a prominent symptom. For individuals with a passive-dependent personality type, assertiveness training may counteract the anxiety reaction in stressful situations. Individual or group dynamic psychotherapy can also be very effective when there are identifiable developmental issues or personality factors that contribute to the patient's serious anxiety. While primary care physicians are not prepared to conduct this therapy themselves, they should recognize that it is available and appropriate to these disorders. If referral to a psychotherapist is considered advisable, it may require considerable reassurance since an anxious patient is usually reluctant to undertake any new experience.

HOSPITALIZATION

It may also prove necessary to consider hospitalization. Treatment in a hospital is rarely necessary for patients with the anxiety disorders described in this chapter. In some panic disorders and those complicated by severe agoraphobia, hospitalization may be necessary simply to reach the patient for a sustained period of time. If alcohol or drug abuse or dependence has developed, hospitalization may prove necessary for detoxification and initiation of the appropriate treatment. Other than in these special situations, however, hospitalization is rarely indicated.

With the above-described approach to management and treatment of the patient with an anxiety disorder, the physician should feel confident that he or she can achieve major symptomatic and functional improvement for this patient.

Case 1. G.R. is a 39-year-old married man seen by his internist for complaints of chest discomfort and tension. His chief complaint was, "I don't like the way I'm feeling and want it to stop." On interview, the patient stated that his illness began approximately five months earlier, when he experienced the sudden onset of severe chest tightness and pain radiating into his left shoulder and arm. He was admitted to the coronary care unit of the local general hospital, where a cardiac evaluation showed no abnormalities. The symptoms recurred intermittently until they increased the following month, leading to a second visit to his internist. The physician did a complete work-up including a cardiac stress test, which again was negative. The patient was put on a weight-reduction diet and sent home.

Within two weeks of stopping his work as a school teacher and football coach for the summer vacation, the symptoms disappeared. In the week before the start of the new school year, the anxiety symptoms recurred with increased frequency and severity. He reported tightness in the chest; arm pain; cold, sweaty extremities; shortness of breath; and subjective feelings of discomfort and fear. The symptoms came to occur almost daily and lasted from minutes to two days. The symptoms were reported to have occurred at any time of the day and under any circumstances. After careful questioning, however, it became apparent that the symptoms tended to occur following some frustration or challenge in the work situation. The patient had become increasingly concerned about his health and was ruminating continually about the possibility of having a severe illness and possibly dying in his sleep. There was no history of a clear-cut panic episode, although anxiety was at times quite severe. The patient denied a feeling of depressed mood, hopelessness, or change in sexual drive or sleep pattern, except that he very occasionally had difficulty falling asleep. Appetite and energy were good. There were no significant changes in the work or family situation, although his job involved long hours and considerable performance pressure. He had been at the same school for 15 years and at precisely the same job for six years.

There was no past psychiatric history and no history of heavy caffeine, alcohol, tobacco, or drug use. There was no family history of psychiatric disorders, but his father had died of an acute myocardial infarction 12 years earlier. Marital adjustment appeared to be quite good, and family relationships with children were excellent. Other life developmental history was unremarkable in any area as far as could be determined. A mental status examination revealed the patient to be within normal limits except for evidence of severe anxiety and tension.

Once this profile was obtained by his internist, the patient was encouraged to talk about his work situation, specifically focusing on those areas that were of greatest concern to him. It appeared that the demands for performance were difficult for him and at the very least exacerbated the symptoms as currently present. It was decided by the patient's physician that these stresses exacerbated but had not caused the anxiety disorder; however, the patient was directed to restrict his work hours somewhat and to delegate more of his duties to the appropriate assistants. He was encouraged to share some of his difficulties with his principal, and the patient did so although reluctantly. The principal turned out to be quite supportive and encouraged the patient to "take it easy" for the next several weeks. The patient was also given oral doses of diazepam, 5 mg three times a day, with good symptomatic relief. The patient was also instructed in deep breathing and muscle relaxation techniques and directed to practice these in the morning and evening daily.

With the above regimen, the patient achieved gradual symptomatic improvement, but several anxiety episodes recurred over the next few weeks. After approximately six weeks of intermittent (but scheduled) visits to his physician, along with utilization of the medication and exercises, the patient was sufficiently recovered to cease regular visits and reported feeling greatly improved. The correct diagnosis in this case appears to be that of generalized anxiety disorder.

Case 2. H.L. is a 48-year-old married woman who was referred to a teaching hospital because of persistent complaints of incapacitating dizziness and fear. The patient had experienced the onset of her symptoms six years earlier, after the death of her mother. She had had similar symptoms for several years in her twenties when she married. Since then the symptoms consisted of sudden attacks of lightheadedness and dizziness, palpitations, rapid breathing, and intense subjective fear. The patient had sought repeated consultation with her local physician and at the emergency room and had been referred for multiple evaluations by an otolaryngologist. The patient had been treated with meclizine (Antivert) for the last several years, with questionable symptomatic benefit. Other repeated medical evaluations, including thyroid function tests, had been within normal limits, but efforts to treat the patient with a variety of antianxiety and antidepressant medications had failed because she complained of massive and intolerable side effects of various types.

The patient had continued in a quite impaired state with progressive loss of ability to travel away from home and function independently because she was afraid of the next symptomatic attack. Her family and husband had tolerated this situation; they accompanied the patient to her place of work and helped with the shopping, until the patient became so frightened that she did not allow her husband even to leave home for his job. Once this occurred, the husband insisted that she be hospitalized for further evaluation and treatment.

In the hospital, a diagnosis of panic anxiety disorder was made and the patient was given oral imipramine, 25 mg four times a day. Initially, the patient protested that this caused her great dizziness and agitation, and the medication was promptly stopped. The patient's functional condition continued to be extremely impaired; she sought constant nursing support even to walk, since she complained constantly of dizziness and fear of falling. After a repeat medical evaluation was within normal limits (including a complete neurologic and otolaryngologic evaluation), the patient was again given imipramine, despite her resistance. Dosage was gradually increased to 50 mg orally, three times a day. After 10 days on this medication regimen, the patient noted the beginning of symptomatic improvement; within four weeks she was free of her symptoms of dizziness and fear of falling. Sessions were held with the patient and her husband to discuss the true nature of her illness and its appropriate treatment.

The patient continued to be quite frightened of traveling or even being left alone. Consequently, a behavioral program was planned that involved graded increases in time alone followed by time at work. With this gradual desensitization to reentering previously avoided situations, the patient became increasingly functional, although she continued to experience some anticipatory anxiety during these periods. At six-month follow-up the patient had regained most, but not all, of her freedom of movement and appeared to be continuing to progress.

The correct diagnosis in this case is agoraphobia with panic anxiety.

Case 3. J.K. is a 67-year-old married man who was admitted to his local general hospital for detoxification from heavy barbiturate addiction—approximately 600 mg of pentobarbital per day. The patient had been dependent on barbiturate medication for nearly 20 years, although at a lower dose, and started using it to help deal with severe anxiety attacks of panic intensity. The patient was quite able to identify the onset and the precise situation around the onset of his anxiety attacks even at this late date. Circumstances around the recent attack were of a totally unstressful type, and it was judged that the environment had made a contribution to the attack. The first attacks started within three months of his mother's death, and he had always been quite close to her. The patient also reported that he had experienced severe anxiety throughout his life when going away from home for prolonged periods, and he had been extremely anxious when he went off to school at age six.

Approximately 20 years earlier, when the anxiety attacks had become quite severe, the patient sought medical treatment. At that time the patient's physician had given him some barbiturate medication, which he had taken intermittently when these attacks occurred. Over the last two years attacks had become more frequent, and the patient had begun to increase his medication intake as well as to combine it with alcohol. His wife was increasingly disturbed at the impairment caused by this combination of medication and alcohol, and she finally induced him to seek further medical help elsewhere. His new general physician recognized the severity of the patient's addiction and the necessity of hospital detoxification. This process was undertaken in the hospital, and psychiatric consultation was sought.

Medical evaluation found the patient to be in excellent physical health despite his chemical dependence; no medical treatment was required other than the detoxification process. As that process proceeded over a period of several weeks, the patient became increasingly agitated over episodic severe anxiety attacks. As he neared completion of his withdrawal schedule, it was determined that he was experiencing a panic anxiety disorder and he was given low doses of imipramine. The medication was increased gradually, and within three weeks the major panic episodes had ceased. The patient, however, complained of continuing lower level, but constant anxiety of a significantly uncomfortable intensity. Because of the patient's previous drug addiction, oral doses of thioridazine (Mellaril), 25 mg three times a day, was begun instead of the more usual benzodiazepine. The combination of imipramine and thioridazine was well tolerated by patient, with major symptomatic relief.

At the time of the patient's hospitalization, he had become so frightened about the possibility of recurrent anxiety attacks that he refused to be left alone at any time. Following discharge, the patient was seen in conjoint therapy with his wife; supportive psychotherapy was used to direct him toward the renewed development of some individual independence. Over a period of several months, the patient gradually came to be able to travel (first with his wife) and then to tolerate being left at home alone for brief periods. Because of his life situation, independent travel was not especially important, and the patient had little motivation to reestablish this ability. His wife, however, found herself able to go about her daily errands and interests without excessive worry felt by her or by the patient.

Over the next two years several efforts were made to help the patient stop using the thioridazine successfully, imipramine was more difficult to discontinue. Each time the latter medication was discontinued, the patient reexperienced severe anxiety attacks, and the imipramine was reinstituted. The patient demonstrated no significant complications from this maintenance medication treatment. Intermittent supportive psychotherapy sessions were scheduled every three months.

The correct diagnosis in this case is agoraphobia with panic disorder, complicated by barbiturate and alcohol abuse and dependence.

References and Further Reading

Agras, S., et al. The epidemiology of common fears and phobia. *Compr. Psychiatry* 10:151–156, 1969.

Benson, H. *The Relaxation Response.* New York: Avon Books, 1975.

Freud, S. On the grounds detaching a particular syndrome from neurosthenia under the description "anxiety neurosis." In *Standard Edition of the Complete Psychological Works of Sigmund Freud,* vol. 3. 1906. Reprint. London: Hogarth Press, 1962, p.90.

Goodwin, D.W., Guze, S. (eds.), *Psychiatric Diagnosis,* 2nd ed. New York: Oxford University Press, 1979.

Klein, D.F. Delineation of two drug responsive anxiety syndromes. *Psychopharmocologia* 5: 397–408, 1964.

Lader, M.H. (ed.), Studies of Anxiety: *British Journal of Psychiatry.* Special Publication No. 3. Ashford, Engl.: Hedley Brother Limited, 1969.

Marks, I.M. The classification of phobic disorders. *Br. J. Psychiatry* 116:377–386, 1970.

Marks, I., and Lader, M. Anxiety states (anxiety neurosis): A review. *J. Nerv. Ment. Dis.* 156: 1–18, 1973.

Noyce, R., Jr., et al. Prognosis of anxiety neurosis. *Arch. Gen. Psychiatry* 37:173–178, 1980.

Quitkin, F.M., et al. Phobic anxiety syndrome complicated by drug dependence and addiction. *Arch. Gen. Psychiatry* 27:159–162, 1972.

Roth, M. The phobic anxiety-depersonalization syndrome. *Proc. R. Soc. Lond.* 52:587–595, 1959.

Wooley, C.F. Where are the diseases of yesteryear? Da Costa's syndrome, soldier's heart, the effort syndrome, neurocirculatory esthenia and the mitral valve prolapse syndrome. *Circulation* 53:749–751, 1956.

Zitrin, C.M., et al. Treatment of agoraphobia with group exposure in vivo and imipramine. *Arch. Gen. Psychiatry* 37:63–72, 1980.

10

Somatoform and Dissociative Disorders
CHARLES SCHWARZBECK III, Ph.D., Ed.M.

Somatoform disorders are a group of mental disorders characterized by physical symptoms that suggest a physical disorder; however, there are no objective organic findings or pathophysiologic mechanisms, and there is positive evidence that the symptoms are probably linked to psychological factors or conflicts, according to the *Diagnostic and Statistical Manual of Mental Disorders,* Third Edition (DSM-III). These disorders, which are not under voluntary control, include somatization disorder, conversion disorder, psychogenic pain disorder, hypochondriasis, and atypical somatoform disorder.

Dissociative disorders are sudden, temporary, reversible alterations in the normal integration of consciousness, identity, or motor behavior. Disturbances in consciousness produce a psychogenic amnesia; in motor behavior, psychogenic fugue results; and changes in identity are manifested either by assumption of a new identity (multiple personality) or by loss of the subjective sense of personal reality and by the presence of a feeling of unreality (depersonalization disorder).

These two diverse groups of disorders, somatoform and dissociative, are covered in one chapter because of their historical association within the category of hysterical disorders. Hysterical disorders were thought to result from psychological conflicts based on early life traumatic memories that have been excluded from consciousness by the defense mechanism of repression. When repression begins to work imperfectly, the conflict may emerge as one of the symptomatic disorders that have been described. This theoretical explanation will be discussed later in the chapter.

Somatoform Disorders
There are three major features of somatoform disorder: (1) the major symptomatology is physical, which implies a physical disorder or medical problem, but there is no objective proof of overt physiologic mechanism underlying the symptoms; (2) the physical symptomatology is likely to be linked to a psychological conflict; and (3) the symptoms are not under voluntary control. The presenting symptoms are, therefore, not willful behavior.

Within the DSM-III system there are five somatoform syndromes: somatization disorder (also called Briquet's syndrome, formerly termed *hysteria*), conversion disorder, psychogenic pain disorder, hypochondriasis, and atypical somatoform disorder.

SPECIFIC SYNDROMES

Somatization Disorder
Patients with somatization disorder have many symptoms that persist or recur. They begin complaining of medical problems as early as the teenage years. Complaints, which are often diffuse, dramatic, or exaggerated, include all medical areas and involve cardiopulmonary difficulties, obstetric and gynecologic symptoms, sexual difficulties, gastrointestinal symptoms, and pseudoneurologic symptoms. In consultation the patient reports a long history of symptomatology and complaints that have caused alteration in daily function, frequent pursuit of medical consultation, or repeated resort to medication. There must have been 12 complaints in men or 14 complaints in women for the diagnosis to be made. Anxiety and depressed mood are frequently associated, and suicidal behavior may occur.

Conversion Disorder
In conversion disorder, which was previously termed *hysterical neurosis, conversion type,* physical funtioning is altered so convincingly that a diagnosis of a physical disorder may be made on initial examination. To diagnose con-

version disorder, the symptoms must not be explicable by a physical disorder or pathophysiologic mechanism. To establish the diagnosis, intensive psychological study must (1) demonstrate a temporal association between the onset of symptomatology and an environmental stimulus, or (2) show that the symptoms allow the patient to avoid an upsetting experience. In many cases there is a strong environmental gain factor in which the patient receives increased support or attention from others because of the symptomatology. The patient classically displays pseudoneurologic symptoms (anesthesias, paresthesias, paralysis, dyskinesia, and altered or defective vision), while less frequently autonomic or endocrine system symptoms, or symptoms having to do with sexuality (such as pseudocyesis, or false pregnancy) are seen.

It is important to remember that there can be an intermixing of organically based and conversion symptomatology; in addition, previously organically generated symptoms may predispose to later conversion symptoms (such as seizure states).

Psychogenic Pain Disorder

In psychogenic pain disorder, the patient reports sensations of pain without adequate physical findings and in association with psychological factors that appear to be etiologically related. The symptomatology relating to the pain is inconsistent with the physician's understanding of neuromuscular and central nervous system function. Usually there is no physiologic mechanism explaining the pain, but when there is, the pain is disproportionate to the injury. Like conversion disorder, psychogenic pain disorder is an expression of psychological conflict; often there is a temporal relationship between a stimulus in the patient's world (or an internal need) and the experience of the pain beginning or increasing. The pain allows the patient to avoid an activity that is conflictual, and the pain experience is therefore externally reinforced.

Hypochondriasis

In hypochondriasis, the patient believes that physical signs or sensations are indicative of serious disease and develops a preoccupation or unrealistic fear of having a serious disease. Such patients are fearful and feel that they cannot rely on medical assurance that they are normal medically. The fear eventually impairs routine function in one or more major areas of life. Hypochondriacal patients are frequently doctor shoppers and often anger practitioners because the disorder prevents the patient from trusting the doctor. Because of the frustrating nature of the complaints and the potential for an almost adversarial quality in the doctor-patient relationship, other truly organic illnesses may be ignored or minimized by family members and physicians. Anxiety and depressed mood are frequently associated features. Paradoxically, when organic disease is present, the patient may actually appear to be less emotionally distressed.

ATYPICAL SOMATOFORM DISORDER

Somatoform disorders that do not meet the criteria for the preceding categories are included in atypical somatoform disorder. An example cited in DSM-III is *dysmorphobia*—an excessive preoccupation with some defect in physical appearance.

DIFFERENTIAL DIAGNOSIS

Follow-up studies have shown that much care must be taken before reaching a diagnostic conclusion that one of the somatoform disorders is present. Studies have shown that there are frequent medical errors with patients who present with what appear to be hysterical symptoms. A study by Slater and Glithero (1965) showed that 22 of 73 patients who were diagnosed as having hysterical disorders were later found to have organic disease that was not detected at hospital admission. The work of Stefansson, Messina, and Meyerowitz (1976) found that 13 percent of patients diagnosed with somatoform disorders were later found to have organic disease, including cancer of the pancreas, brain tumor, and ureteral stone. Similarly, Raskin, Talbott, and Meyerson (1966) found that 14 percent of patients referred with a working diagnosis of conversion reaction had organic pathology either as their main problem or in addition to the conversion reaction. From these studies of hospital patients, it is suggested that between 12 and 30 percent of those who receive the diagnosis of a somatoform disorder have organic illness that has been incorrectly overlooked.

Multiple sclerosis, systemic lupus erythematosus, porphyria, and hyperparathyroidism seem to be special risks for oversight given the multiplicity and anatomic diversity of their presentations.

Somatoform disorders may occur in association with other psychiatric disorders such as schizophrenia, panic anxiety, and depressive disorders. A somatoform disorder should not be diagnosed if the somatic concern is a direct result of a pathologic process integral to the other diagnostic group. Examples might include somatic delusions of schizophrenia or depression with psychotic features.

Dissociative Disorders

The primary characteristic of dissociative disorders is a sudden and temporary change in the mind's ability to integrate the function of consciousness, identity, or motor behavior. Functions that pertain to coordination of affect with thought organization and of cognition with sensory processes are also called *synthetic functions,* and they are crucial to the patient's well-being. When there are abrupt changes in synthetic functioning, the patient's experience of self and others is often distorted while memory or motility may also be changed. With the rapid alteration of cognitive functions, there is usually a limitation of memory—especially with regard to personal happenings. If a change in personal identity occurs, the patient complains of feeling like a different person or of not feeling real. The patient's experience of the surrounding world may be described as disconnected or unreal. Changes in motor behavior are always accompanied by changes in conscious cognitive functioning or identity. This is typically presented as an involuntary behavior involving an alteration of memory or subjective experience around the behavior.

The five dissociative disorders in DSM-III are psychogenic amnesia, psychogenic fugue, multiple personality, depersonalization disorder, and atypical dissociative disorder.

SPECIFIC SYNDROMES

Psychogenic Amnesia

Psychogenic amnesia is characterized by a sudden inability to recall significant personal information in the absence of any organic brain impairment. The loss of recall must exceed ordinary forgetfulness and must not be associated with features of a psychogenic fugue state.

There are three types of memory losses possible with pyschogenic amnesia. (1) In localized or circumscribed amnesia, the most common subgroup, the individual loses recall of all events occurring during a circumscribed period of time after a traumatic, disturbing event (for example, an automobile accident). (2) Selective amnesia is limited in the duration of the amnesia but only involves loss of recall of some, not all, events after a sudden emotional stress. For example, a patient might recall an argument that occurred between her parents, but she might fail to recall sexual violations or physical injuries that took place at exactly the same time. (3) Generalized amnesia is infrequently seen, because stressors that trigger amnesia are specific either to content or to time. In this disorder, memory loss is total and encompasses the individual's entire life up to and including the present.

Unlike patients with psychotic disorders and many organic disturbances, these patients are usually aware that there is a disturbance with recall. There may be a relative indifference to the amnesia despite disorientation, perplexity, or aimless wandering.

Psychogenic Fugue

Psychogenic fugue most frequently takes place after some life-threatening disaster has occurred. Its primary characteristics are the person's sudden departure from the usual home, school, or work site and an assumption of a new identity without memory of the previous identity. Following this occurrence and the individual's return to regular day-to-day functioning and locale, usually within hours to days, there is no recollection of what occurred during the fugue state. This diagnosis is not used when there is an organic mental disorder. Psychogenic fugue differs from the somewhat similar schizophrenic behaviors in that the new identity taken on during this transient dissociative disorder is rarely outlandish and frequently does not annoy other people. The patient often displays rather isolated and seemingly goal-oriented behaviors, rather than the confused and purposeless actions characteristic of severe schizophrenic illnesses. This amnestic disorder can be differentiated from temporal lobe epilepsy, by the facts that in epilepsy the patient does not take on a new identity, emotion is dysphoric in quality, and stress does not always precipitate the epileptic episode. The psychogenic fugue is not a seizure disorder, and there is no brain wave abnormality.

Multiple Personality

In multiple personality, the individual possesses two or more distinct, fully integrated personalities (as documented in the well-known best-sellers *Three Faces of Eve* and *Sybil*). Stress often causes patients to move rapidly between different personalities, and the subpersonalities are usually not recognized by the original personality. These subpersonalities are generally quite distinct in their traits; they often seem quite opposite, and may even have different sexual identities. The personalities may have had an historical connection. Sometimes a patient may report that one of the personalities is unaware of another personality. On other occasions patients report that the different personality states are known to each other. Patients with this disorder usually do not spontaneously state at the time of the episode that they have "lost time"; when the examiner asks about this, however, they answer affirmatively.

This disorder is typically a chronic one, as it exists with greater frequency over a lifetime than is true of the other dissociative disorders. The subpersonalities may carry on internal "conversations" that may be difficult to distinguish from auditory hallucinations.

Depersonalization Disorder

The basic feature of depersonalization disorder is a rapid change in the patient's perception or experience of the self so that the usual sense of one's own reality is disrupted, resulting in impairment of routine daily function. When this disorder occurs, patients may report perceiving changes in their anatomy, feeling like "robots made out of an erector set," and "seeing myself from a distance as though I were looking down from an airplane or dreaming about myself." There patients frequently acknowledge fears of going insane, feelings of dizziness, and a sense of having a tenuous hold on their control of emotions and actions. Even though this disorder is rather dramatic with its rapid onset, reality testing remains essentially intact and the symptoms are experienced as alien. Depersonalization disorder may be accompanied by significant difficulty in memory, sensory anesthesias, transient speech disturbances, or loss of reality of surroundings. The initial onset may be as early as adolescence. Its course is more chronic than that of some other dissociative disorders. Of note is the fact that depersonalization symptoms may accompany major affective disorders, personality disorders, psychotic reactions, and seizure disorders; they also commonly occur in normal individuals (30 to 70 percent of young adults), although without the impairment in function.

Atypical Dissociative Disorder

The dissociative states that do not meet criteria for the previous disorders are included in the residual category of atypical dissociative disorder.

DIFFERENTIAL DIAGNOSIS

The reactions described in this section are often difficult to diagnose because they frequently resemble the appearance of borderline, schizoid, or psychotic disorders. Hallucinations, delusions, and often a progressive deterioration in intellectual processing and functioning are paramount in psychotic disorders, but these rarely exist with dissociative disorders. While patients with dissociative disorders such as amnesia or multiple personality present with bizarre content, the form of thought is not as profoundly disordered as it is in psychotic reactions. Nevertheless, the boundary between hysterical reactions and psychotic illness seems less distinct as we discover that a patient with an underlying hysterical disorder can subsequently develop psychotic pathology.

Many of the symptoms seen in dissociative disorders are found in patients with histrionic personality disorder (see Chapter 13). Diagnostic psychological testing is frequently used to establish the diagnosis. The use of the tests can provide an index of whether medications are indicated and, if so, whether antianxiety (glycerol or benzodiazepine derivatives) or antipsychotic medicines (phenothiazines, butyrophenones, or thioxanthene derivatives) should be prescribed.

It is also quite important to recognize that partial seizure states, usually of temporal lobe origin, can lead to dissociative symptoms indistinguishable from those caused by primary dissociative states. Repeated and special electroencephalographic studies may be required to identify such seizure states.

Etiology of Somatoform and Dissociative Disorders

The precise etiology of somatoform and dissociative disorders is not known. As has been noted previously, however, these disorders have been encompassed within the older concept of hysterical phenomena, which are among the most investigated of all mental disturbances. Beginning in the mid-1800s, Jean-Marie Charcot, Pierre Janet (1907), and Sigmund Freud (1892; 1893; 1896) undertook to demonstrate the psychological basis of hysterical conditions such as amnesias, fugues, paralyses, and anesthesias. Freud eventually emerged with the most comprehensive theory, which remains prominent as an explanatory hypothesis for the disorders in this chapter. Acknowledging that there might be constitutional (that is, physically based) underlying factors, Freud stated that these factors were unknown and went on to examine psychological causes. It was Freud's great contribution to recognize that early life developmental events could predispose towards adult-onset disorders. Freud focused on emotionally traumatic childhood events, primarily those of a sexual nature. Infantile sexual impulses were believed to pose significant problems to the child's personality development. Failure to resolve these problems or conflicts adequately could lead to later vulnerabilities to life events and stresses. Disturbances in core relationships between the child and his or her parents were considered crucial to these developmental failures or arrests. If the disturbances occurred at particular periods in the child's life, there would be a tendency for the child to *repress* the emotional conflict and pain from awareness into the portion of the mind that Freud termed the *unconscious*. Repression would become the dominant psychological defense mechanism (see Chapter 13) in later life as well. When this defensive maneuver broke down under stress in adulthood, various derivative symptoms might appear. Somatoform and dissociative states were the most typical.

Since Freud's work, later theorists have offered many additions and alterations to this hypothesis. It has been recognized, for example, that deprivation of basic security needs and nuturing in the first three years of a child's life may form the basis for some of the more severe forms of the disorders that have been described. Inconsistent mothering and deprivation of key caring persons may produce later disturbances of interpersonal relationships, heightened anxiety levels, and inadequate self-quieting resources. External stresses, thus, prove more threatening and overwhelming in adolescence and adulthood.

The importance of the *cognitive* style associated with many of the preceding disorders has also been noted. Individuals with certain somatoform and dissociative disorders have a characteristically diffuse, global form of thinking, and they have difficulty feeling affection and recognizing detail and cause-and-effect relationships. This difficulty leads them to experience external stresses as overwhelming, inexplicable, and out of control, and it also contributes to repression of memories into unconsciousness. When events are not available for recall and resolution, the person's internal state is more likely to remain in turmoil and various symptoms eventually develop.

Finally, it seems likely that certain family situations might contribute to these disorders. The later development of some somatoform conditions (as well as medical disorders subject to psychological influence, such as asthma) may be encouraged by an anxious mothering figure who is overly attentive to the infant's physical functions and any disturbance of those functions.

Managment and Treatment of Somatoform and Dissociative Disorders

Treatment of somatoform and dissociative disorders can be quite difficult and lengthy, but sometimes dramatic results may occur with brief interventions. War-time experiences have demonstrated that interviews using hypnosis or amytal can lead to swift resolution of dissociative states precipitated by intense stress. Rapid interventions seem able to prevent more chronic impairments in patients with these conditions.

In general, however, the treatment of choice for these patients is insight-oriented psychotherapy, which seeks to assist them in regaining control of the emotions and thought processes made unavailable by repression. Emphasis may be placed on restructuring cognitive processes to improve their ability to integrate memories with present experiences. They must progress to more independent adaptation and coping as well as alter interpersonal relationships toward more consistent, nurtural, less dependent stances. The psychotherapy may often involve sessions several times per week, and the patients may experience intense attachment and have unrealistic expectations. They may be angry when the dependence is noted and alternatives are suggested. The therapist must, however, anticipate such experiences because they are central to the process of emotional growth and change.

Other psychological therapies should not be overlooked either. Family therapy may be quite useful when family dynamics are encouraging or perpetuating the patient's illness (this is especially true for adolescents). Group therapy may also prove beneficial by exposing the patient to a multiplicity of figures from whom he or she can learn different aspects of interpersonal relating. Excessive dependence may be diffused and more direct confrontation of defenses or immature behaviors facilitated.

Pharmacotherapy is usually of secondary importance but may be important in some patients. If manifest anxiety is quite high or dissociative states prolonged, antianxiety medication may give some relief. Benzodiazepines should be used first, but they should be well monitored to prevent abuse. Low doses of neuroleptic medication can be effective for prolonged dissociative conditions if the benzodiazepines are inadequate.

Antidepressants, which are often used when depressive signs and symptoms are prominent, are probably more useful when neurovegetative changes are part of the total clinical picture. There have been special claims made for the monoamine oxidase inhibitors in what has been labeled *hysteroid dysphoria,* which occurs in immature, self-dramatizing, and highly dependent people who may have very high levels of anxiety, including diverse phobic symptomatology. The dysphoria is a mixture of depression and anxiety. Lithium carbonate may also be indicated when dissociative or somatoform disorders occur in association with rapid mood shifts of shorter duration than required for diagnosis of bipolar disorder. These mood shifts may resemble overreactions to external events rather than purely internally caused. Hysteroid dysphoria may, of course, be a variant of cyclothymic disorder but the presentation can be quite different from clear-cut mood swings.

Case 1. R.L. is a 48-year-old married woman who was referred for psychiatric evaluation and subsequent treatment because of persistent difficulty in swallowing. The patient reported a sensation that food (more than liquids) was sticking in her throat and that she might choke (which never occurred). Repeated gastrointestinal evaluations (including barium swallows and esophagoscopy) were normal. On psychiatric interview, it was learned that the patient had experienced the onset of her symptoms in close relation to a visit to her mother's home in a distant city four months earlier. The symptoms had worsened on her return to work. Furthermore, it was learned that R. had experienced gastrointestinal symptoms at various stressful times of her life only to have them subside gradually; some of those symptoms were similar to but milder than the current ones. The patient indicated that she believed her difficulties had a psychological basis although she could not venture even a vague guess as to what it was. Her mood was rather anxious, and she achieved good results on intelligence and reality testing. The patient indicated that she had difficulty trusting others and tended to lead a very isolated existence outside of work, where her performance was excellent.

Over a series of individual interviews it was learned that the patient had had a rather deprived, anxious childhood. Her father had abandoned her mother soon after R.'s birth. The mother had been a critical, demanding woman who put R. in a boarding school for several years starting when R. was four. R. had grown up anticipating criticism, denigration, and the unavailability of help. Any expression of emotion was ridiculed or punished. Assertiveness and displays of anger were not tolerated.

The patient gradually recognized that she had long been enraged with her mother but was either unable or afraid to express it. Her visit home had revived her anger, which could be only partially repressed. On her return to work, R. had encountered problems with an older female supervisor who did not, according to R., recognize R.'s abilities. This supervisor fit closely with R.'s image of her mother, and this problem only aggravated the unresolved and unexpressed fury toward the mother.

Recognition and verbalization of these issues did not at first help R. resolve her swallowing problem (similar to globus hystericus). In fact, R. at first felt more anxious and distressed over her feelings. With several months of continued exploration and connection to other internalized conflicts, R.'s symptoms resolved completely. Interestingly, after her swallowing normalized, R. visited a sister and developed severe nausea during the visit. This, too, resolved through an analogous therapeutic process.

Case 2. V.R. is a 28-year-old white woman who was referred for study following a gynecologic consultation. This mother of two children had recently separated from her husband following a turbulent marriage of seven years. The marriage had been characterized by her husband's gambling, frequent trips out of town, and numerous affairs that were never spoken about directly.

The patient had had a long history of medical involvement with idiopathic headaches as a teenager; irregular menstruation in her late teenage years; difficult pregnancies that required long periods of being restricted to bed; and frequent consultations with specialists in internal medicine and obstetrics and gynecology for numerous symptoms, which initially involved every organ system. Most recently, she had presented with a bloated abdomen and cramping, although her mood and other aspects of overt psychiatric functioning were seemingly unaffected and normal. All diagnostic studies showed no abnormalities.

In consultation, V. showed no remarkable symptomatology, and her mental status examination was essentially normal. She described herself as a "victim" in her marriage, and she explained that she had been a devoted mother and wife but had always been misunderstood by her husband. With some indifference, she jokingly described her physical complaints as "more of the same," and then in a rather cavalier way explained that the examiner need not worry about her. She continued to refer to her physical complaints, however, and discussed the restrictions of mothering as it affected her autonomous functioning, such as continuing her education, pursuing employment, or moving on to a more constructive and positive lifestyle. She recalled "being forced to go out on my own when the children needed me so much" several months earlier, but that she had become overly tired, that she had "problems with my coordination," and "when I heard the doctor might put Petey in the hospital to check him out, I kept getting sick with a lot of vomiting." She added that the physicians in her small town could not agree on what was wrong. By the second interview, a rather flattering and flirtatious style became recognized as the patient characteristically described relationships within a dependency model.

The patient had three older brothers. V. described her mother as a "passive woman who put up with so much from my father . . . even as cute as he was." As she talked about her past, she frequently broke into tears, explaining that she did not know why she felt upset. When an interpretation was made that it had not been safe to compete with her mother and that it sounded as though she were more special to her father than her mother was, she suddenly became saddened and wept again. At this point, there developed a pattern in which she would flatter the examiner only to discredit what had been agreed on moments earlier. When asked about early sexual history, she strikingly described her interest in the examiner's style and then exclaimed that she was "fun-loving. . . and all the men I get mixed up with have sexual problems themselves in the end." Whenever internal upset was considered in consultation, she always referred to her victim status—either with regard to misunderstanding others or in relation to how her short-duration medical symptomatology "paralyzes me."

This patient received the diagnosis of somatization disorder. The medical complaints functioned effectively in keeping this woman's upset "outside" of her. Indeed, she presented with a positive and joking manner; the only exception occurred when an interpretation dealt with the way she used her complaints.

The patient was treated with insight-oriented psychotherapy on a twice-a-week basis for approximately three months. After 23 sessions, it became clear that V.'s complaints, her excessive concern about whether her doctor really cared for her, and her inability to remember material from one appointment to the next were preventing therapeutic gain. Interpretations of resistant strategies only resulted in her introducing new "tragedies" in her life. A recommendation for more intensive and more frequently attended psychotherapy was made so that this woman's overwhelming symptomalogic picture could be kept within bounds. A move to psychoanalysis and emphasis on the transference relationships precipitated a marked depression; she was hospitalized very briefly after a globus hystericus reaction occurred at about the fourth month of treatment. Treatment was pursued four times weekly over a course of 32 months with the patient becoming free of all conversion symptomatology, which she explained was "nothing more than my same old stupid self. . . I just figure out what's wrong inside when it happens now."

References and Further Reading

Freud, S., Breuer, J. On the physical mechanism of hysterical phenomena. 1892. Standard edition, vol. 2, pp. 3–17.

Freud, S. Some points in a comparative study of organic and hysterical paralyses. 1893. *Collected Papers,* vol. 1. New York: Basic Books, pp. 42–58.

Freud, S. Heredity and the aetiology of neurosis. 1896. *Collected Papers,* vol. 1. New York: Basic Books, pp. 143–156.

Freud, S. *Complete Psychological Works of Sigmund Freud.* 24 vols. London: Hogarth Press, 1953.

Greenspan, S.I., Lourie, R.S. Developmental structuralist approach to the classification of adaptive and pathologic personality organizations: Infancy and early childhood. *Am. J. Psychiatry* 138: 725–735, 1981.

Guntrip, H. *Psychoanalytic Theory, Therapy, and the Self.* New York: Basic Books, 1971.

Janet, P. *L'antomatisine psychologique: essai de psycholigie experimental sur les formes inferieures do l'activite humaine.* 1899. From the fourth edition of La societe Pierre Janet and Le laboratorie de psychologie pathologique de la Sorbonne, Paris, 1973.

Janet, P. Psychological treatment of hysteria: Importance of *l'idee fixe.* 1899. In Goshur, C. (ed.), *Documentary History of Psychiatry: A Source Book on Historical Principles.* New York: Philosophical Library, 1967, pp. 883–888.

Janet, P. *The Major Symptoms of Hysteria.* 1907. Reprint. New York: Hafner, 1965.

Janet, P. Psychoanalysis. *J. Abnorm. Psychol.* 9:1–35, 1914–1915.

Klein, D.F. Psychopharmacological treatment and delineation of borderline disorders. In Hartocollis, P. (ed.), *Borderline Personality Disorders.* New York: International Universities Press, 1977, pp. 365–383.

Klein, D.F., David, J.M. *Diagnosis and Drug Treatment of Psychiatric Disorders.* Baltimore: Johns Hopkins University Press, 1969.

Raskin, M., Talbott, J.A., Meyerson, A.T. Diagnosed conversion reactions. *J.A.M.A.* 197: 530–534, 1966.

Schwarzbeck, C. The discharged adolescent patient. *Interaction* 1:43–47, 1979.

Schwarzbeck, C. Identification of infants at risk for child abuse: Observations and inferences in the examination of mother-infant dyad. In Williams, G.J., Money, J. (eds.), *Traumatic Abuse and Neglect of Children at Home.* Baltimore: Johns Hopkins University Press, 1980, pp. 240–246.

Shapiro, D. *Neurotic Styles.* New York: Basic Books, 1965, pp. 108–133.

Slater, E., Glithero, E. Follow-up of patients diagnosed as suffering from "Hysteria." *J. Psychosom. Res.* 9:0–13, 1965.

Stefansson, J.G., Messina, J.A., Meyerowitz, S. Hysterical neurosis, conversion type: clinical and epidemiologic considerations. *Acta Psychiatr. Scand.* 53:119–138, 1976.

Torgerson, S. The oral, obsessive, and hysterical personality syndromes. *Arch. Gen. Psychiatry* 37:1272–1277, 1980.

Psychosexual Disorders
CHERYL T. DUNN, M.D.

This chapter discusses the sexual disorders in which psychological issues are the primary factors contributing to the impairment. Excluded from this chapter are sexual difficulties thought to be primarily or solely of biologic etiology. The *Diagnostic and Statistical Manual of Mental Disorders,* Third Edition (DSM-III) divides the psychosexual disorders into the following four major groups—gender identity disorders, paraphilias, psychosexual dysfunctions, and other psychosexual disorders—which will be further elaborated later in the chapter.

Three clinical aspects of the psychosexual disorders are included in this chapter: the sexual history, classification and diagnosis, and treatment.

The Sexual History

Sexual information can be obtained as part of the presenting complaint or from the later review of systems. All too often, however, this area is abbreviated or omitted entirely because the patient is reluctant to bring it up or because the interviewer is uncomfortable with the subject. A good physician must resolve this personal discomfort first if he or she is to help the patient be at ease and give a meaningful, thorough sexual history. The following is a guide to gathering a sexual history.

Questions about sexual function should be introduced either when the patient alludes to problems in this area or at the interviewer's initiative in the review of genitourinary tract signs and symptoms. Relevant sexual questions can easily follow inquiries about urination or vaginal symptoms. In this manner, one will be asking *natural questions about natural functioning.* The fact that one is addressing this issue as part of the review of systems indicates that it is as legitimate and comfortable a part of the history as is any other part. At this point, it is useful to pause in the interview and give the patient a chance to think about what is probably an emotionally charged subject. If the patient is given a moment of silence to contemplate, one will be more likely to elicit the concerns that are really there instead of an abrupt "No."

When the patient does ask a simple question about sexual information, it should be acknowledged and answered if known. In just a few seconds one may be able to dispel a myth that has probably been the source of considerable anxiety on the patient's part. One should start out by reassuring the patient that there is much misunderstanding about sex and that the particular concern is a common one. One must be certain not to give patients the wrong information; they may carry misinformation given to them for many years before checking it out again. This is true for any area of medicine, but especially so with sex because, until recently, factual knowledge about sex has not been available. If the clinician does not know the answer, he or she should say something like, "That is a good question and I simply don't know [or remember] the answer, let's look it up together," or, "Let me get back to you on our follow-up visit and we can talk about it further." Having a handy desk reference will help, or the question can be answered at a later appointment. Patients do not expect instantaneous answers about sexuality, and they will greatly appreciate candor.

It is also possible that a patient will ask about a more complex problem than a simple informational answer can satisfy. The patient might say, "Well, my wife and I have not had sex for six months and I cannot get an erection. I don't know what to do and I feel terrible about it." This type of question can catch the examiner off guard. It is appropriate to say simply, "Tell me more about the problem." Ask the patient for elaboration, just as one would for any other symptom.

By the time one has discussed the problem to this point, the 20 minutes that have been allotted to the patient for this appointment have been used up, and the interview must end rather abruptly. One does not want the patient to go away upset at being cut off after a painful subject has just been brought up. The process of ending the interview comfortably is made easy with the acknowledgment to the patient that it would be advisable to continue talking further about the problem. This offers the hope that by talking about these issues, new ways of dealing with the problem can emerge.

Two interviewing techniques can help alleviate the patient's anxiety. One is the use of the universal statement, which indicates that the problem is widespread; it lets the patient know that everyone has sexual concerns at times, and these concerns are perfectly natural. Second is the use of reassuring statements, which can give the patient hope that help is available to deal with this problem, and that a resolution can probably be found. Another appointment can be scheduled with the patient at a time when the physician will be able to spend a full session discussing this sexual problem. When the patient returns for follow-up visit, one should take a structured sexual history.

THE STRUCTURED INTERVIEW

The structured sexual history is a set of sequentially related questions. To illustrate, one could assume that the previously mentioned patient is coming back for follow-up visit. Before one can be of further help, more information is needed about him. What is his sexual background? How did sex figure into his childhood, adolescence, young adulthood, and adulthood? How did it develop in his marriage? One can tell him from the outset that these things need to be discussed in order to begin with a clear-cut background of information.

The structured interview may begin in various ways with an open-ended question. For example, "Tell me how you were first introduced to sex in your very young years." Or, "What is your earliest childhood memory having to do with sex? Do you remember when you first became aware of sex?" Proceeding from this kind of question and touching on the major topics throughout the patient's life, the structured interview can help elicit the patient's sexual background. One may use universal statements to help reduce tension throughout the interview; the patient could be asked, for example, "Most children masturbate either alone or with other children. What are your own memories about masturbation as a young child?" "In your adolescent years, when do you remember beginning to date; how much sexual experience did you have before marriage?" Another universal statement may be helpful, "Many men feel guilty about masturbating during marriage; what are your own views about it?"

The interviewer will want to include questions about how the patient's sexual attitudes and behaviors were affected by a variety of influences such as parental attitudes and behavior, religious influence, and experiences with persons of the same sex. For example, this universal statement might be helpful, "Many people have sexual experiences with members of the same sex; how has that been for you?" This a very general, nonthreatening way to show both interest in and acceptance of these matters. Finally, it will be essential to determine if there have been any medical problems that have interfered with sexual activity during the patient's life. High-risk times should be specifically sought out; for example, one should elicit the patient's memories about first intercourse, the first marital experience with sex, the reaction to the birth of the first child, and the first recognition of a sexual problem.

The structured interview should, then, lead naturally to more specific information about the current sexual problem. For example, one will want to ask this patient to describe the onset of the problem specifically, including emotional precipitants, job-related problems, or family changes. The patient must elaborate on exactly what he means by the different words he uses to describe his sexual problem. For example, if the patient says that he has "premature ejaculation," this should be described more precisely. Is the patient saying that he ejaculates before he wishes to or before his partner wishes him to, or does he have some other specific meaning to those words? If the patient says that he has difficulty with erection, is he saying that he has difficulty obtaining an erection or difficulty maintaining it? He should be asked whether this problem occurs only under specific circumstances (such as when he is highly anxious about something else nonsexual), or is related to heavy alcohol consumption or the use of other drugs. One will want to help the patient remember whether he is taking any prescribed medications that might be interfering with his sexual functioning.

With this type of specifically structured interview, the historian will be less likely to miss important information in the patient's life that may well relate to the current problem.

If the patient has a spouse or partner, another session should be scheduled to gather further history in an unstructured interview in which views of both the patient and the partner are clarified. Often important differences are revealed. The interview should begin with a brief summary statement of prior contact and an open-ended statement to set the agenda—for example, "Mrs. Brown, during his last office visit, your husband and I spoke about his concerns over his difficulty maintaining an erection during sexual activity. Today I would like to ask both of you to share your views on this problem." In an informal, unstructured way, the couple can be guided into questions of when the problem began, what precipitants can be identified, what the emotional relationship was like at the onset of this problem, what events relevant to this problem finally brought the patient to the doctor, how are they both feeling about each other, and what the problem is at this time. At the end of this session, or perhaps after another conjoint session to gather more information, the clinician is ready to offer a tentative diagnosis and referral for further diagnostic evaluation or treatment (or both).

Classification and Diagnosis

In DSM-III, the psychosexual disorders are classified into four major groups—the gender identity disorders, the paraphilias, the psychosexual dysfunctions, and other psychosexual disorders. These groups and their subclassifications are listed in Table 11-1.

GENDER IDENTITY DISORDERS
According to John Money (1977), a child has formed an identification with his or her anatomic sex by the age of 12 to 18 months. This identification with anatomic sex, known as

Table 11-1. Classification of Psychosexual Disorders

Gender identity disorders
   Transsexualism
   Gender identity disorder of childhood
   Atypical gender identity disorder
Paraphilias
   Fetishism
   Transvestism
   Zoophilia
   Pedophilia
   Exhibitionism
   Voyeurism
   Sexual masochism
   Sexual sadism
   Atypical paraphilia
Psychosexual dysfunctions
   Inhibited sexual desire
   Inhibited sexual excitement
   Inhibited female orgasm
   Inhibited male orgasm
   Premature ejaculation
   Functional dyspareunia
   Functional vaginismus
   Atypical psychosexual dysfunction
Other psychosexual disorders
   Ego-dystonic homosexuality
   Psychosexual disorder not elsewhere classified

Table 11-2. Diagnostic Criteria for Transsexualism

A. Sense of discomfort and inappropriate about one's anatomic sex.
B. Wish to be rid of one's own genitals and live as a member of the other sex.
C. The disturbance has been continuous (but not limited to periods of stress) for at least two years.
D. Absence of physical intersex or genetic abnormality.
E. Not due to another mental disorder, such as schizophrenia.

Reproduced with permission from *Diagnostic and Statistical Manual of Mental Disorders,* 3rd ed. Washington, D.C.: American Psychiatric Association, 1980, pp. 263–264.

gender identity, is the individual's own subjective sense of his or her anatomic sex. If a man, with male genitalia, experiences himself as a male, then diagnostically he is said to have a normal gender identity. A gender identity disorder, according to DSM-III, is diagnosed when the individual feels very strongly that his sexual anatomy is wrong. For example, if a man with male anatomic genitalia experiences himself as a female and wishes to change his male sexual characteristics, he is diagnosed as having transsexualism. The diagnostic criteria for transsexualism are presented in Table 11-2.

No exact statistics are known but an estimated 10,000 transsexuals live in the United States (Feinbloom, 1976). Approximately 2,000 of this group have had sex-conversion surgery. Most of the people who are transsexuals are physiologically and chromosomally normal. Of those who undergo sex-conversion surgery, the vast majority consider themselves heterosexual in orientation postoperatively.

The other major disorder in this category, gender identity disorder of childhood, has basically the same criteria with an onset prior to puberty. In children, this disorder is accompanied by behavior, dress, speech, and play patterns of the opposite sex. *Gender role* is the term applied to such manifestations of one's gender identity.

PARAPHILIA

Paraphilia refers to a disorder in which sexual arousal is dependent on an act or fantasy other than one involving a consenting partner of the opposite sex. The pathognomonic aspect is that an unusual stimulus is necessary for sexual excitement.

Paraphilias may be benign or malicious and dangerous. The DSM-III defines a number of them (which are listed in Table 11-1); the most common ones are fetishism, transvestism, pedophilia, exhibitionism, sexual masochism, and sexual sadism. These behaviors may feel comfortable or distressing to the individual, as well as to the partner. In some cases the individual may be apprehended by the law and face serious consequences.

The paraphilia most often identified in psychiatric practice is probably transvestism. In this disorder, sexual arousal is achieved when the person dresses in clothing normally worn by members of the opposite sex. Those affected are nearly always male and usually have a primarily heterosexual orientation other than the transvestism. The diagnostic criteria for transvestism are presented in Table 11-3.

PSYCHOSEXUAL DYSFUNCTION

Psychosexual dysfunctions represent psychological inhibitions of normal sexual response and are widely prevalent disorders. These disorders must be understood within the framework of normal psychosexual function, which has two aspects: (1) sexual desire and (2) the

Table 11-3. Diagnostic Criteria for Transvestism

A. Recurrent and persistent cross-dressing by a heterosexual male.
B. Use of cross-dressing for the purpose of sexual excitement, at least initially in the course of the disorder.
C. Intense frustration when the cross-dressing is interfered with.
D. Does not meet the criteria for transsexualism.

Reproduced with permission from DSM-III, p. 270.

Table 11-4. Primary Changes During Physiologic States of Sexual Response

	Excitement	Plateau	Orgasm	Resolution
Men	Erection Scrotal-testicular retraction	Heightening of sexual tension with continued enlargement and retraction of structures	Rhythmic contractions of penis and urethra Ejaculation	Loss of erection Return to normal size and position of structures Refractory period (variable)
Women	Vaginal lubrication Clitoral swelling Labia and breasts engorge Vagina expands Uterus pulls up and back	Formation of orgasmic platform Clitoris retracts under hood Labia minora deepen in color and signify impending orgasm	Rhythmic contractions of orgasmic platform Contractions of uterus	Disengorgement and return to normal position of clitoris, nipples, labia, orgasmic platform, and uterus No refractory period Continued stimulation can result in multiple orgasms

Abstracted from W.H. Masters and V.E. Johnson, *Human Sexual Response.* Boston: Little, Brown, 1966.

sexual response cycle, a set of distinct physiologic occurrences. Through the work of William Masters and Virginia Johnson the human sexual response was first researched, identified, and delineated. They provided the foundation, as well as the impetus, for contemporary understanding of human sexuality and sex therapy. Masters began his extraordinary pioneering work in sexual physiology 30 years ago, in St. Louis, Missouri, two years before the death of Kinsey.

Masters and Johnson divided the sexual response into the four phases of excitement, plateau, orgasm, and resolution (the DSM-III description of the four phases of sexual response has evolved from the work of Masters and Johnson). The mediators of these changes were described primarily as increased blood flow (vasocongestion) and secondarily as increased muscle tension (myotonia). Male and female sexual responses are analogous but differ in detail. In the male, the excitement phase includes erection and scrotal-testicular retraction. In the plateau phase, sexual tension is heightened and tissue blood flow increased; structures enlarge and retract. Orgasm involves rhythmic contractions of penis and urethra, followed by ejaculation. In the resolution phase, the erection is lost, the structures return to normal size and position, and there occurs a refractory period during which the male is not sexually arousable (see Table 11-4).

In women, the excitement phase involves vaginal lubrication and clitoral swelling analogous to erection in the male. The labia and breasts engorge, the vagina expands, and the uterus pulls up and back. The plateau phase is characterized by the swelling of the outer area of the vagina, forming the orgasmic platform; the clitoris retracts under its hood; and the labia minora deepen in color, which signifies impending orgasm within the next 60 to 90 seconds. In orgasm, rhythmic muscular contractions of the orgasmic platform occur from three to 12 times or more; the uterus contracts simultaneously. Resolution is characterized by immediate disengorgement and return to normal position of clitoris, nipples, labia, orgasmic platform, vagina, and uterus. There is no refractory period, and continued stimulation can produce multiple orgasms in the female.

The DSM-III retains a description of sexual response in terms of four phases. However, it characterizes the first phase as the appetitive stage, and their version of the excitement stage combines Masters and Johnson's first two stages, excitement and plateau.

Thus the DSM-III four-phase cycle includes the following: (1) The appetitive phase includes the stage of desire to experience sexual arousal, and the fantasies about it. (2) The excitement phase begins with a sense of heightening sexual tension. In men, erection and scrotal-testicular retraction occur. In women, vaginal lubrication occurs, accompanied by clitoral swelling, swelling of the other sexual organs, and formation of the orgasmic platform, as well as lengthening and widening of the inner two-thirds of the vagina. (3) The orgasm phase is experienced by men as the rhythmic contractions of the penis and the urethra as well as ejaculation. Women experience orgasm as rhythmic contraction of the orgasmic platform and of the uterus (there is usually not subjective awareness of the latter). (4) The resolution phase consists of a general sense of relaxation and feeling of well-being. In men the erection is lost and the structures return to their normal size and position; a refractory period occurs during which the man is not able to achieve another orgasm. In women, disengorgement occurs and the sexual organs and the orgasmic platform return to their normal position. There is no refractory period in women, and continued stimulation may result in multiple orgasms.

The dysfunctional physiologic responses can be inferred from the normal ones. At any point in the four phases of the human sexual response, an impairment may occur (a given individual may experience more than one impairment). The impairments specifically described in the DSM-III are inhibited sexual desire, inhibited sexual excitement, inhibited female orgasm, inhibited male orgasm, premature ejaculation, functional dyspareunia, functional vaginismus, and atypical psychosexual dysfunction (this category is for dysfunctions that have not been included in the other specific diagnoses). The specific DSM-III criteria for each of the psychosexual dysfunctions are listed in Tables 11-5 through 11-11.

Table 11-5. Diagnostic Criteria for Inhibited Sexual Desire

A. Persistent and pervasive inhibition of sexual desire. The judgment of inhibition is made by the clinician's taking into account factors that affect sexual desire such as age, sex, health, intensity and frequency of sexual desire, and the context of the individual's life. In actual practice this diagnosis will rarely be made unless the lack of desire is a source of distress to either the individual or his or her partner. Frequently this category will be used in conjunction with one or more of the other psychosexual dysfunction categories.

B. The disturbance is not caused exclusively by organic factors (e.g., physical disorder or medication) and is not due to another axis I disorder.

Reproduced with permission from DSM-III, pp. 278–279.

Table 11-6. Diagnostic Criteria for Inhibited Sexual Excitement

A. Recurrent and persistent inhibition of sexual excitement during sexual activity, manifested by:

In males, partial or complete failure to attain or maintain erection until completion of the sexual act, or

In females, partial or complete failure to attain or maintain the lubrication-swelling response of sexual excitement until completion of the sexual act.

B. A clinical judgment that the individual engages in sexual activity that is adequate in focus, intensity, and duration.

C. The disturbance is not caused exclusively by organic factors (e.g., physical disorder or medication) and is not due to another axis I disorder.

Reproduced with permission from DSM-III, p. 279.

Table 11-7. Diagnostic Criteria for Inhibited Female Orgasm

A. Recurrent and persistent inhibition of the female orgasm as manifested by a delay in or absence of orgasm following a normal sexual excitement phase during sexual activity that is judged by the clinician to be adequate in focus, intensity, and duration. The same individual may also meet the criteria for inhibited sexual excitement if at other times there is a problem with the excitement phase of sexual activity. In such cases both categories of psychosexual dysfunction should be noted.

Some women are able to experience orgasm during noncoital clitoral stimulation, but are unable to experience it during coitus in the absence of manual clitoral stimulation. There is evidence to suggest that in some instances this represents a pathological inhibition that justifies this diagnosis whereas in other instances it represents a normal variation of female sexual response. This difficult judgment is assisted by a thorough sexual evaluation, which may even require a trial of treatment.

B. The disturbance is not caused exclusively by organic factors (e.g., physical disorder or medication) and is not due to another axis I disorder.

Reproduced with permission from DSM-III, p. 279.

Table 11-8. Diagnostic Criteria for Inhibited Male Orgasm

A. Recurrent and persistent inhibition of the male orgasm as manifested by a delay in or absence of ejaculation following an adequate phase of sexual excitement. The same individual may also meet the criteria for inhibited sexual excitement if at other times there is a problem with the excitement phase of sexual activity. In such cases both categories of psychosexual dysfunction should be noted.

B. The disturbance is not caused exclusively by organic factors (e.g., physical disorder or medication) and is not due to another axis I disorder.

Reproduced with permission from DSM-III, p. 280.

Table 11-9. Diagnostic Criteria for Premature Ejaculation

A. Ejaculation occurs before the individual wishes it, because of recurrent and persistent absence of reasonable voluntary control of ejaculation and orgasm during sexual activity. The judgment of "reasonable control" is made by the clinician's taking into account factors that affect duration of the excitement phase, such as age, novelty of the sexual partner, and the frequency and duration of coitus.

B. The disturbance is not due to another axis I disorder.

Reproduced with permission from DSM-III, p. 280.

Table 11-10. Diagnostic Criteria for Functional Dyspareunia

A. Coitus is associated with recurrent and persistent genital pain, in either the male or the female.

B. The disturbance is not caused exclusively by a physical disorder, and is not due to lack of lubrication, functional vaginismus, or another axis I disorder.

Reproduced with permission from DSM-III, p. 280.

Table 11-11. Diagnostic Criteria for Functional Vaginismus

A. There is a history of recurrent and persistent involuntary spasm of the musculature of the outer third of the vagina that interferes with coitus.

B. The disturbance is not caused exclusively by a physical disorder, and is not due to another axis I disorder.

Reproduced with permission from DSM-III, p. 280.

Etiology

As with almost all of the psychosexual disorders, there are many etiologic theories about psychosexual dysfunction, but they are primarily divided into the psychoanalytic and the behavioral.

Psychoanalytic theory emphasizes the origin of psychosexual disorders in childhood sexual conflicts. Although quite complicated, analytic theory focuses on unresolved childhood sexual attraction toward the parent of the opposite sex; this attraction has been forbidden by the conscience and repressed into the unconscious mind. There the conflict (wish-inhibition) continues to operate at times of expected sexual arousal, interfering partially or totally.

Behavioral theorists might point more to heightened anxiety experienced during early sexual experiences. The anxiety becomes linked with arousal and thereafter impairs normal sexual response.

Kaplan (1974) best reconciles these polar views by arguing for combined effects of both remote and immediate experience and learning in creating adult psychosexual disorders. She presents a multicausal philosophy in which relative importance of different causative factors varies from patient to patient. Before treatment, the clinician can attempt to assess these factors by interview, history, and psychological testing. On the other hand, the significance of intrapsychic resistances and transference may become evident only when treatment has begun, activating older issues (treatment is discussed later in the chapter).

OTHER PSYCHOSEXUAL DISORDERS
While homosexuality itself is not considered a mental disorder, it may in some persons be associated with enough anxiety that a psychiatric disturbance is diagnosable. Judd Marmor (1971), an expert in the study of homosexuality, defines a person with a homosexual orientation as "one who is motivated in adult life by a definite preferential erotic attraction to the same sex, and who usually (but not necessarily) engages in overt relations with them." Sexual orientation refers to overt behavior, to fantasy life, or to both areas. Anxiety can relate to either of these factors. In other words, a person who has not exhibited homosexual behavior but who has a predominantly homosexual fantasy life can experience as much anxiety as a person who engages in overt homosexual relationships. It is only in the individual who has a persistent and marked concern about changing sexual orientation that the diagnosis of ego-dystonic homosexuality is made.

The most important element in the diagnosis of ego-dystonic homosexuality (Table 11-12) is the presence of a homosexual orientation for a continuing period of time, usually over the space of years, as opposed to a brief period precipitated by a specific situation. In addition, these individuals wish to achieve sexual arousal heterosexually but are unable to do so and thus do not pursue active heterosexual relationships. People with ego-dystonic homosexuality have strongly negative and disturbing feelings about their homosexual orientation and behavior. At times the homosexual arousal has been so negatively experienced that it has been relegated to the fantasy life only and not to overt relationships.

Table 11-12. Diagnostic Criteria for Ego-Dystonic Homosexuality

A. The individual complains that heterosexual arousal is persistently absent or weak and significantly interferes with initiating or maintaining wanted heterosexual relationships.
B. There is a sustained pattern of homosexual arousal that the individual explicitly states has been unwanted and a persistent source of distress.

Reproduced with permission from DSM-III, p. 282.

The incidence of ego-dystonic homosexuality is not known for either males or females. However, the task force on homosexuality set up by the National Institutes of Health has estimated that about 4 percent of white, college-educated adult males are predominantly homosexual and that approximately 1 to 2 percent of the total adult female population are predominantly homosexual (Livingood, 1972). It is not known what proportion of either of these groups would be categorized as ego-dystonic in their homosexual orientation.

Etiology
There is very little published work that discusses the distinctions between *homosexuality*, which is not a disorder, and *ego-dystonic homosexuality*, which is categorized as a psychosexual disorder. Investigators have primarily focused on the understanding of homosexual behavior and its development. Theories abound as to the development of homosexuality, and definitive statements cannot yet be made.

Briefly, some data support the notion of a hormonal basis for homosexuality; a number of sex steroids, such as testosterone, continue to be researched. It seems clear that there are many patients whose sexual interests and activity are highly influenced by hormones, and controlled studies with a larger population of patients are needed. At least one genetic study provides evidence of a very high concordance rate of homosexuality in monozygotic male twins.

Psychological theories of homosexuality have had many adherents. Freudian theory postulates that each individual carries a basic bisexual potential and that normal development leads to heterosexuality; homosexuality reveals a fixation or impairment in the usual maturational process, although everyone is thought to have latent homosexual feelings. Part of the theory describes homosexuality as an expression of unconscious conflict resulting in marked self-preoccupation; within this preoccupation a male may be looking for a love object symbolizing himself. In addition, the development of castration anxiety may produce the fear and avoidance of heterosexual relationships. Within Freudian theory there are multiple and complex psychodynamic mechanisms postulated.

Other psychological theories concern family dynamics. There has been a widespread general clinical impression that homosexual males have a history of an unusually close relationship with the mother and a distant relationship with the father. However, there are no definitive data to establish causation or even clarify the contribution of these relationships to the development of sexual orientation. It is clear that many males experience this kind of parental relationship without developing a homosexual orientation, and the distinguishing factors between the two groups have not been delineated.

The behavioralists use learning theory to explain homosexuality. According to learning theory, a person's behavior is progressively shaped by the environment, which supplies rewards and punishments. Homosexuality is viewed as a learned response—a behavioral pattern that may be strengthened or weakened by the factors that affect learning in general.

Many investigators have tried to study personality traits, neuroticism, and character of dyadic relationships, as well as functional disability in homosexuals as compared with heterosexuals. At this time, two conclusions can be drawn from the literature: (1) the similarities between homosexuals and heterosexuals are much greater than the differences, and (2) a large percentage of adult homosexual males show significant female-oriented behaviors by the preadolescent years. These behaviors include strong relationships with girls in preadolescence, an aversion to males, dislike of aggressive boys' games, and fondness for doll play, as well as a preference for girls' dress and female roles in games.

Treatment

TREATMENT OF TRANSSEXUALISM
There is no known cure for transsexualism. Psychoanalysis and other forms of psychotherapy were the only treatments available until the 1950s. Since that time, sex reassignment has become another approach; it is considered a rehabilitation process, not a "cure," and the entire process takes several years. The usual assessment involves a sweeping psychiatric evaluation with corroborative data from the family; the primary goal of assessment is to confirm the patient's long-standing conviction of having the wrong anatomic sex and his or her utter commitment to sex reassignment. There are no other diagnostic tests for confirmation. Other major disorders may be ruled out, but even if any are present, they may not be a contraindication for surgery.

According to John Money (1977), the most important presurgical procedure is the "real life test"—a two-year period of time in which the patient lives as a member of the opposite sex in every conceivable aspect of life short of surgery. An anatomic male, for example, would dress as a woman publicly and at work, as well as privately and socially. He would undergo demasculinizing procedures, such as hormonal treatment and beard electrolysis. He would spend the two years approximating, as closely as possible, the experience of being a woman, and he would be monitored psychiatrically over this period of time.

If the sex reassignment surgery is agreed on, then a variety of surgical procedures are possible. Postoperative follow-up care must be quite comprehensive for a successful outcome.

These unusual procedures in the rehabilitation of the transsexual have made possible the alleviation of great suffering in the person who feels himself or herself imprisoned in the wrong body. The treatment remains controversial, however, and its final place in the therapeutic approach is unsettled.

A number of group studies have been reported in the treatment of gender identity problems. One study by Green and Fuller (1973) is particularly noteworthy; that study focused on young boys, defined as "feminine boys," who had such attributes as dressing in women's clothes, fantasizing interest in girls' activities (such as "playing house"), displaying feminine gestures, and at times expressing the wish to be a girl. A treatment program was designed for these boys and their families. The fathers of these boys were treated in one group, and the mothers were treated together in another group. The boys were positively reinforced for male behavior and negatively reinforced, with a comment, for each feminine gesture. Each parents' group dealt with common feelings, hope for change, and ways of encouraging and discouraging feminine behavior, as well as didactic information about normal development. The therapists examined outcome, which showed reduction in feminine behaviors; long-term outcome is pending.

TREATMENT OF PARAPHILIAS

Most data about treatment of paraphilias relate to therapy for affected individuals whose sexual behavior has resulted in legal difficulties. It is not known how applicable the experience is for other people with similar difficulties.

Aversive Techniques

Aversive conditioning is a behavioral technique that shows increasing success in altering behavior such as fetishism, exhibitionism, and pedophilia; this technique has also been used to help homosexuals who are uncomfortable with their sexual preference. The patient or the therapist administers an unpleasant stimulus, such as a bearable but uncomfortable electric shock. In one model the stimulus is presented at the same time as a representation of an undesirable behavior. For example, a fetishistic man who wishes to change his sexual preference is presented with a picture of the fetish object; at the same moment, the picture is paired with a shock. In another technique, the shock would be administered only when the patient began to experience sexual arousal.

Aversion relief is another procedure in which the undesired behavior and the aversive stimulus are presented together; they are both terminated when the desired sexual behavior is presented. For example, in treatment of a pedophile, the child figure and the shock would be presented together and both would be stopped when an adult figure was presented.

Clearly, with these kinds of procedures, the benefit must outweigh the pain caused by the undesirable sexual behavior, as well as the discomfort of the procedure itself. The choice would be that of the informed patient.

Group Therapy

Group therapy has been used for many different types of sexual problems in the past two decades. Imprisoned sex offenders have been treated in groups when individual therapy was not available. Pedophiles have participated in groups with the goal of controlling or sublimating sexual impulses. Outpatient groups have been used in treatment of exhibitionists to help them become aware of feelings (such as low self-esteem) that preceded the impulse to exhibit themselves. Lectures and other didactic techniques have also been used in these groups to help patients deal with feelings around the interpersonal aspects of sex.

Group therapists for sex offenders have worked with both homogeneous and heterogeneous groups in dealing with exhibitionists, pedophiles, and assaultive sexual offenders, as well as with homosexuals who wish therapy. The group atmosphere was uniformly characterized as one of cohesion and support for a common goal. Group members were highly effective in confronting each other's denial as well as in promoting openness, problem-solving attitudes, and the positive value of changing behavior.

Follow-up studies of these groups have revealed fewer problems and fewer subsequent arrests for antisocial behavior than occurs in untreated comparison groups.

TREATMENT OF PSYCHOSEXUAL DISORDERS
There are basically four main approaches to the treatment of the other sexual disorders: (1) psychodynamic psychotherapy; (2) behavior modification; (3) the combination approach of Masters and Johnson and derivative schools, which uses psychotherapeutic and behavioral techniques together; and (4) group therapy.

Psychodynamic Psychotherapy
In psychodynamic psychotherapy, the presenting symptoms are considered to result from an underlying personality disturbance that needs to be dealt with through insight, an understanding of defenses, and active reflection on past traumatic experiences. (For a discussion of individual psychotherapy, see Chapter 20.)

Behavior Modification
In behavior modification, the presenting problems are considered learned behaviors that can be modified by direct relearning or retraining. Behavioral techniques include systematic desensitization and aversion techniques.

Systematic desensitization, a major behavioral tool used in sex therapy, is based on the idea that one overcomes a fear by approaching it on a step-by-step basis in an anxiety-free atmosphere. Anxiety is decreased through the use of a *specific sequential process*. The fearful event is clarified, a set of steps is established from the least to the most anxiety-provoking, and the patient is then taught a method of learning to relax. During the procedure the patient first enters into a state of relaxation and then is exposed to the least anxiety-provoking event in the hierarchy, then to the next step, and then the next, and so on. Each step in the hierarchy is added only when it can be accomplished without an increase in the patient's anxiety. If anywhere along the way the patient becomes anxious, then the process is stopped and the patient returns to a state of relaxation again before proceeding.

In 1958, Wolpe demonstrated success with this procedure for male patients with premature ejaculation or difficulties with erection. Patients were encouraged to carry out the hierarchical techniques with their partners, progressing to the next step only when they were free of anxiety. Most of the behavioral techniques or exercises used today are based on this model.

Combination Therapies
Masters and Johnson developed a blend of psychotherapy and behavior modification; many other sex therapy programs grew as derivatives or modifications of their basic ideas. In Masters and Johnson's original treatment program, therapy consisted of a 14-day period. Each couple worked with one male and one female therapist who helped them as a team. Detailed histories were taken in individual sessions, and a medical history and examination were performed. Then "round-table discussions" among the four people were used as a format for providing information and correcting misunderstandings. After the problems were clarified, sensate-focus exercises were assigned in which the couple was asked not to have intercourse, but rather to spend time touching and stroking each other and to communicate what experiences were pleasurable. The object was to shift the focus from performance to pleasure. Daily discussions followed in which the problem-specific strategies were

discussed. In this manner the therapy progressed until the specific dysfunction was resolved.

The unique feature of Masters and Johnson's therapeutic approach is the use of sensate focus in addition to specific strategies. The purpose of sensate focus is to change the goal of sexual encounter from orgasmic performance to sensual erotic pleasure, which provides a way of decreasing inhibiting anxiety around performance. When sexual contact becomes enjoyable, then specific strategies are employed to correct the individual dysfunction.

Many variations on this treatment model are found in the literature. The complexity of time scheduling in individual practice, the demands of clinic scheduling, and the cost of a two-therapist team are just a few of the considerations that influence the treatment contract. Helen Singer Kaplan (1974) describes success with a traditional appointment schedule, with sessions once a week or several times a week. Sometimes an agreement is made calling for a certain number of sessions, and other times the therapy is continued until the problem is resolved. Some therapists will work only with the couple; some will work with the symptomatic person alone.

Much controversy surrounds the prescription for a male-female team. Masters and Johnson feel that it is important to have such a team providing treatment; in their view it leads to the dilution of transference issues and the seeming ease and speed with which rapport can be established between each therapist and the marital partner of the same sex. Kaplan (1974) points out that no outcome studies have analyzed this factor and that two therapists per session double the cost of the therapy. She describes suggestions used in her clinic for dealing with problems that arise from the use of a single therapist and offers the flexible option of a therapist team if this becomes an issue that interferes with the therapy.

The therapist may perform the physical examination for the patients, refer the patient for examination, or require examination only if the history reveals possible medical problems. This brings up the issue of the background of the therapist. It has not been established whether it is essential that one member of the team be a medical doctor to conduct successful therapy, and it is uncertain what the background training should be.

Finally, after sensate focus is accomplished, the strategies for the specific problems are chosen, but the choice may differ to some extent depending on the therapist. For example, Masters and Johnson use the "squeeze" method to treat premature ejaculation; in this method, the wife squeezes the penis when the husband signals impending ejaculation. Kaplan recommends the start-stop technique, in which the woman manually stimulates the man's penis until he signals an impending orgasm. Then she stops until he signals return of control; with practice, the man becomes aware of the sensation of "inevitability" and is gradually able to exert control over ejaculation. After extravaginal ejaculatory control is mastered, then the start-stop procedure is employed during intercourse, with the man controlling the woman's thrusting. Finally the start-stop technique is practiced with the man thrusting and controlling his own orgasm. This procedure is highly effective up to 98 percent of the time in teaching control of ejaculation.

The exact curative strategies for other sexual dysfunctions have not been completely defined; thus they vary depending on the therapist and the nature of the patient's problem. The paradigm of sensate focus plus specific strategy has had great acceptance in the treatment of psychosexual dysfunction.

This form of sex therapy has been shaped by psychotherapy and behavior modification. Traditional dynamically oriented psychotherapeutic treatment of sexual disorders has aimed at the resolution of intrapsychic and marital conflicts through the medium of talking, within the doctor-patient relationship; therapy is confined to the doctor's office. Traditional behavior modification treatment of sexual disorders has focused on isolated symptoms using desensitization and relaxation techniques.

For many years, therapists felt that sexual problems were always a sign of psychopathology. Today the view has changed; sexual difficulty can be an isolated symptom as well as a more global psychiatric one. In either case, sex therapy alone can frequently yield immediate improvement in sexual dysfunctions. Kaplan (1974) conceptualizes sex therapy as a specialized form of treatment that integrates psychotherapy and behavior modification. It is this integration that she labels "the new sex therapy." More analytical psychotherapy is used in Kaplan's treatment approach only when specific issues become so conflictual that they obstruct symptom-oriented work.

Group Therapy

A group model of sex therapy is reported by Lonnie Barbach (1975) in the treatment of women who have not experienced orgasm. Barbach's premise is that a woman can and should take as much responsibility for her own sexual pleasure as possible, and that, in fact, most women can teach themselves to reach orgasm. Barbach describes several unique aspects of her program; she worked with women only (as opposed to couples), in a group situation, in which a combination of therapeutic techniques, in a low-cost, brief treatment program—10 sessions, each 90 minutes long, over the space of five weeks. Briefly, each group included five to seven women, ages 18 to 58, with two women serving as leaders. The treatment program involved group sessions with discussions of sexual anxiety; in addition, members agreed to do one hour of homework per day, including a step-by-step masturbation program. Physiologic information about female anatomy and sexuality was also discussed. Individual instruction was given under certain circumstances.

Barbach's outcome statistics are striking. A group of several hundred women had participated in the group over the years. The women either had never experienced orgasm or were erratic in performance. At the end of five weeks, 93 percent of these women were experiencing orgasm consistently with self-stimulation. Within three months, more than 50 percent were experiencing orgasm with partners.

The reported success rates of the various sexual therapies are impressive. Most studies using a combination of psychotherapeutic techniques plus specific behavioral strategies report rates of substantial alleviation that are far greater than those of traditional individual psychotherapy alone. Human sexuality is now being understood as a natural function. Treatment of sexual dysfunction is available in an increasing number of modalities. Progress in this area has led to the clinician's ability to decrease anxiety and impairment as well as increase sexual responsiveness and pleasure.

TREATMENT OF EGO-DYSTONIC HOMOSEXUALITY

There continues to be great variability of opinion as to the preferred treatment of ego-dystonic homosexuality. Individual, long-term dynamic psychotherapy was and may remain the most frequently used technique. Outcome statistics are conflicting and results, therefore, are uncertain.

Aversive behavioral therapy and aversion relief have also been employed; the homosexual fantasy or image forms the undesired stimulus to be conditioned away. The long-term outcome and adjustment are unknown.

Homosexuality has been treated with significant success through group therapy. Some groups are explicitly run with the goal of preference reversal. These groups include an exploration of early life experiences that shaped sexual behavior as well as specific group exercises meant to examine interpersonal feelings. Other therapy groups seek to treat maladaptive thought and feeling patterns in the individual members.

Bibliography

Barbach, L.G. *For Yourself: The Fulfillment of Female Sexuality.* New York: Doubleday, 1975.

Feinbloom, D.H. *Transvestites and Transsexuals.* New York: Delacorte/S. Lawrence, 1976.

Fischer, J. *Handbook of Behavior Therapy with Sexual Problems.* New York: Pergamon Press, 1977.

Green, R. *Sexual Identity Conflict in Children and Adults.* New York: Basic Books, 1974.

Kaplan, H.S. *The New Sex Therapy.* New York: Brunner/Mazel, 1974.

Livingood, J.M. *Task Force on Homosexuality.* National Institutes of Health. Washington D.C.: Government Printing Office, 1972.

Marmor, J. Homosexuality in males. *Psychiatr. Ann.* 1(4):45–59, 1971.

Masters, W.H., Johnson, V.E. *Human Sexual Response.* Boston: Little, Brown, 1966.

Masters, W.H., Johnson, V.E. *Human Sexual Inadequacy.* Boston: Little, Brown, 1970.

Money, J.W. *Handbook of Sexology.* Amsterdam: Elsevier/North Holland Biomedical Press, 1977.

12

Psychological Factors Affecting Physical Condition

JESSE RUBIN, M.D.

An estimated 50 to 80 percent of all visits to physicians are prompted by stress-related symptoms. A relatively small percentage of patients with such symptoms are treated by psychiatrists; most medical care for psychological factors affecting physical condition (PFAPC) is supplied by family doctors, internists, pediatricians, gynecologists, and general surgeons. It is important, then, for all primary-care physicians to understand how psychological factors impinge on health, which physical illnesses are likely to have an emotional component, and what forms of treatment are available when PFAPC is diagnosed.

No specific disorder or group of disorders is characterized by PFAPC. Rather, according to the *Diagnostic and Statistical Manual of Mental Disorders,* Third Edition (DSM-III) the diagnosis is used when "psychologically meaningful environmental stimuli are temporally related to the initiation or exacerbation of a physical condition;...[when] the physical condition has either demonstrable organic pathology...or a known pathophysiological process;...[and when] the condition is not due to a Somatoform Disorder." (See Table 12-1.)

The situations that in DSM-III are called "psychologically meaningful environmental

Table 12-1. Diagnostic Criteria for Psychological Factors Affecting Physical Condition

A. Psychologically meaningful environmental stimuli are temporally related to the initiation or exacerbation of a physical condition (recorded on axis III).
B. The physical condition has either demonstrable organic pathology (e.g., rheumatoid arthritis) or a known pathophysiological process (e.g., migraine headache, vomiting).
C. The condition is not due to a somatoform disorder.

Reproduced with permission from *Diagnostic and Statistical Manual of Mental Disorders,* 3rd ed. Washington, D.C.: American Psychiatric Association, 1980, pp. 303–304.

stimuli" include important interpersonal transactions, such as loss of a loved one or persistent conflict at home or at work. DSM-III also notes that the full emotional impact, or meaning, of the stimuli are often not apparent to the patient and may even be entirely out of his or her awareness.

The diagnosis of PFAPC is not, in the strictest sense, a medical one. Rather, it should be considered a notation in the patient's chart that serves to alert the treating physician, consultants, and future physicians that the patient's emotional state affects the course of his or her illness and needs to be taken into account when formulating treatment plans. Inadequate attention to psychological factors invites treatment failure, medical and surgical complications, and chronicity of illness.

While any illness may have psychological components, certain specific conditions are particularly responsive to stress. These conditions, the presence of any one of which should alert the physician to the possibility of PFAPC, include the "classic seven" illnesses investigated by Franz Alexander and his associates (1968)—bronchial asthma, rheumatoid arthritis, ulcerative colitis, essential hypertension, peptic ulcer, neurodermatitis, and thyrotoxicosis. Other stress-responsive syndromes are obesity, tension headache, migraine headache, angina pectoris, painful menstruation, sacroiliac pain, acne, tachycardia, arrhythmia, cardiospasm, pylorospasm, nausea and vomiting, regional enteritis, and frequency of micturition. In addition, psychological factors may be important in patients who, regardless of the specific presenting illness, (1) have high levels of recent life-change events, including interpersonal loss, (2) possess certain personality traits or profiles, (3) have severely strained psychological defense mechanisms, (4) have a history of important recent alterations in lifestyle or behavior, or (5) have inadequate family and social support systems.

In this chapter, we will briefly trace the history of psychosomatic theory in order to provide a framework for understanding patients in whom psychological factors are important. Current concepts about stress, life change, and illness will then be reviewed. Finally, diagnostic issues and treatment strategies will be discussed.

Theories About Psychosomatic Illness
A number of theoretical models have been developed in the last 60 years to explain how personality type and emotional conflict contribute to the initiation of illness. Each of these attempts to bridge the gap between emotional stress and physical response. While none is universally correct, each helps our understanding and treatment in some individual patients.

SYMBOLIC REPRESENTATION MODEL
During the 1920s, Groddeck said that emotional state is identical to physical state because both derive from the same deep "vital force." Therefore, physical illness directly and symbolically expresses emotional conflict, and there is no basic difference between psychological and physical disease. Groddeck described, for example, the symbolism inherent in an accidental fall and leg fracture. He referred to the act of falling as a symbol of being childlike and unable to stand up for oneself, while the bedridden convalescence was a symbolic expression for the wish to retreat from life.

PERSONALITY PROFILE MODEL
Flanders Dunbar, writing in the 1930s and 1940s, concluded that each psychosomatic illness is due to a specific kind of defective personality organization. She believed, for example, that patients with hypertension experience chronic rage and an inordinate need to be liked. Such patients have a life-long conflict in the area of relationship to authority and sensitivity to criticism. They feel that criticism is unjust, but they will not do anything about it for fear of provoking dislike.

Each specific defective personality type leads to a final common pathway of poor integration between mind and body, resulting in the dissipation of energy, which is then no longer available to maintain health. Her concept of dissipation of energy foreshadowed current thinking about inadequacy of psychological defenses as central to the development of psychosomatic conditions (this concept is discussed more fully in the following section).

The personality profile approach was followed by Friedman and Rosenman, who wrote in 1974 that people predisposed to coronary artery disease possess a specific personality, which they labeled *type A*. They described the type A personality as "Any person who is aggressively involved in a chronic, incessant struggle to achieve more and more in less and less time, and is required to do so, against the opposing efforts of other things or other persons.... Persons possessing this pattern also are quite prone to exhibit a free floating but extraordinarily well rationalized hostility....For Type A behavior pattern to explode into being, the environmental challenge must always serve as the fuse." Type A personality has been implicated in the development of coronary artery disease generally, as well as in fatal heart attacks in particular.

Bahnson has used the personality profile method to characterize patients at risk for cancer. He states that the cancer patient has experienced disappointment, loss, and despair in his or her parental relationship, leading to mistrust and hostility in adult interpersonal relationships. Such persons, according to Bahnson, develop a personality marked by self-containment, inhibition, rigidity, repression, and regression (see Case 4).

SPECIFICITY MODEL
From 1932 until 1968, Franz Alexander and his associates (1968) postulated the following

sequence for the seven illnesses (mentioned earlier) that they studied:

> Predisposing emotional conflict (specific and unresolved), called the "central nuclear conflict" + constitutional factors + specific life stress events ⟶ specific psychosomatic illness. For example, in thyrotoxicosis, the presumed sequence is: Precocious and conflicted self-sufficiency and a need to care for others + (unknown) constitutional factors + blocking of capacity to care for others by life events ⟶ thyrotoxicosis.

REGRESSIVE INNERVATION MODEL
Margolin, Grinker, and (more recently) Reiser hypothesized that psychological stress nonspecifically contributes to the development of physical illness by inducing a regression to infantile, poorly regulated autonomic nervous system discharge.

Stress, Life Change, and Illness

The four models that have been described assume that psychological factors are important chiefly in the etiology of a few well-defined illnesses. Another, more recent, psychosomatic approach looks at how stress and the individual's defenses against it affect health in general. (While stress has been used to denote both adverse environmental stimuli and also the bodily responses they induce, we will use stress as a collective term that includes both stimulus and response.) Selye's work in the early 1950s emphasized the nonspecific nature both of environmental stressors and of the stress response. Selye believed that the body's response to *any* environmental stress consisted of three stages: alarm, resistance, and exhaustion.

A number of studies have confirmed that severe, general environmental stress has this nonspecific effect on health. For example, Reiser quoted one study in Wales showing that the mortality rate for recently bereaved persons was 700 percent higher during the year after the loss of a close relative than that of a control group. During a major flood in Bristol, there was a 50 percent higher mortality rate among people whose homes had been flooded than in those who had no such disaster. In London, patients with the diagnosis of tuberculosis reported significantly more life stress than did a control group.

Holmes and Rahe and co-workers, in attempting to quantify the relationship between life stress and illness, have focused on the stressful effects of change of any sort on health. Their central thesis is that any life change, good or bad, involves stress. They developed an empirically derived life-change scale, in which life events are rated for degree of stressfulness. The major life-change stressor is the death of a spouse, which is rated at 100 points; other life changes are scaled down from that anchor point. Marriage, for example, is rated at 50 points; retirement, 45 points; trouble with one's boss, 23 points; and vacation, 13 points. The higher the score of life-change events within a given period of time, the higher the vulnerability to illness (see Cases 1–3). Subsequent studies have born out this general relationship between life change and illness. However, as Rahe points out, this is an epidemiologic, statistical relationship and does not necessarily hold for any given individual.

PSYCHOLOGICAL DEFENSES AND STRESS
DSM-III notes that it is not simply the number and severity of changes but rather "the meaning ascribed to (them) by the individual" that contributes to illness. Selye's initial general formulation of stress has been refined; we now know that the same stress will have different meanings and therefore induce different specific reaction patterns in different individuals. For example, Rahe and co-workers studied serum levels of uric acid, cholesterol, and cortisol in men undergoing training for Navy underwater demolition work. The results indicated that periods of training involving stress and novelty correlated with elevation of serum cortisol; elevations of serum uric acid tended to

occur when the subjects were eagerly and confidently preparing to take on new, challenging, and often physically complicated activities; and cholesterol was elevated when individuals felt overburdened and nearly overwhelmed. In these experiments, physiologic reactions were specific both in terms of the meaning ascribed to the stress and also in terms of the response profile.

In a similar experiment, Rubin found a difference in cortisol and urinary MHPG levels during aircraft carrier landing training as between pilots (who were active) and radar intercept officers (who were passive) during the experience. Miller subjected yoked (that is, wired together) teams of rats to an electric shock, but allowed one rat (the "executive" rat) to press a lever that would avoid a shock. On postmortem examination, he found that the executive rats had less gastrointestinal ulceration than the passive rats. However, when the executive rats had to take a shock in order to turn off a longer train of shocks (a situation more comparable to the pilots in Rubin's study), then the executive rats had more stomach lesions. Miller states, "Apparently, in a simple situation, it is a great advantage to be in an executive position, but in a conflict-inducing one, it can be a great disadvantage." That is, insofar as one can cope, one can avoid serious stress reactions. But when a stimulus implies an overwhelming threat or conflict, vulnerability to pathology increases.

The meaning of a stressor is a direct function of the adequacy of the psychological defense mechanisms it evokes (see the discussion of ego defenses in Chapter 13). Defense mechanisms (or simply defenses) are "unconscious intrapsychic processes serving to provide relief from emotional conflict and anxiety" (*A Psychiatric Glossary*, 5th ed., Washington, D.C.: American Psychiatric Association, 1980). When these defenses are adequate, stressors by and large will not cause somatic problems. As Rahe puts it, "Certain defense mechanisms appear capable of 'defracting away' the impact of life change events."

Adequacy of Psychological Defenses

A number of studies have focused on intactness of psychological defenses as a specific indicator of resistance to stressors. For example, parents whose children had leukemia but who used strong psychological defenses (such as denial, repression, intellectualization, and isolation) showed less adrenal response to the stress of their children's illness than those who had weaker defense mechanisms. Stein and coworkers (1976) showed that husbands whose wives were dying of cancer but who had adequate psychological defense mechanisms, including being able to express and share grief, showed less impairment of the immune systems during and after their wives' death than did those judged to be using less adequate defenses. J. Rubin measured esophageal motility in healthy young adults during psychiatric interviews and found that nonperistaltic (spastic) esophageal activity occurred within the interview when defensive mechanisms were inadequate.

Defensive Inadequacy

One class of stress—loss—and one type of defensive inadequacy—giving up and given up—have been singled out by Engel (1954) and Schmale as uniquely predisposing to illness. Schmale feels that loss predisposes to illness by precipitating the *giving up/given up syndrome,* which (as summarized by Kimball) consists of: (1) a feeling of helplessness and hopelessness; (2) a sense of inadequacy; (3) a feeling of impoverishment of relationships; (4) a diminished sense of the future; (5) a preoccupation with the past; and (6) a perception of the present environment as alien and lacking in guidelines for behavior (see Cases 2–4).

Sifneos (1973) used the term *alexithymic* to describe another type of defensive inadequacy. Alexithymia means "unable to read feelings"—that is, an inability (1) to sense feelings (affects); (2) to describe the psychologic accompaniment of feelings; and (3) to communicate feelings (see Case 5).

Reiser feels a breakdown of psychological defenses is one of the essential steps leading to psychosomatic illness. According to Reiser, illness develops in three stages: In step 1, a perception of external danger interacts with nonspecific physiologic mobilization to produce a breakdown of defenses and psychological alarm. This leads to excessive nonspecific psychoneuroendocrine mobilization and an altered condition of the central nervous system. In step 2, there occur altered levels of consciousness and also altered central nervous circuitry, which leads to step 3, changes in visceral function. The third stage then combines with other necessary factors, such as genetic predisposition, exposure to allergens, and other precipitants, and produces activation of disease.

Minuchin extends the idea of defensive inadequacy from the individual to the family. He writes that psychosomatic illness (especially anorexia nervosa) evolves from a family characterized by enmeshment (lack of boundaries), overprotectiveness, rigidity, and lack of conflict resolution. When, through therapy, the family develops adequate defense systems, the index patient improves.

STRESS, THE BRAIN, AND THE BODY
What events in the brain correspond to the mental perception of stress? Miller's experiments with rats indicate that when they can cope with a stress, they have higher levels of norepinephrine in the brain than when they are in a hopeless situation. Miller postulates the following alternative chain of events: (1) stress ⟶ coping ⟶ increased brain norepinephrine ⟶ decreased brain dopamine ⟶ decreased steroids ⟶ fewer gastric ulcerations. This is in contrast with: (2) stress ⟶ noncoping ⟶ decreased brain norepinephrine ⟶ release of brain dopamine ⟶ increased steroids ⟶ increased gastric ulcerations. Similarly, Antelman and Caggiula present evidence that "behavioral responses to stress involve the activity of brain catecholamine and, particularly, dopamine-containing systems, and their interaction with other neurotransmitter systems such as norepinephrine and serotonin." They hypothesize that the nigrostriatal system is the most important dopamine system involved in acute behavioral responses to stress, and that "the mesolimbic dopamine system, with its connections to the limbic forebrain areas traditionally linked to emotional and motivational functions, may ...regulate the degree to which particular emotions gain ascendancy and compel the individual's attention...and [may] reflect the effects of prolonged stress."

Brain and Body
We will focus on four of the many feedback systems between the brain and the rest of the body: the voluntary nervous system, the autonomic nervous system, the endocrine system, and the immune system.

Voluntary Nervous System. This is the fast feedback and feed-forward brain-body connection (Mayfield) and is significantly involved in many psychosomatic illnesses. For example, chronic spasm of the striated musculature is a major component of most chronic pain syndromes.

Autonomic Nervous System. This is the intermediate-speed (moderately slow) brain-body feedback system. Simple autonomic reactions like blushing with shame, tachycardia and sweating with anxiety, and urgency of micturition with excitement all indicate the intimate connection between the autonomic nervous system and the emotions. Autonomic imbalance is prominent in such illnesses as asthma and pylorospasm.

Neuroendocrine System. During the past decade, attention has focused on the neuroendocrine system as a key area in psychosomatic relationships. Because the neuroendocrine system is a slow feedback system, its integrity is essential for long-term health. Reiser, for example, states, "Effective ego defenses may protect against sudden endocrine activation; or increased endocrine activity may come into play when ego defenses are inadequate or failing."

As currently understood, the final common neuroendocrine pathway is through the hypothalamus, which secretes releasing and inhibiting factors that influence secretion of pituitary hormones. Some of these factors have direct effects on nonendocrine organs (examples are prolactin and melanocyte-stimulating hormone), but most, in turn, influence other endocrine organs, including the thyroid, primary sexual organs, and adrenal gland, which in turn influence the brain and mind. Persky found that "when cortisol, corticosteroids and placebo were each administered intravenously to the same subjects in a balanced design, the order of anxiety enhancement was as follows: corticosterone > cortisol > placebo." Persky also noted that those glucocorticoid substances generally tend to be mood elevating while the mineralocorticoids tend to produce dysphoria. Neuroendocrine responses, particularly ones involving the adrenal glands, influence reactivity to antigens, resistance to infection, and virtually all other regulatory networks.

Immunologic System. Keller, Stein, and associates showed that lesions of the anterior hypothalamus suppress humoral and cell-mediated immune responses. The effects of grieving on the immunologic system have already been noted. Weiner (1977) reviewed evidence for the involvement of the immune system in such diseases as allergic rhinitis, bronchial asthma, eczema, thyroid disease, rheumatoid arthritis, and ulcerative colitis. The tendency to form the antibodies involved in these illnesses is largely inherited, and whether their formation is augmented or diminished by environmental factors is as yet unclear; however, these conditions are all stress-reactive.

Biologic Rhythms
All of the feedback systems that have been described are subject to ultradian, circadian, and longer rhythmic patterns, so that environmental stimuli will have different impacts at different times. The stability of some of these rhythms (sleep cycles and patterns of rapid eye movement, or REM) has been shown to have a direct effect on depression in man. Since depression and the giving up/given up syndrome are related, biologic rhythmic activity is inferred to have an effect on resistance to illness.

DIFFERENTIAL DIAGNOSIS
DSM-III states, "This category [PFAPC] should not be used for conversion disorders, which are regarded as disturbances in which the specific pathophysiological process involved in the disorder is not demonstrable by existing standard laboratory procedures and which are conceptualized with psychological constructs only" (see Table 12-1). In dramatic forms of conversion disorder, such as hysterical blindness or limb paralysis, the differential diagnosis is clear. Conversion disorders typically occur in patients with a high level of emotionality and fluctuating dramatic affective response. While the classic attitude of *la belle indifference* in conversion is rare, its presence will help establish that diagnosis. The basic aspect of the differential diagnosis is that a discrete physical illness *must* be present in patients with PFAPC, while patients with conversion reactions by definition do not have such diagnoses or phenomena.

The differentiation between PFAPC and hypochondria or psychogenic pain may be difficult. Clinical electromyographic techniques, for example, have demonstrated the presence of muscle spasm in many patients whose pain was considered psychogenic. In addition, while hypochondriacal patients often recite a long list of symptoms and are typically complaining, hostile, and demanding, a careful examination will sometimes uncover a chronic physical condition exacerbated by psychological factors. Still, by definition, PFAPC depends on positive evidence of a physical illness; in the absence of such evidence, one must resort to one of these other diagnoses.

Chronic factitious disorder with physical symptoms (CFDPS; also known as Münchausen syndrome) may initially present as PFAPC, and the two may be indistinguishable for a time. The differential diagnosis depends on an initial suspicion (and later confirmation) that physical illness in CFDPS is compulsively self-induced and lacks apparent motive. The diagnosis of CFDPS is suggested by the patient's repeated dramatic presentation of apparently severe and critical illness, along with a lengthy medical and surgical record. CFDPS is a very rare condition, while PFAPC is common.

In malingering, there is an obvious, conscious, noncompulsive gain hoped for from physical complaints.

Material presented in preceding sections of this chapter should alert the physician to those clinical situations in which PFAPC needs to be considered. Such situations include patients with any of the following:

1. One of the seven classic psychosomatic diseases (see p. 175; Weiner estimates that 50 percent of patients with these illnesses fit Alexander's specificity model)
2. Type A personality
3. A high Holmes-Rahe score
4. Alexithymia, the giving up/given up syndrome, or other evidence of defensive strain, especially in the absence of adequate family and social support systems
5. A recent change of habitual life-style behaviors (such as eating, drinking, sleeping, and drug-taking)

TREATMENT

The purpose of noting PFAPC is to alert the physician to the treatment strategies available. Whatever treatments are instituted, they must be directed toward keeping patients in an *active* role in their illness. They must keep as their long-term goal the achievement of mastery over their lives. Physical and emotional passivity are to be tolerated only insofar as the patients' physical condition absolutely requires it. To induce this active state in patients (and their families), physicians must communicate a willingness to work with the patients actively over long periods. Physicians must also optimistically communicate the fact that there are a number of treatments available, and that they are willing to try any or all of them in an appropriate sequence.

Placebos

Administering a placebo means inducing in patients an act of faith that they will get better. A necessary, but not sufficient, condition of successful placebo therapy is that physicians themselves believe that they can help the patients, and that the patients have some power to heal themselves. In placebo therapy, the physician and patient agree on an approach toward healing; the nature of the approach is irrelevant so long as (1) they are honest with each other and (2) the therapy will do no harm. Some placebo therapies are the optimistic administration of medication; education, which can involve imparting one's positive experiences in treating similar patients; frequent induction of laughter; and mobilization of religious faith. Disingenuous administration of an inert substitute for another medication is contraindicated and represents a poor clinical approach.

*Behavioral Change
and Behavioral Techniques*

Therapeutic behavioral change flows from the uncovering of recent pathogenic behavior patterns. For example, patients can be simply counseled to return to regular living habits after the death of a spouse. This advice may help them fend off infections at a time when their immune system is weak. There are also complex techniques available for specific illnesses—for example, Fordyce described the use of behavioral modification techniques in the treatment of pain, and Ferster outlined behavioral schedules in the treatment of obesity. It must be kept in mind that behavioral instruction, however simple or sophisticated, will be followed only to the extent that the relationship between the physician and the patient is a supportive one.

Reinforcement of the Social Network
The physician should support and guide the patient's family. Time spent with them may be as important as time spent with the patient.

Psychotherapeutic Techniques
At the simplest level, all physicians should be capable of offering supportive psychotherapy to their patients. All that is involved is listening and generating useful, common-sense advice. If a patient with a physical illness has had a high frequency of major recent life changes, just allowing the patient to ventilate his or her feelings about them will help.

Intensive psychotherapy, particularly psychoanalytic therapy, is curative in many patients with psychosomatic illness if those patients are adequately verbal (see Case 5). Alexithymia can be reversed and the patient "reconnected" to his affective state. Careful psychoanalysis of faulty, strained defense mechanisms leads to the gradual disappearance of psychosomatic illness, which is usually replaced by neurotic symptoms. These symptoms in turn are responsive to further analytic intervention.

Klagsburn has reported that group therapy resulted in prolongation of life and improvement of its quality in women with cancer. He attributed these results to mutual support, encouragement of patients to be active and to take responsibility for their treatment, and expression of their rage at having the illness.

Medication
If a specific intercurrent psychiatric diagnosis (in addition to PFAPC) is made, appropriate psychotropic medications should be given in a patient with physical illness unless there is a contraindication. In the absence of a specific concomitant psychiatric diagnosis, drug therapy is sometimes useful but must be approached empirically.

A trial of either benzodiazepines or tricyclic antidepressants may be considered even in the absence of symptomatic anxiety or depression. If benzodiazepines are tried, they should be given in doses similar to those required for control of moderate anxiety, and they should be prescribed on a regular basis for at least four weeks. Before beginning a trial of benzodiazepine, the patient should be evaluated to assess his or her potential for addiction. After a trial, benzodiazepines must be discontinued slowly over a period of weeks or months. Too sudden a discontinuance may lead to withdrawal symptoms, anxiety, and exacerbation of physical illness. Trials of tricyclic antidepressants (Cases 4 and 6) also involve the use of full therapeutic doses for one month. With these agents, addiction is not a problem, but one must be sensitive to drug interactions and potential toxicity. Failure of treatment with either of these drugs may be related to inadequate trial or patient noncompliance. Lithium, antipsychotic medications, and monoamine oxidase inhibitors are not useful in patients with PFAPC unless there are other specific psychiatric indications.

Autoregulatory Techniques
The autoregulatory techniques can powerfully, although slowly, help to reestablish healthy psychological regulation in the face of pathophysiology. There are a number of autoregulatory techniques available, all of which can be augmented by biofeedback instrumentation. Each technique produces one or more of the following: deep muscle relaxation, autonomic balance, and altered mind/brain states.

Deep Muscle Relaxation. In the 1920s, Jacobson introduced progressive relaxation (or self-operations control), which consists of instructing the patient to lie supine, assume a passive attitude, and progressively focus on relaxing each muscle group in the body. Jacobson's techniques have been used successfully in a number of psychosomatic syndromes.

Autonomic Balance. After becoming skilled at progressive relaxation, the patient can be taught autonomic balance. The most reliable system for achieving this is autogenic therapy. In this treatment, the patient repeats to himself or herself, on a prescribed schedule, a standard set of *autogenic phrases* (such as, "My arms are heavy," "My legs and arms are warm," "My breathing is regular"). Once these are mastered (usually within two to six months), the patient experiences an *organismic shift* into a relaxed, light autohypnotic state. The therapist then prescribes additional, individually tailored phrases for the patient's use (for example, "My chest is warm" for asthma).

Altered Mind/Brain State. When muscle relaxation and autonomic balance are achieved, a number of autoregulatory techniques lead to altered, deeply relaxed mental states. Techniques for achieving this include transcendental meditation, yoga, open focus (Fehmi), repeated prayer, mind-body expansion (Shealy), and autogenic meditation and neutralization (Luthe). Any of these techniques can be combined with mental imagery (Simonton).

Biofeedback. Biofeedback instrumentation is a useful adjunct to the autoregulatory therapies. Biofeedback instruments show patients that they are able to achieve control of their muscles and circulation before they have any such proprioceptive and enteroceptive experience.

In order for autoregulatory therapies to succeed, they must be prescribed in sufficient dosage and for a long enough time. For some patients, they must be practiced initially as often as 12 times a day, 10 to 20 minutes at a time, for six weeks (Shealy). Usually, four to six times a day for two months is adequate initially. The initial intensity can be tapered off slowly. Because autoregulatory therapies work slowly, interpersonal support and biofeedback instrumentation can help with patient compliance.

Case 1. M.W. is a 36-year-old man with acute symptoms of bleeding ulcer. His past history was significant in that he had always been excessively dependent on his mother and on his wife, a somewhat hysterical and immature woman 12 years his junior. Just prior to the onset of M.'s illness, his wife had had a psychotic episode in which she threatened to harm their children and revealed that she had been having an extramarital affair. On psychiatric and psychological evaluation, M. appeared to be shut in, rigid, bitter, and overtly angry, as well as intolerant of his own impulses and feelings. Collaboratively the psychiatrist and internist were supportive of the patient in his attempts to deal with his wife, to be effective with his children during his wife's illness, and to find other family and friends who would be helpful to him. His ulcer symptoms diminished considerably and were of only minor importance for approximately six years, when his mother died suddenly. At that time M. again had active ulcer disease. He returned to psychotherapy where he dealt extensively with his relationship to his mother and to her death, his wife's recurrent threats to leave him, and his phobia about cancer. Psychotropic medicine was not used.

Case 2. J.B. is a 21-year-old man admitted to the hospital with an acute flare-up of lupus erythematosus of eight years' standing. Just prior to admission, J. underwent several life stresses, including the pregnancy of his girlfriend (which resulted in a hurried marriage) and an inability to carry on with work that was appropriate to his level of technical training. Two days prior to admission, he began acting strangely and praying excessively. While the history was difficult to take, there was some question of his ingesting up to three times his prescribed dose of steroids. He became confused, erratic, and disorganized. On admission, he was withdrawn, made inappropriate responses, and had difficulty with recent memory.

In reconstructing the events leading up to his hospitalization, the following was important: he had been taking too large a dose of steroids because he thought he would not be able to perform at his job and he had prematurely taken on the responsibility of fatherhood and marriage. These factors led to a defensive breakdown, which in turn increased his panic and multiplied the pressure he was living under. At that time a physical setback occurred and lupus flared up, manifested by joint severe inflammation. Treatment in this case was relatively successful through a combination of psychological, physical, and environmental manipulations. Adjustment of the steroid level led to remission of the memory loss, which had probably been due to a toxic state. Work with J.'s wife and parents has led to better a structure of his personal life and the alleviation of financial pressures. He has also been able to return to his technical training.

Case 3. H.N. is a 20-year-old college student. At the age of 16, at a time when he had to make several important decisions concerning his relationship with his parents, H. developed mild ulcerative colitis. A second, moderately severe bout a year later seemed related to an operative procedure and to difficulty in his studies. A third, very severe bout, occurred when H. returned home after his first year of college, when he was in conflict over sexual feelings and thought his parents would reject him because of this. He was admitted to the hospital in poor condition, but he improved significantly after a few psychiatric interviews and changes in his medication.

After his discharge from the hospital, H. was seen in psychotherapy, first once a week, then every other week. Treatment was marked by depression centering about fears of failure at school. The patient returned to college and suffered a transient episode of depersonalization. After another year of psychotherapy both his physical health and his psychological condition were relatively good. His management was marked by good cooperation of the attending physician, the consulting gastroenterologist, and the psychiatrist.

Case 4. V.L., a 24-year-old woman, has been diagnosed as having Hodgkin's disease. She became preoccupied with the thought that the Hodgkin's disease was God's punishment for an abortion she had had about a year before the disease was diagnosed. She did well for two years, when radiation therapy was prescribed. While she was undergoing the first treatment, she had a panic attack and refused further treatment. The refusal to continue with radiation therapy led to psychiatric consultation.

Since her family had been supportive in the past, they were called to help in this situation. In addition, in psychotherapy, she began to understand her sense of helplessness and powerlessness both in general and specifically when alone in the room with the radiation equipment, and she was able to face further treatment. The treatment led to a remission of the disease. However, anxiety became more pervasive in her life and threatened her capacity to function. She increased the intensity of psychotherapy and began exploring the connections between her feeling of having been deserted as a child, with repressed strong rage, and her current need to isolate herself and not develop strong sexual or interpersonal relationships. Her anxiety attacks were well controlled by tricyclic antidepressants, and the conflicts described were worked through in long-term psychotherapy. The patient became able to cooperate in her medical regime, although she needed some intermittent psychotherapy each time that intensive chemotherapy or radiation was reinstituted. On eight-year follow-up she is married and working successfully; her disease is under good control.

Case 5. E.L., a 30-year-old woman, reported occurrence of persistent abdominal cramps and diarrhea within a month of her marriage. E. had always been something of a prodigy and had worked extremely hard to please both her parents. They in turn were indulgent and protective toward her. After graduating from law school, E. got a high-level, high-pressure, demanding job with a law firm. She did well and enjoyed her work as well as her social life.

While the temporal connection between her marriage and the symptoms was rather striking, E. maintained that the marriage was a good one. Her internist found that diazepam (Valium), 5 mg four times per day, had been effective in supressing the symptoms, which he diagnosed as severe spastic colon.

The patient was seen for two years in psychoanalysis. During that time, underlying rage at her parents and siblings was explored, as were her perfectionistic, rigid defenses and her inability to feel affect. It seemed that under the stress of a successful career as well as the need to establish a marital relationship, E.'s habitual rejection of her own feeling state and her rigid defenses had come under a great deal of strain. During the first year of analysis the medication was very slowly discontinued. Two years after the end of analysis, follow-up shows that she is somewhat more vulnerable to depression and anxiety than previously, but is also more open to a variety of feelings and had no somatic symptoms.

Case 6. S.C. is a 50-year-old woman who reported a four-year history of mixed migraine and tension headaches. She had a history of severe depression, which had been successfully treated by psychotherapy. Prior to the onset of the headaches she experienced increased job pressure and was concerned about her husband's escalating drinking. The patient was mildly anxious but showed no remnants of the prior depression. The patient was found to have chronically cold extremities and very high frontalis, masseter, and trapezius muscle tension, which she could not at first voluntarily relieve. She was treated with autoregulatory therapies combined with biofeedback and was able to abort the migraine attacks within a few months. At the same time, she decreased her medication—which consisted of methysergide maleate (Sansert) and ergotamine tartrate with caffeine (Cafergot)—by 75 percent. However, tension headache was more resistant to autoregulatory therapy, and after four months, a trial of imipramine was begun. With a combination of autoregulatory therapy and imipramine, the patient was symptom-free within a few months; the imipramine was discontinued, with no rebound in symptoms and no recourse to headache medication. No exploration was made of the pressure at work, the prior depressive episode, or her marital situation.

References and Further Reading

Ader, R. (ed.). *Psychoneuroimmunology.* New York: Academic Press, 1981.

Alexander, F., French, T., Pollock, G.H. *Psychosomatic Specificity.* Chicago: University of Chicago Press, 1968.

Cousins, N. *Anatomy of an Illness.* New York: Norton, 1979.

Engel, G.L. Studies of ulcerative colitis. III. The nature of the psychological processes: a review and formulation. *Am. J. Med.* 16(3):416–433, 1954.

Gaarder, K., Montgomery, P. *Clinical Biofeedback: A Procedural Manual.* Baltimore: Williams & Wilkins, 1977.

Globus, G., Maxwell, G., Savodnick, I. (eds.). *Consciousness and the Brain.* New York: Plenum, 1976.

Gunderson, E.K., Rahe, R. (eds.). *Life Stress and Illness.* Springfield, Ill.: Charles C Thomas, 1974.

Kaplan, H., Freedman, A., Sadock, B. (eds.). *Comprehensive Textbook of Psychiatry/III.* Baltimore: Williams & Wilkins, 1980.

Kaplan, H., Knapp, P.H., Cheren, S., et al. (eds.). Psychological Factors Affecting Physical Conditions. In Kaplan, H., Freedman, A., Sadock, B. (eds.), *Comprehensive Textbook of Psychiatry/III*, vol. 2. Baltimore: Williams & Wilkins, 1980, pp. 1843–1985.

Monat, A., Lazarus, R. (eds.). *Stress and Coping.* New York: Columbia University Press, 1977.

Ransom, J.A. Life change and illness studies: past history and future directions. *J. Human Stress* 4(1):3–15, 1978.

Schultz, J.H., Lothe, W. *Autogenic Methods,* vol. 1. *Autogenic Therapy.* New York: Grune & Stratton, 1969.

Sifneos, P. The prevalence of alexithymic characteristics in psychosomatic patients. *Psychother. Psychosom.* 22:255, 1973.

Stein, M., Schiaui, R. D., Camerino, M. S. Influence of brain and behavior on the immune system. *Science* 191:435–440, 1976.

Stroebel, C. Biological Rhythms in Psychiatry. In Kaplan, H., Freedman, A., and Sadock, B. (eds.), *Comprehensive Textbook of Psychiatry/III*, vol. 1 Baltimore: Williams & Wilkins, 1980, pp. 221–228.

Usdin, G. (ed.). *Psychiatric Medicine*. New York: Brunner/Mazel, 1977.

Weiner, H. *Psychobiology and Human Disease*. New York: Elsevier, 1977.

13

Personality Disorders
SYD BROWN, M.D.

"I really don't know why I was brought here. I don't have any problems, and I don't need to see a shrink! It's my parents who have the problems—you should be seeing them, not me!"

"Look, I only agreed to come here because my wife insisted on it, so let's not get into *everything,* okay?"

"Yeah, okay, I've been taking some drugs lately, but, hell, everyone does it—I bet you take drugs, too, don't you?"

"Well, I really don't know why people treat me like I'm special, they just do."

"My God, I just can't believe what was going on! I said to him, 'How dare you speak to me like that, who do you think you're talking to?' And then he had the total and complete gall to insist that he was right! Well, I never heard of such a thing. I tell you, I was so upset!"

"Of course I've got friends, plenty of friends. My best friend? Well, I've got a lot of friends, plenty of friends."

The preceding quotations represent typical statements that clinicians hear when they interview patients in clinics, schools, or their private offices; such statements serve as indicators that a personality disorder may be present. Obviously, a diagnosis is never made on the basis of a single statement, but the statements demonstrate some of the diagnostic keys to recognizing personality disorders: a refusal to admit that one has problems, evasiveness, rationalizing behavior problems, perceiving themselves as special, a histrionic flair, and a shallowness that equalizes all interpersonal relationships, with the effect that close relationships are not developed or maintained. This chapter will examine these clinical phenomena, which are often more difficult to treat than are other psychiatric disorders because the affected patients are frequently unwilling to accept help or engage in treatment. These patients are often brought to the therapist by others and frequently state that they were coerced into coming for treatment by their parents, spouses, teachers, employers, court workers, or other authority figures; they openly express their disdain for treatment.

Patients with personality disorders are often manipulative and, in the attempt to avoid responsibility for their actions, will lie or distort situations, trying to place themselves "in a good light" or to impress the clinician. They rarely show symptom-related anxiety, typically stating that someone else is bothered by their behavior, but that they are not. In addition, they often arouse strong countertransference in the clinicians attempting to treat them. Few patients can be as frustrating as those with personality disorders, and few make it harder for the clinician to avoid judging the patient. While individuals with personality disorders may be dissatisfied with the impact of their behavior on others (and particularly with the way this impact then reflects back onto themselves), it is rare that they are concerned with the presence of the traits. However, while the traits may be ego-syntonic, the individual may still be concerned about the effect they have on others. What might bring such an individual to seek treatment is a disturbance of mood that results from the ongoing social difficulties and tensions.

The Concept of Personality Disorders
The *Diagnostic and Statistical Manual of Mental Disorders,* Third Edition (DSM-III) defines personality disorders as follows:

> Personality *traits* are enduring patterns of perceiving, relating to, and thinking about the environment and oneself, and are exhibited in a wide

range of important social and personal contexts. It is only when *personality traits* are inflexible and maladaptive and cause either significant impairment in social or occupational functioning or subjective distress that they constitute *Personality Disorders*. The manifestations of Personality Disorders are generally recognizable by adolescence or earlier and continued throughout most of adult life, though they become less obvious in middle or old age.

Many of the features characteristic of the various Personality Disorders, such as Dependent, Paranoid, Schizotypal, or Borderline Personality Disorder, may be seen during an episode of another mental disorder, such as Major Depression. The diagnosis of a Personality Disorder should be made only when the characteristic features are typical of the individual's long-term functioning and are not limited to discrete episodes of illness. (p. 305)

The major features of personality disorders are as follows:

1. Enduring, long-standing patterns of behavior are characteristic of the individual with a personality disorder. In stressful situations the inflexibility and maladaptiveness will often result in a rigid style of coping and problem-solving that will seriously alienate the individual from others, even those who might be of assistance.

2. Significant impairment in social or occupational functioning is present in those who manifest personality disorders, and they have great difficulty in establishing and maintaining close interpersonal relationships. They often value others for their material value rather than as partners in a shared experience. Social relationships tend to be somewhat shallow, and work relationships are often distorted by the manipulativeness of these individuals. While people with personality disorders may be competent workers, may generate ideas and be able to develop them, or may even be geniuses, it is likely that at some point they will have substantial difficulty with colleagues, subordinates, or superiors.

3. Individuals with personality disorders often elicit strong responses, frequently hostile, from others, leading to difficulty in the social context of relationships with others. While they may be creative, interesting people, and may even have qualities that cause others to seek them out as companions, their style of relating to others, particularly their manipulativeness and self-centeredness, wears thin and often generates resentment.

4. The clinical features of personality disorders are generally recognizable by adolescence. By mid-adolescence, people have developed a characteristic style of coping with and adapting to life; this style is fairly apparent in interviews with individual patients and with others who know them—parents, siblings, and those close to them. Remembering the DSM-III specification that the features are "typical of the individual's long-term functioning," one cannot diagnose a personality disorder unless the patient's history confirms that the currently maladaptive functioning represents a long-standing pattern.

CLASSIFICATION, DIAGNOSIS, AND CLINICAL FEATURES

Certain features are common to most, if not all, patients with personality disorders. In working with these patients, the therapist must try to understand them, a task often made difficult by their defiance of the therapeutic work and of the therapist. It is important for the therapist to understand what these patients are defending against—that is, the source of the pain, anxiety, or conflict they are unable to acknowledge that they are experiencing.

There are several aspects to the initial task of diagnosing a personality disorder. First, an axis I diagnosis must be insufficient to explain the presenting problems. (Axis I diagnoses describe the specific clinical syndromes of mental disorders, as discussed elsewhere in this text. For example, a patient who presents with a depressive disorder must also exhibit other persistent difficulties for the clinician to identify the presence of a personality disorder; these difficulties might include a paranoid personality disorder that is present even when the patient is not depressed.) Second, the patient's presenting problems must be representative of a long-standing pattern of maladaptive behavior toward social or work relationships. Finally, other conditions that could result in the same symptoms, especially neurologic disorders, must be ruled out. Alcoholism and malingering must also be considered as possible contributory factors.

Personality Disorders and Psychopathology
DSM-III includes a separate category, axis II, for personality disorders (and specific developmental disorders) to ensure adequate consideration of these clinical entities in people who also have more apparent axis I disorders. While the interrelationships of axis I and axis II disorders are complex and open to much debate, it is essential to appreciate the psychopathology of personality disorders. While specific organic factors have not been identified (although such factors are considered important in schizophrenia and the affective disorders, they are not thought likely to be involved in personality disorders), and while these disorders are not included among the axis I disorders, which are identifed as the *clinical psychiatric syndromes,* patients who present with personality disorders are suffering nevertheless. Their lives are often unstable and unsatisfying, their relationships are shallow, they have little ability to improve their lives appreciably, and they are often depressed. While many of these patients will contend that they are not depressed, particularly if they are referred for treatment by someone else, one can see evidence of their depression in the way they discuss their relationships with others, their hopes for the future, and their consideration of their current status. Good therapeutic work may enable them to admit that what they presented as anger was in fact depression and their fight against that depression.

Another important factor in personality disorders and psychopathology is the role these disorders play when in patients who present with axis I disorders. The treatment of a patient with a dysthymic disorder may be quite different from that of one who has that diagnosis and additionally has a borderline personality disorder. In the second patient, concerns about suicide must be heightened, and the clinician must make adjustments in the general therapeutic strategies when these powerful disorganizing forces are present. The same holds true for many of the other personality disorders as they coexist with—and complicate the treatment of—other disorders. These patients sorely test therapists' skills and personal strengths, and also teach us much about our own limitations as healers. It is perhaps this combination of factors, together with the countertransference reactions, that makes this heterogeneous and disparate group of patients so difficult to work with, but it is also successes with these patients—and there are successes—that can teach us so much about personality and human functioning, both healthy and pathological.

THE PERSONALITY DISORDERS
According to DSM-III, the personality disorders can be divided into three clusters:

1. The paranoid, schizoid, and schizotypal personality disorders include the patients who often appear odd or eccentric. They tend to avoid relationships and exhibit restricted affect. These patients share many of the clinical features of schizophrenics.
2. Patients with histrionic, narcissistic, antisocial, and borderline personality disorders are often dramatic, emotional, or erratic. They tend to be manipulative in their relationships, and typically relate to others as material objects rather than as people with whom to share experience.

3. The avoidant, dependent, compulsive, and passive-aggressive personality disorders are found in patients who are often anxious and fearful. They tend to have great difficulty in achieving a sensible balance of relationships, tending to be either extremely demanding and clinging or resistant and aloof.

There is also a residual category for atypical, mixed, and other personality disorders.

Paranoid Personality Disorder
The essential feature of a paranoid personality disorder is, according to DSM-III, a long-standing pattern of "pervasive and unwarranted suspiciousness and mistrust of people, hypersensitivity, and restricted affectivity."

Clinical Features. Patients with this disorder are often rigid in their interpersonal style and are rarely willing to compromise. They frequently adopt a moralistic stance and are quite critical of others, particularly those whom they view as weak or defective. They tend to externalize and use projection as a characteristic defense. Issues of dependency are critical, and they are hypersensitive to any indication that someone else may have some control or influence over them. Because they want to avoid ambiguity and ambivalence, they prefer that relationships be tightly structured, and they are keenly aware of hierarchical relationships. They are often interested in mechanical devices, electronics, and automation. When they express affect, it is likely to be in a humorless and serious manner. If this disorder is stable, impairment may not be too severe, and patients with paranoid personality disorder rarely come to clinical attention. However, in more disturbed patients, all relationships are grossly impaired, and transient psychotic symptoms may occur during periods of extreme stress. An additional note of interest is that individuals with this disorder are, not infrequently, leaders of esoteric religions, cults, or fringe political groups, because of their grandiosity and moralistic charisma and because some may view them as energetic, ambitious, and capable.

Differential Diagnosis. There is some indication that this disorder in some persons may precede the development of paranoid disorders and schizophrenia, paranoid type, the two major differential diagnoses for paranoid personality disorder. The primary differential issue is the lack of persistent psychotic symptoms, such as delusions and hallucinations, in the paranoid personality disorder.

Schizoid Personality Disorder
The essential feature of a schizoid personality disorder is a long-standing pattern of "a defect in the capacity to form social relationships, evidenced by the absence of warm, tender feelings for others and indifference to praise, criticism, and the feelings of others" (DSM-III, p. 310).

Clinical Features. Patients with this disorder display little motivation or capacity for social involvements and relationships. They have few, if any, friends, and are often characterized as "loners." They are often noticeably awkward in situations that demand social interaction. These patients engage in excessive daydreaming but do not lose the ability to recognize reality. Their fantasies, which are often of a compensatory nature, may involve imagining themselves as socially successful. They evidence great difficulty with the direct expression of affect, including aggression, and the astute clinician can detect a fearful note behind this aversion to feelings. These patients tend to prefer solitary activities and occupations in which they may focus their energies on interests and activities that do not require interaction with other people. They may often be successful in these activities as long as the pressure for interaction is minimal; it is demands for interaction with others that arouses their anxiety. In clinical interviews, these patients engage in little eye contact with the interviewer. Their responses tend to be short and they engage in little spontaneous conversation.

Differential Diagnosis. There are some indications that this disorder is a precursor for the development of schizophrenia, but this is largely based on reconstructive histories of schizophrenic patients, who frequently displayed schizoid characteristics at earlier stages of their illness. Predictive studies have not verified this to be the case for most patients. The principal differential diagnoses are (1) schizotypal personality disorder, in which patients display eccentricities of communication or behavior, and (2) avoidant personality disorder, in which patients are socially isolated due to their hypersensitivity to rejection (but those with avoidant personality disorder do show a desire for social interaction). Schizoid disorder of childhood or adolescence predisposes to the development of schizoid personality disorder, and it is the appropriate diagnosis for patients under the age of 18.

Schizotypal Personality Disorder

The essential feature of a schizotypal personality disorder is a long-standing pattern of "oddities of thought, perception, speech, and behavior that are not severe enough to meet the criteria for Schizophrenia" (DSM-III, p. 312).

Clinical Features. Patients with this disorder often display magical thinking, ideas of reference, illusions, and derealization, although no single feature is invariably present. These patients have great difficulty communicating their own thoughts and feelings, yet are highly sensitive to what others are feeling, and are often suspicious of others. Social interaction is very difficult for these patients, and they tend to avoid interaction, perhaps understanding that they may appear odd even to laymen; they may also be reacting to the way that others have responded to them in the past. They are often anxious or depressed. Transient psychotic symptoms may appear briefly under extreme stress. It should be noted that this is a new diagnostic classification, and further study is necessary to determine its validity and utility.

Differential Diagnosis. This disorder more closely resembles schizophrenia than do any other personality disorders. Indeed, under earlier diagnostic systems, many of these patients would have been classified as borderline, latent, or simple schizophrenics. The differentiation of this disorder from schizophrenia, residual type, is based on identifying a history of a previously active phase of schizophrenia with psychotic symptoms (see Chapter 6). Schizoid and avoidant personality disorders lack the oddities of behavior, thinking, and perception that are seen in the schizotypal personality disorder. Additionally, schizotypal patients often have family histories of schizophrenia. Schizotypal patients may also meet the requirements for borderline personality disorder; in such cases, both should be diagnosed.

Histrionic Personality Disorder

The essential feature of a histrionic (formerly *hysterical*) personality disorder is a long-standing pattern of "overly dramatic, reactive, and intensely expressed behavior and characteristic disturbances in interpersonal relationships" (DSM-III, p. 313).

Clinical Features. These patients typically are dramatic, overreactive, and overly emotional in their responses. They are often flamboyant in social situations, and quickly draw attention to themselves, both through their overly dramatic style and also by virtue of their powerful reactions, including tantrums, to minor irritations. While they may display a certain degree of warmth and charm, one senses their shallowness and superficiality, and evidence of the way that the disorder impairs their interpersonal relationships is readily available from their histories as well as from their present situations. In general, they make friends quickly but have difficulty maintaining meaningful relationships, as they are often demanding, manipulative, egocentric, and inconsiderate. Their affective displays are typically aimed not only at gaining attention but also at avoiding responsibility for their behavior. The lability that these patients display is often frustrating to those who deal with them, leading many—acquaintances, friends, and even some clinicians—to yield to their demands. These patients are often seductive, both in their dress and mannerisms as well as in their verbal style. They typically deny the provocative nature of their behavior, or rationalize it with statements such as, "I can't help it, I'm an emotional person." In clinical interviews these patients appear to enjoy the attention of the clinician, and their behavior is rarely toned down. They may display *la belle indifference,* appearing not to be affected by certain situations while overreacting to others. Despite their general emotionality, they have difficulty articulating their own feelings. Repression and dissociation are typical defenses in these patients.

Differential Diagnosis. Somatization disorder, featuring complaints of physical illness, may coexist with this disorder. Borderline personality disorder may also be present in patients with histrionic personality disorder, although histrionics do not typically display the feelings of emptiness, the identity confusion, or the brief psychotic episodes of the borderline patient. Narcissistic personality disorder may also be present. The clinical presentation may also include major depression, dysthymic disorder, brief reactive psychosis, and conversion disorder.

Narcissistic Personality Disorder

As characterized in DSM-III, the essential feature of a narcissistic personality disorder is a long-standing pattern of "a grandiose sense of self-importance or uniqueness; preoccupation with fantasies of unlimited success; exhibitionistic need for constant attention and admiration; characteristic responses to threats to self-esteem; and characteristic disturbances in interpersonal relationships" (DSM-III, p. 315).

Clinical Features. Patients with this disorder present as self-centered, vain, and unconcerned with the feelings of others. They tend to exaggerate their own abilities and achievements; when reality interferes too harshly with this view (for example, getting a lower grade than expected or not getting a desired promotion), they tend either to feel like a failure or to blame others for their inability to achieve to their own expectations. Patients with this disorder manifest poor interpersonal relationships, often created by their self-absorbed demandingness, sense of entitlement, and lack of empathy for others. They are, in a sense, too concerned with their own agenda to be genuinely concerned with others, except as these others help the patients present themselves as being successful and worthy of admiration or provide the patients with some other advantage. Because much of their interest in others is exploitive, persons with this disorder rarely have close interpersonal relationships. Those they do have tend to alternate between idealized and devalued, a manifestation of their inability to accept a balance of both the positive and negative characteristics of others (*splitting*). The self-esteem of these patients is fragile, and they typically respond to challenges to their self-esteem either with a cool indifference or with marked feelings of rage. Depression is a common feature.

Differential Diagnosis. Narcissistic personality disorder is a new diagnostic category, and differential issues have yet to be clearly defined. Perhaps the clearest differential features are the sense of entitlement and the quality of the grandiosity apparent in the patient with narcissistic personality disorder; these qualities are not as predominant in the persons with histrionic or borderline personality disorders, which often coexist with the narcissistic personality disorder. The clinical presentation may also include dysthymic disorder, major depression, and brief reactive psychosis. Alcohol and drug abuse disorders are often seen in the narcissistic patient.

It must be noted that this diagnostic category is not only new but also controversial. While the psychiatric literature (especially works with psychoanalytic orientation) has often discussed problems of narcissism, this is the first inclusion of narcissism as a formal diagnostic entity, and there are many who feel it is not well enough articulated as a discrete clinical syndrome to warrant a classification distinct from histrionic or borderline personality disorders.

For some, this diagnosis, more than any other, represents a moral judgment concerning the individual's expression of narcissism. Because an element of narcissism is an important feature in healthy personalities—all of us need to view ourselves as being worthwhile and successful—the distinction between healthy narcissism and pathologic narcissism then becomes a moral judgment rather than a clinical one. Psychoanalysts would counter this argument by pointing to the quality of the pathologic narcissism, its developmental significance, and the implications for treatment as reasons for maintaining this as a separate diagnostic classification. Further research to determine its validity and clinical utility is required.

Antisocial Personality Disorder

An antisocial personality disorder involves, according to DSM-III, "a history of continuous and chronic antisocial behavior in which the rights of others are violated, persistence into adult life of a pattern of antisocial behavior that began before the age of 15, and failure to sustain good job performance over a period of several years" (DSM-III, pp. 317–318).

Clinical Features. Several types of behavior predictive of the development of an antisocial personality disorder are often present in childhood, and, by definition, are present in adolescence. In childhood, typical symptoms include lying, stealing, fighting, truancy, and resisting authority. In adolescence, patients typically engaged in substance abuse or unusually early, aggressive, or promiscuous sexual behavior. Attention deficit is also frequently a precursor of antisocial personality disorder. Much of this behavior continues into adulthood, with the additional difficulties of inconsistent occupational, marital, and parental functioning. From this discussion, it is clear that historical information is crucial in the diagnosis of this personality disorder. These patients are typically brought to clinical attention against their will, often because of court referral. Their mental status is generally normal; they do not display symptoms of major thought disorder or of affective illness. In fact, they often appear glib and nonchalant, tending to downplay the seriousness of their behavior and to externalize responsibility. Underlying dysphoria may surface if the opportunity for acting out is restricted (for example, by incarceration); the risk of suicide is increased, as are somatic complaints. While many of these patients gradually improve their functioning during adulthood, the development of depression and of hypochondriacal concerns may occur.

Differential Diagnosis. Conduct disorder of childhood and adolescence, which predisposes to the development of antisocial personality disorder, is the appropriate diagnosis if such behavior occurs before age 18. An adult who engages in illegal behavior but does not present with the other difficulties that constitute a personality disorder should be described as having a condition not attributable to a mental disorder. Substance use disorder is also a frequent feature and can complicate the diagnosis. If the antisocial behavior is related to the substance use disorder (for example, selling illegal drugs to support one's own addiction), the diagnosis of antisocial personality disorder is not made unless the behavior associated with a personality disorder was present continuously for at least five years between the age of 15 and adulthood. Mental retardation or schizophrenia is diagnosed rather than antisocial personality disorder when both are present. While manic episodes may be present, differentiation in this case is relatively easy, because it is based on historical information.

Borderline Personality Disorder

The essential feature of a borderline personality disorder is a long-standing pattern of instability in a variety of areas, including interpersonal behavior, mood, and self-image" (DSM-III, p. 321).

Clinical Features. Predictable unpredictability is the hallmark of the borderline personality disorder, along with intense and unstable relationships, impulsive behavior, and intensity of affect. These patients will tend to move quickly from relationship to relationship, exaggerating the significance of each, almost as though they were trying to prove that the relationships are satisfying even when their needs are clearly not being met. These relationships are often of a dependent nature, and borderline patients are typically very demanding in such relationships. This dependency can quickly turn into hostility if they feel frustrated by the other person, and that hostility is as intense, and as intensely expressed, as was the dependency. Patients with borderline personality disorder seek out relationships as an antidote to the acutely painful emptiness and loneliness that they experience; hence they will even involve themselves in relationships in which they are exploited if doing so can help them avoid being alone.

Borderline patients often complain of a sense of identity diffusion, often expressing depression and confusion when discussing their plans for themselves (for example, career goals), and often achieve less than their potential might have allowed them to. In clinical interviews these patients typically project responsibility for their difficulties onto others. Psychotic symptomatology may appear, but such episodes are usually brief.

Avoidant Personality Disorder
The essential feature of an avoidant personality disorder is a long-standing pattern of "hypersensitivity to potential rejection, humiliation, or shame; an unwillingness to enter into relationships unless given unusually strong guarantees of uncritical acceptance; social withdrawal in spite of a desire for affection and acceptance; and low self-esteem" (DSM-III, p. 323).

Clinical Features. These patients are hypersensitive to rejection and humiliation, and equate the two. Hence, for them, rejection is humiliation, and the slightest sign of disapproval can be viewed as catastrophic. As a defensive maneuver, these patients then withdraw from opportunities to develop close relationships rather than risk disapproval. These people may have a few close friends, but they require constant reassurance that they are approved of. Low self-esteem is an obvious feature of such people. They often tend to misinterpret social interaction as being a negative reaction to them. These people try to keep out of the spotlight so as not to be noticed, as another defensive maneuver to avoid disapproval. An obvious consequence of this is that they take few risks in their personal or occupational activities. In clinical interviews they appear anxious and vulnerable, and they may misinterpret the interviewer's comments, nonverbal gestures, or facial expression as indicating disapproval.

Differential Diagnosis. The social isolation that characterizes the patient with avoidant personality disorder is also present in someone with schizoid personality disorder; however, the latter has no desire for social involvement and is indifferent to criticism—qualities that serve as ready differential features. Similarities also exist with social phobias, as both are concerned with humiliation in social situations, but in social phobias the concern is usually related to a specific situation rather than social relationships in general. However, social phobias may coexist with avoidant personality disorder. If the patient is under 18 years of age, the appropriate diagnosis is avoidant disorder of childhood or adolescence. Avoidant behavior and excessive sensitivity to rejection may be seen during depressive episodes, especially in adolescents.

Dependent Personality Disorder
The essential feature of a dependent personality disorder, as described in DSM-III, is a long-standing pattern "in which the individual passively allows others to assume major responsibility for major areas of his or her life...; the individual subordinates his or her own needs to those of others on whom he or she is dependent" (DSM-III, p. 324).

Clinical Features. These patients are typically dominated by others—usually parents or spouse—on whom they rely for decision-making in virtually all spheres of their lives. They externalize responsibility and are always the passive members of relationships. They are followers rather than leaders and are rarely willing to assert themselves for fear of jeopardizing their dependent relationships and having to accept responsibility for themselves. They are low in self-esteem, are pessimistic, and tend to belittle their own abilities and potentials.

Differential Diagnosis. Patients with agoraphobia also exhibit dependent behavior, but they take an active role in insisting that others assume responsibility for them; a patient with dependent personality disorder passively maintains a dependent relationship. Dependent personality disorder frequently coexists with other personality disorders, typically histrionic, schizotypal, narcissistic, or avoidant disorder. The clinical presentation may also include dysthymic disorder and major depression.

Compulsive Personality Disorder

The essential feature of a compulsive personality disorder is a long-standing pattern of "restricted ability to express warm and tender emotions; perfectionism...; insistence that others submit to his or her way of doing things; excessive devotion to work and productivity to the exclusion of pleasure; and indecisiveness" (DSM-III, p. 326).

Clinical Features. Compulsive people are extraordinarily concerned with orderliness, and routines; they want to make sure that everything is done "just right," in strict accordance with stated rules and procedures. Such people are not comfortable in unstructured situations, and seek out structure whenever possible. Their rigidity extends to their superego functioning, and they tend to be moralistic. They are rarely if ever spontaneous, particularly in the expression of affect. Their expression of affect tends to be somewhat constricted, and, while they may describe feeling states, they rarely do so with any affect as they talk. However, they can describe incidents or situations with a wealth of facts that can be both impressive and diagnostic. They tend to pay such close attention to detail that they can have great difficulty making decisions, because they get wrapped up in endlessly examining the details and repeatedly weighing all the alternatives. They also tend to be somewhat obstinate and resentful of attempts to change the way things are done; in such situations they tend to be oblivious to the feelings this arouses in other people.

Compulsive people also tend to be somewhat withholding of both personal affection and material goods; they are, in a word, cheap when it comes to giving of themselves. When in occupations that capitalize on these attributes, particularly the demand for orderliness and routine, compulsives can do quite well. They can also participate in stable marriage relationships, but they tend to have few friends. In clinical interviews compulsive patients tend to be neatly dressed and to present in a somewhat stilted manner. They are quite concerned that the interviewer understand all the facts that they bring up, and they are likely to ask many questions about details of recommendations, arrangements, and similar matters. Affect is constricted, and their mood is usually serious, although they may display some anxiety or depression. Typical defenses are isolation, intellectualization, displacement, reaction formation, and undoing.

Differential Diagnosis. Patients with compulsive personality disorders lack the obsessions and compulsions that are the defining characteristics of the obsessive-compulsive disorder, although some patients do present with both disorders. The major differential feature is the significant impairment in social functioning of the patient with personality disorder. Schizoid and paranoid personality disorders may coexist with compulsive personality disorder, as may paranoid disorder. The clinical presentation may also include hypochondriasis, dysthymic disorder, and major depression.

Passive-Aggressive Personality Disorder
The essential feature of a passive-aggressive personality disorder, according to DSM-III, is a long-standing pattern of "resistance to demands for adequate performance in both occupational and social functioning; the resistance is expressed indirectly rather than directly" (DSM-III, p. 328).

Clinical Features. The name of this disorder is based on the assumption that the patient's passivity is an expression of covert aggression. Hence, a student who delays completing assignments, a worker who "forgets" to read the latest procedural directives, and a spouse who is always late for appointments are all expressing covert hostility to these responsibilities, rather than directly confronting the source of their hostility. When pressed for increased or improved productivity, they feel resentful but do not express it directly; instead, they sabotage the demands by procrastinating, forgetting, dawdling, or other maneuvers that either prevent the work from being finished or make the result unsatisfactory. This sabotage has obvious deleterious consequences in both social and occupational functioning. When confronted with their behavior, these patients are likely to rationalize it or project the responsibility outward onto others. They frequently generate anger and resentment, because the responsibilities that they do not accept are assumed by others, who must do the work, complete the errands, or follow through on other obligations; when these patients are late, others must wait for them, also causing resentment. These patients lack self-confidence and tend to be pessimistic about the future. They have little insight into their behavior and are even unable to associate their sometimes conscious resentment against authority figures with their passive-resistant behaviors.

Differential Diagnosis. Oppositional disorder of childhood or adolescence may present a similar clinical picture, and that is the appropriate diagnosis if the patient is under 18 years of age. The nature of the passivity differentiates these patients from patients with dependent personality disorder. There may also be passive-aggressive features in histrionic and borderline personality disorders. The clinical presentation may include major depression, dysthymic disorder, and alcohol abuse or dependence.

Atypical, Mixed, or Other Personality Disorder
The residual category of atypical, mixed, or other personality disorder is to be used when a clinician decides that a personality disorder is present but cannot make a determination about the specific category. Note that, as stated above, more than one personality disorder may be noted as coexisting; in addition, a patient may have one personality disorder and also have features of one or more other personality disorders. The three classifications in this residual category are: (1) atypical personality disorder, for use when a personality disorder is present but a more specific designation cannot be made; (2) mixed personality disorder, for use when the patient manifests a personality disorder that includes features of several of the specific personality disorders but does not meet enough criteria that any individual personality disorder can be diagnosed; and (3) other personality disorder, for use when a personality disorder is present but is different from the classifications included in the standard DSM-III nomenclature (for example, masochistic, impulsive, or immature personality disorder).

Figure 13-1 presents a decision tree, which may assist the reader in comparing personality disorders.

ETIOLOGY
Little firm information is currently available about the etiology of the personality disorders, and there is no generally accepted consensus, on one basic cause of personality disorders. For many years the concept of personality disorders has been evolving, and DSM-III represents an attempt to classify these disorders more systematically than has been done before. It is only with the advent of DSM-III, for example,

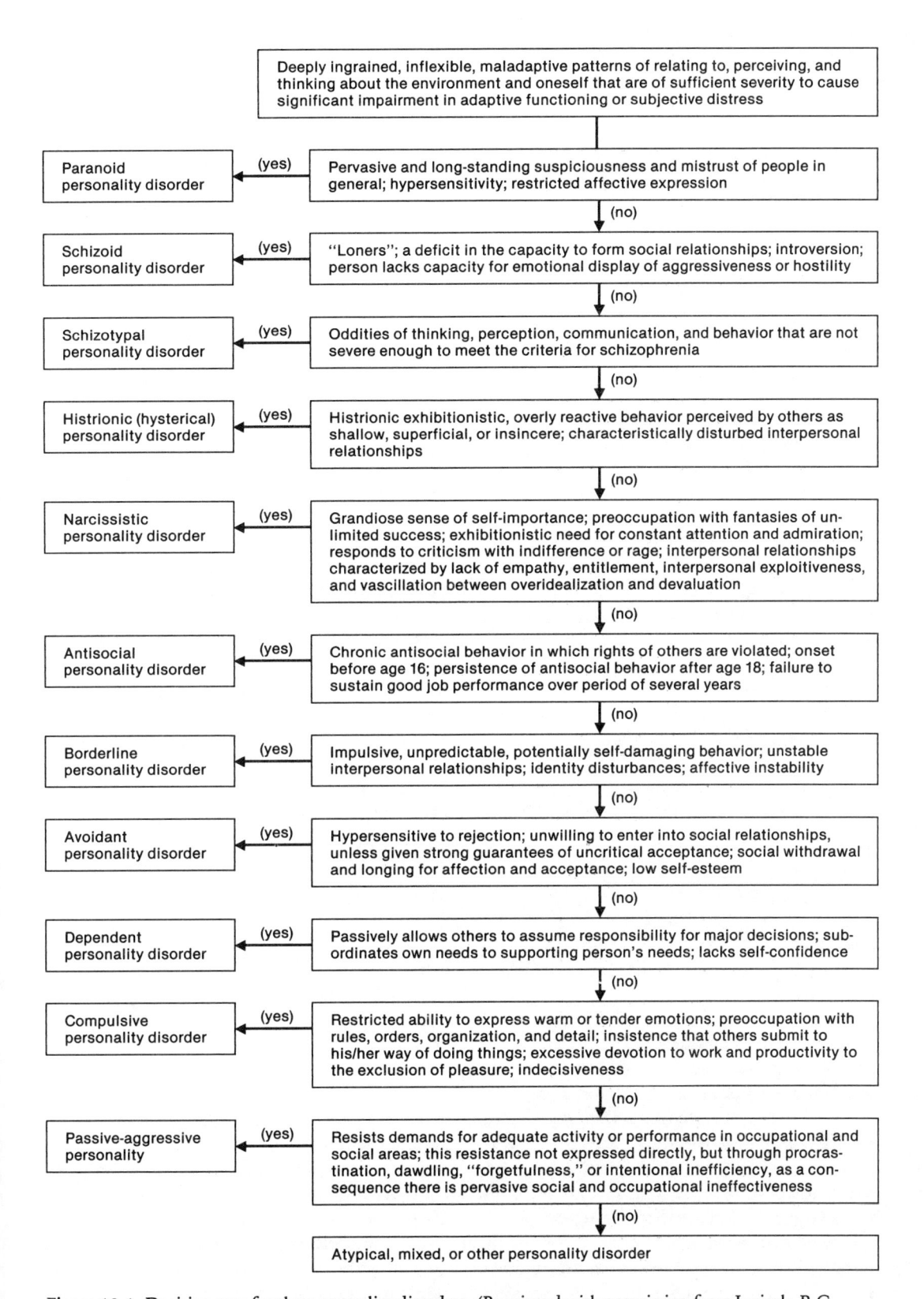

```
                    ┌─────────────────────────────────────────────────────────┐
                    │ Deeply ingrained, inflexible, maladaptive patterns of   │
                    │ relating to, perceiving, and thinking about the         │
                    │ environment and oneself that are of sufficient severity │
                    │ to cause significant impairment in adaptive functioning │
                    │ or subjective distress                                  │
                    └─────────────────────────────────────────────────────────┘
                                                │
```

Paranoid personality disorder	←(yes)	Pervasive and long-standing suspiciousness and mistrust of people in general; hypersensitivity; restricted affective expression
		↓(no)
Schizoid personality disorder	←(yes)	"Loners"; a deficit in the capacity to form social relationships; introversion; person lacks capacity for emotional display of aggressiveness or hostility
		↓(no)
Schizotypal personality disorder	←(yes)	Oddities of thinking, perception, communication, and behavior that are not severe enough to meet the criteria for schizophrenia
		↓(no)
Histrionic (hysterical) personality disorder	←(yes)	Histrionic exhibitionistic, overly reactive behavior perceived by others as shallow, superficial, or insincere; characteristically disturbed interpersonal relationships
		↓(no)
Narcissistic personality disorder	←(yes)	Grandiose sense of self-importance; preoccupation with fantasies of unlimited success; exhibitionistic need for constant attention and admiration; responds to criticism with indifference or rage; interpersonal relationships characterized by lack of empathy, entitlement, interpersonal exploitiveness, and vascillation between overidealization and devaluation
		↓(no)
Antisocial personality disorder	←(yes)	Chronic antisocial behavior in which rights of others are violated; onset before age 16; persistence of antisocial behavior after age 18; failure to sustain good job performance over period of several years
		↓(no)
Borderline personality disorder	←(yes)	Impulsive, unpredictable, potentially self-damaging behavior; unstable interpersonal relationships; identity disturbances; affective instability
		↓(no)
Avoidant personality disorder	←(yes)	Hypersensitive to rejection; unwilling to enter into social relationships, unless given strong guarantees of uncritical acceptance; social withdrawal and longing for affection and acceptance; low self-esteem
		↓(no)
Dependent personality disorder	←(yes)	Passively allows others to assume responsibility for major decisions; subordinates own needs to supporting person's needs; lacks self-confidence
		↓(no)
Compulsive personality disorder	←(yes)	Restricted ability to express warm or tender emotions; preoccupation with rules, orders, organization, and detail; insistence that others submit to his/her way of doing things; excessive devotion to work and productivity to the exclusion of pleasure; indecisiveness
		↓(no)
Passive-aggressive personality	←(yes)	Resists demands for adequate activity or performance in occupational and social areas; this resistance not expressed directly, but through procrastination, dawdling, "forgetfulness," or intentional inefficiency, as a consequence there is pervasive social and occupational ineffectiveness
		↓(no)
		Atypical, mixed, or other personality disorder

Figure 13-1. Decision tree for the personality disorders. (Reprinted with permission from Janicak, P.G., Andreiukaitis. DSM-III: Seeing the forest through the trees. Decision trees. *Psychiatr. Ann.* 10:297, 1980.)

that *narcissistic disorder* and *borderline disorder* actually represent diagnoses rather than clinical descriptions of patients. In general, however, there is some evidence that genetic, constitutional, environmental, and developmental factors all play a role in the etiology of personality disorders. It appears to be the full interaction of all these factors—both nature and nurture—that results in personality disorders.

Genetic and Constitutional Factors
The study of genetic factors in personality disorders has tended to look for evidence of any genetic transmission of the disorder, rather than focusing on specific factors, such as biochemical or metabolic factors. In general, studies have noted some evidence for the presence of a genetic factor in those personality disorders that most closely resemble schizophrenia (that is, paranoid, schizoid, and schizotypal personality disorders).

Constitutional factors play a role in the development of some personality disorders. Hyperkinesis ("Attention deficit disorder with hyperactivity" in DSM-III), learning disabilities, and other neurologic "soft signs" that were diagnosed in children, and have been found to be correlated with the later diagnosis of personality disorders in the same individuals when they were adolescents. There has been some suggestion that the presence of minimal brain dysfunction in children might predispose them to develop a personality disorder.

Environmental and Developmental Factors
Few dispute the statement that early childhood experience has a major impact on a person's development, but strong evidence has yet to be found to corroborate this statement with regard to personality disorders. Prospective studies that examine these issues by following children into adolescence and adulthood have not found any actual correlation between the development of personality disorders and the presence of early experiences that had been postulated as being significant to the development of these disorders. A major confounding variable in all such research is that, in most cases, the genetic factors (nature) and the environmental factors (nurture) have the same source: the child's parents and family. As an additional environmental influence, sociocultural factors also affect the developing child. The way that the cultural environment—that is, the community—rewards or punishes impulse control (or lack of impulse control), concern for others (or disdain for others), limit-testing, social involvement, deviance, and so on, will play a major role in what the individual learns about how to cope and adapt. It is equally obvious that this environmental influence is not absolute, as shown by the numerous people who dramatically improve their sociocultural status—or do something that deteriorates it.

Developmental factors—the way the child grows and matures both in the same way and at the same rate as others around him or her, resolving developmental issues—have a profound impact on the personality and hence on personality disorders. An examination of developmental factors that uses the *biopsychosocial* model focuses on the interplay of all the factors affecting the child's progress at each stage of development. The biologic, psychological, and social factors are all seen as influencing the child's progress through the developmental stages and the tasks that must be mastered at each stage of growth.

The most cogent discussion of developmental issues from a psychoanalytic perspective is Erik Erikson's concept of the "eight ages of man." This conceptualization, which closely corresponds to Sigmund Freud's (1937) model of psychosexual development, focuses on the developmental tasks that must be resolved in each of the stages of life. Whereas Freud primarily emphasized intrapsychic development, Erikson describes the psychosocial tasks that must be mastered. Briefly, these stages, named for the different outcomes that result if the tasks are mastered or not, are:

1. Basic trust versus basic mistrust (the first 18 months of life): The child comes either to trust that the environment will consistently provide gratification of his or her basic needs or to doubt that it will.
2. Autonomy versus shame and doubt (18 months to three years): The child, while learning to control muscular coordination, develops a sense of himself or herself as being able to exert self-control without loss of self-esteem or does not develop this self-confidence.
3. Initiative versus guilt (three to five years): The child develops a sense of pleasure in exploration or a sense of guilt about the goals of exploration and the fantasies of aggressive attack and conquest that can accompany this exploration.
4. Industry versus inferiority (six to 12 years): The child enters school and develops a sense of being able to master the fundamentals of technology or a sense of inferiority because he or she cannot do this.
5. Identity versus role confusion (puberty and adolescence): The youth develops a sense of integration of an ego identity or a sense of confusion about his or her appropriate role.
6. Intimacy versus isolation (young adulthood): The individual develops a sense of being able to commit himself or herself to specific affiliations and partnerships or a sense of being distant from others.
7. Generativity versus stagnation (adulthood): The individual achieves satisfactory levels of productivity and creativity, particularly in the task of establishing and guiding the next generation, or does not and displays a sense of stagnation, of being unable to continue growing.
8. Ego integrity versus despair (maturity): The individual reviews his or her life and experiences a sense of satisfaction at achievements, both personal and occupational, or feels dissatisfaction and a sense of despair.

From a developmental perspective, a personality disorder would develop during the second 18 months of life, when the child must master issues of control and yield to parental controls on impulses and behavior. In bowel training and control, the child is asked to assert control over behavior he or she had not been expected to control earlier. Situations that are analogous to this control issue may be seen in later conflicts as the child matures. When control becomes a struggle between the child and the parents, other situations that also require the control of impulses may well become a struggle between the child and parent or (later on) between the adolescent or adult and society.

Social learning theorists would certainly agree that early environment has a major impact on one's development, and they would also agree that the child's relationship with his or her parents is an important point of focus. However, they would examine this relationship in terms of the reinforcement of behavior and learning that takes place, rather than focusing on the nurturant issues of this relationship. For these theorists, the development of a personality disorder—or any psychopathology—results from the reinforcement of behavior that is later deemed to be undesirable. The reinforced behavior is strengthened, becoming a permanent part of the individual's behavioral repertoire; if it receives substantial reinforcement, it may constitute a prominent or even predominant part of the person's characteristic style of life.

EGO DEFENSES

Everyone utilizes defenses to mediate the anxiety we all experience in life. These defenses—unconscious mental processes—assist us in resolving conflicts so that we can carry on our lives. They often serve us well in the occupations we choose. For example, it is helpful for a scientist to use the fairly sophisticated defense of intellectualization so that he or she may examine data objectively. Difficulties arise, however, when the defenses serve to deflect rather than resolve conflict. The deflected conflict is avoided, leaving the conflict unresolved, only to rise again. This avoidance is especially important in pathologic defenses, which can be emotionally crippling. Perhaps the most obvious case of this is the withdrawn psychotic patient, who avoids conflict by totally withdrawing from interaction with the environment. Defenses that are intractable, as is often true in people with personality disorders, can seriously impair patients' ability to carry on their lives successfully.

Therapists must be extremely careful when confronting the defensive structure of patients with personality disorders. The *defensive structure* represents the combination of several defensive mechanisms, with varying degrees along the continuum of mature, immature, and pathologic; the specific mechanisms used may vary in any given situation. Most people use one or more of these defenses, but in patients with personality disorders the use of these defenses tends to be rigid, and hence brittle. The type of interpretation that may assist neurotic patients may only serve to enrage those with personality disorders, who use their defenses not only to ward off anxiety, but also to maintain distance between themselves and others. The following sections briefly summarize the key defense mechanisms one is likely to encounter in work with these patients.

Specific Defense Mechanisms

Acting Out. An overworked and often misused phrase, *acting out* means the expression of affect or impulses through motor behavior rather than more appropriate expression of the affect. It typically involves aggressive or sexual impulses and can occur in all categories of personality disorders. Acting out is one of the most difficult defenses to deal with, as the motor behavior may often provoke strong reactions (for example, anger or fear) in other people, and intervention must be prompt so these patients do not do irreparable damage to themselves or to others. Limits need to be set both in the interview room and in the patients' environment, so that the acting out can be controlled; they can then be helped to understand what the feeling was that they were acting out.

Splitting. In splitting, patients divide people into *good people* and *bad people* rather than accepting both the good and the bad features of all individuals. Splitting is characteristic of the way that narcissistic and borderline patients attempt to resolve the natural ambivalence about accepting individuals, particularly authority figures, with both their positive and negative attributes.

Isolation. The defense of isolation removes the affective component from an experience. Such patients tend to be orderly and compulsive; for them, control issues are paramount in treatment as in all other parts of their lives.

Undoing. Undoing is an effort to change the behavior or its consequences after the fact, and may accompany isolation in the compulsive's defensive maneuvers.

Reaction formation. In reaction formation, the emotional impulse is essentially reversed. Instead of an outburst of rage, for example, exaggerated formality and politeness emerge. Compulsive personalities demonstrate this defense.

Intellectualization. A relatively high level (that is, developmentally late in its appearance) defense, intellectualization allows internal impulses to be distanced or diminished in intensity.

Repression and Dissociation. The defense of repression and dissociation allows patients to acknowledge unpleasant or even dangerous experiences, but they reverse the affect and seem not to be upset by that experience. *La belle indifference* is most often seen in patients with histrionic personality disorder.

Fantasy. Some patients, particularly those with schizoid personality disorder, replace unpleasant realities with fantasy, allowing them to view themselves as friendly, successful, social, and so on, achieving a satisfaction they do not enjoy in reality. Where they are too fearful of genuine intimacy to engage in close relationships, they create, in fantasy, imaginary relationships that provide them with a sense of satisfaction without making them confront their own worst fears.

Passive Aggression. Patients who utilize passive aggression are seen as turning anger back onto themselves. Unable to accept or express their anger directly, they do so indirectly, typically in a passive manner. Hence, they will procrastinate completing responsibilities despite obvious school, work, or social consequences.

Hypochondriasis. The presentation of unsolvable and unrelievable complaints, hypochondriasis is an attempt to render helpers incompetent and to make them feel as helpless as the patient does. This is most often seen in borderline, dependent, and passive-aggressive patients.

Projection. Projection involves attributing to other persons emotions that exist in the person utilizing the defense. In the process, the unacceptable impulse is distanced by experiencing it as outside rather than inside the mind. This is the primary defense of patients with paranoid personality disorder or psychosis.

Introjection or Identification. A person can assimilate the external source of anxiety by using introjection or identification. These maneuvers occur in normal development but may be seen in some personality disorders such as paranoia.

Repression. Persons utilizing repression essentially push out of awareness the whole impulse or emotion being defended against. Historically, this defense was one of the first mechanisms observed and is employed in histrionic (formerly *hysterical*) disorder.

Denial. Denial is common in patients with personality disorders but is a particularly central defense in those with substance abuse disorders. Its power can hardly be imagined until it is encountered in experience.

Regression. At times of internal or external stress, any person may regress to an emotionally earlier level of adaptation. This process is more likely in certain personality disorders than in others. The patient with borderline personality disorder will commonly employ this defense.

Sublimation. One final mechanism of defense, sublimation, is not usually seen in pathologic disorders. This defense is the healthy process by which emotions and impulses are channeled into socially approved or encouraged activities and behaviors.

Treatment

TREATMENT STRATEGIES

As already stated, the countertransference that patients with personality disorders frequently arouse in therapists can present a major difficulty in their treatment, and many therapists prefer not to work with them at all. The therapist who does work with these patients should attempt to be aware of these feelings and try to avoid becoming angry at such patients or defensive with them. One must acknowledge one's reactions and then attempt to continue developing the therapeutic alliance. Making moral judgments of these patients is a sure way to defeat the therapeutic process.

In psychotherapy, the therapist should attempt to maintain the focus on the patients' behavior rather than on their explanations of that behavior. As is true for therapists working with adolescents—who are similar to adults with personality disorders in many ways—the therapist should encourage patients to talk about their feelings and to reflect on their behavior and others' reactions to them. The therapeutic relationship should be seen as a joint alliance between the patient and the therapist. The therapist needs to set limits on what is acceptable and what is not, and to provide appropriate structure for the patient. The therapist should also encourage the patient to develop social support systems in addition to the therapy.

There are numerous pitfalls the therapist must be wary of. It is critical to avoid defensiveness, as patients with personality disorders often attempt to cope with their own anxiety by making others anxious, and this can weaken the therapeutic alliance. The therapist should also avoid encouraging the dependency of the patient and beware of any rescue fantasies in which the therapist sees himself or herself as the patient's savior.

The therapist must attempt to hold patients responsible for their behavior without blaming or punishing them. These patients often view interpretations as accusations, and the therapist must be careful about interpretations, particularly early in the therapeutic process. It is important that communications between the therapist and patient be kept clear, and the therapist must be acutely aware of the nonverbal messages he or she is communicating in addition to the content and manner of verbal statements. Patients with personality disorders are keenly aware of others' behavior, and they may tend to distort nonverbal cues—as well as direct verbal statements—and interpret them in a way quite different from the message intended by the therapist. Because the classic passive "blank screen" approach, which is helpful to neurotics, may well arouse distrust in patients with personality disorders, the therapist should be responsive to these patients as people.

Group therapy is often valuable in the treatment of patients with personality disorders. Like adolescents, these patients are often more effective in confronting each other with their behavior than a therapist is, and they are often more likely to accept direct confrontation from someone they view as a peer from someone they view as an authority figure. With adolescents whose acting out becomes severe enough, milieu therapy, in either a hospital or a residential treatment center, is often the treatment of choice. This allows a varied therapeutic approach and can include individual, group, family, and milieu therapy; the environment can be structured with clear, consistent limits, and the patients provided with almost constant feedback concerning the way that their behavior affects others. Behavior modification programs (for example, token economies) are often part of the milieu and can be extremely valuable in helping the patient learn to adapt and cope within a social system.

Psychoactive medication may be used with these patients, but only for the relief of specific target symptoms. One cannot cure a personality disorder through medication, although medications can help the patient be more available for psychotherapy by relieving his or her anxiety, depression, or other symptoms. When the personality disorder is one part of an overall illness—for example, schizophrenia or a major affective illness—then medication is indicated. However, since many patients with personality disorders, particularly adolescents and young adults, also present with histories of abuse of numerous illicit drugs, therapeutic medication is exceptionally complicated. The patients might, for example, overdose on medication; the more seriously disturbed patients may well have already attempted suicide with some of these same medications.

TREATMENT OF SPECIFIC PERSONALITY DISORDERS

Paranoid Personality Disorder

Therapeutic work with the paranoid patient should be characterized by a professional, not overly warm style in which the therapist conveys respect for the patient. The therapist must be aware that he or she is being closely scrutinized by the patient, and all dealings must be straightforward, nondefensive, and courteous. Trust and intimacy are major difficulties for paranoid patients, and this problem will be shown in the therapeutic relationship and the therapeutic work. Interpretations, particularly those that concern issues of dependency, sexual concerns, and a desire for intimacy, are extremely threatening to these patients, and a therapist who is too determined to interpret these issues, or does so too early in the development of the therapeutic relationship, will jeopardize the therapeutic process.

Low doses of neuroleptic medication may prove helpful, but even the suggestion of such an invasion is likely to set off much anxiety and suspiciousness in a paranoid person. The recommendation must be carefully timed and the patient allowed to consider the possibility and discuss his or her reactions.

Schizoid Personality Disorder

Treatment for the patients with schizoid personality disorder parallels treatment for those with paranoid personality disorder, although there may be a somewhat better potential for the slow establishment of a therapeutic relationship. Schizoid patients tend to be more introspective than paranoid patients; with the development of trust, the former group can make good use of therapy. While they may be silent for much of the time in individual or group therapy, the clinician may see signs of involvement, and note that these patients may be able to use therapy, especially group therapy or activities therapy, as an important social support.

Schizotypal Personality Disorder

Treatment of schizotypal patients parallels treatment for the previous two categories of patients. It is often difficult to understand the inner experience of these patients, and therapists need to be wary of confronting and ridiculing—or appearing to ridicule—their belief systems. The neuroleptics may be useful in the treatment of these patients, but further study is required. Dosages should be lower than those necessary for actively psychotic patients.

Histrionic Personality Disorder

The key to therapy with histrionic patients is assisting them to recognize and understand their own feelings and needs. This may be undertaken in individual or group therapy: the approach in either case involves helping the patient to examine his or her own feelings, reactions, and behavior. The therapeutic relationship is likely to be a stormy one, because the transference reaction in these patients is often powerful. The therapist needs to be particularly wary about sexual issues, as these patients tend to be seductive and to exaggerate the therapist's responses to them. The less experienced therapist must be acutely aware of the nonverbal messages that are communicated to these patients, as these messages are often misinterpreted.

A subgroup of histrionic patients that is even more dramatic and reactive reports a persistently dysphoric mood. These patients have appropriately been called *hysteroid dysphorics,* and there is evidence that antidepressant medication, especially the monoamine oxidase inhibitors, may be quite helpful to them.

Narcissistic Personality Disorder

Because the clinical syndrome of narcissistic personality disorder has been discussed primarily by psychoanalysts, most therapy with these patients has involved psychoanalysis or psychoanalytically oriented pychotherapy. The focus of this treatment is the development of the therapeutic relationship and the use of insight achieved through the therapy as a means of resolving the pathology. The analytic process explores issues basic to the parent-child relationship. The transference developed in this work is particularly strong and is often characterized by a *transference psychosis* (in which the patient acts as if the therapist were the original psychological object, the parent), rather than a *transference neurosis* (in which the patient reports having feelings about the therapist that are similar to those that he or she had about the parent).

Antisocial Personality Disorder

In working with antisocial patients, one must understand that they are frightened by intimacy because they have had no genuine experience with it. They did not experience the sustained, caring relationships with their parents (or parent substitutes) that allow most people to accept intimacy with others. Frequently, in fact, their parents were neglectful, abusive, or rejecting. Hence, the pain and anxiety that most people learn to accept as part of intimacy, along with the warmth and caring they seek, is overwhelming for these patients. Many internalize negative self-images from these experiences; to avoid the pain this engenders, they act out to externalize the pain onto others. The dysphoria they display when they cannot act out demonstrates the depth of their anxiety and their rigid, if often ineffective, conscience.

Individual psychotherapy is not as effective with these patients as are peer groups and structured programs. In fact many would argue that traditional psychotherapy is usually ineffective with adult antisocial personalities. Firm limits must be established, and the patient must be held responsible for his or her behavior. Group support is helpful in dealing with the patient's self-destructiveness and also for overcoming the fear of intimacy. When the acting out behavior has come under control, membership in the group, and identification with the group, can provide an experience in sharing and intimacy; this process provides these patients with some of the parenting experience they did not receive as children. Examples of programs that have shown some success are self-help groups for convicts, structured halfway houses, and wilderness schools, all of which are variants of milieu therapy. Many of these programs also utilize encounter group therapy, typically led by participants rather than by mental health professionals, who most typically serve these programs in an advisory, rather than direct-service, role.

Borderline Personality Disorder
As already noted, the transference relationship in psychotherapy with borderline patients tends to be extremely powerful, and therapists must be always aware of their own countertransference reactions. Therapists working with these patients may often find themselves idealized one week as the greatest person or the most understanding and empathetic therapist, only to find themselves thoroughly devalued and demeaned the following week. The overwhelming anger these patients present, combined with their impulsivity, can result in major management problems in psychotherapy; their self-destructive behavior, perhaps aimed more at manipulating the therapist than at actual self-destruction, can result in suicide. Deciding how to respond in such situations is often difficult and can have profound implications for further therapeutic work. These patients tend to regress in psychotherapy, especially unstructured psychoanalysis. Psychoanalysts treating these patients have adopted a modified psychoanalytic approach that aims at the resolution of pathologic internalized representations of interpersonal relationships while also utilizing special support systems when necessary. Another approach features a more supportive, reality-oriented relationship and more limited therapeutic goals. In either case, the therapist must be concerned with the potential for regression and manipulation; backup support systems, including hospitalization, must be available.

Avoidant Personality Disorder
The primary task of a therapist working with avoidant patients is to develop a supportive therapeutic alliance so that they can begin to feel more comfortable and able to accept feedback. Assertiveness training may be very helpful to these patients, but care must be taken to provide support for them, and the work may well go slowly. Group therapy is also useful for these patients. Evidence of persistent depression should result in active psychopharmacologic intervention.

Dependent Personality Disorder
Assertiveness training can be quite useful for these patients; however, as is true in treating patients with avoidant personality disorders the therapist must be careful not to push the

patients too quickly. It is important to avoid challenging dependent relationships even when they are pathologic; these relationships are vitally important to the patient, and if the therapist challenges them too quickly or too harshly the therapeutic alliance could be damaged.

Compulsive Personality Disorder

In contrast to other patients with personality disorders, compulsive patients are able to admit their suffering. The lack of spontaneity and emotional freedom results in little pleasure, and they are affected by the criticism of their "cheapness" from people they value. These problems are ego-dystonic, and can lead the patient with compulsive personality disorder to seek treatment. These patients can also utilize nondirective therapeutic techniques (psychoanalysis or psychoanalytic psychotherapy) to explore areas and issues that they cannot otherwise approach.

A major issue in therapy with compulsive patients is control—the issue that dominates the clinical picture discussed previously. Therapists may find themselves in seemingly endless discussions of technical arrangements for the therapy, or they may find themselves hearing the same statements over and over, including a great deal of minutiae. Therapists may also find their interpretations being challenged. The countertransference that this challenge may engender needs to be carefully watched, particularly because the compulsive traits being discussed here are necessary for successful completion of training to be a therapist, and it is likely that these traits still are part of the therapist's personality. The major therapeutic strategy with such patients is to focus on the patient's feelings. Behavior therapy can be very useful for these patients, because it can provide opportunities to interrupt compulsive rambling and to focus on specific behavior. This approach arouses anxiety, which can leave patients open for learning. Group therapy can also be helpful for compulsive patients, because group members can provide direct feedback on the effect of their behavior.

Compulsive patients may become quite depressed. At such times, the compulsive features usually worsen and psychotherapy becomes quite ineffectual until the depression is alleviated. Antidepressant medication may be beneficial.

Passive-Aggressive Personality Disorder

Psychotherapy with passive-aggressive patients is often a difficult task. Direct interpretations of their behavior are often ineffective with these patients; a more successful tactic involves a focus on the patient's behavior and its probable consequences. The therapist must be wary about walking a thin line between accepting their demands for dependency, which are pathologic, and refusing their dependency, which is tantamount to rejection. The therapist may expect the patient to cover his or her resentment, expressing it indirectly and covertly—for example, by being late for appointments, missing appointments, confusing technical arrangements, and so on.

References and Further Reading

Erikson, E. *Childhood and Society*. New York: Norton, 1963.

Freud, A. *The Ego and the Mechanisms of Defense*. London: Hogarth Press, 1937.

Grinker, R.R., Werble, B., Drye, R. *The Borderline Syndrome*. New York: Basic Books, 1968.

Gunderson, J.G., Singer, M.T. Defining borderline patients: an overview. *Am. J. Psychiatry* 132: 17-24, 1975.

Hall, C.S., Lindzey, G. *Theories of Personality*. New York: Wiley, 1978.

Kernberg, O. *Borderline Conditions and Pathological Narcissism*. New York: Jason Aronson, 1975.

Kernberg, O. *Object Relations Theory and Clinical Psychoanalysis*. New York: Jason Aronson, 1978.

Lion, J.R. *Personality Disorders: Diagnosis and Management*. Baltimore: Williams & Wilkins, 1974.

Loevinger, J. *Ego Development*. San Francisco: Jossey-Bass, 1976.

Mack, J.E. *Borderline States in Psychiatry.* New York: Grune & Stratton, 1975.

Mahler, M. A study of the separation-individuation process and its possible application to borderline phenomena in the psychoanalytic situation. *Psychoanal. Stud. Child* 26:403–424, 1971.

Masterson, J.M. *The Narcissistic and Borderline Disorders.* New York: Brunner/Mazel, 1981.

Perry, J.C., Klerman, G.L. The borderline patient. *Arch. Gen. Psychiatry* 35:141–150, 178.

Shapiro, D. *Neurotic Styles.* New York: Basic Books, 1965.

Shapiro, E.R. The psychodynamics and developmental psychology of the borderline patient: A review of the literature. *Am. J. Psychiatry* 135:1305–1315, 1978.

Sloan, R.B., Staples, F.R., Krystol, A.H., et al. *Psychotherapy Versus Behavior Therapy.* Cambridge: Harvard University Press, 1975.

Spitzer, R.L., Williams, J.B.W., Skodol, A.E. DSM-III: The major achievements and an overview. *Am. J. Psychiatry* 137:151–164, 1980.

Stone, M. *The Borderline Syndrome: Constitution, Personality, and Adaptation.* New York: McGraw-Hill, 1980.

Vaillant, G.E, Perry, J.C. Personality disorders. In Kaplan, H.I., Freedman, A.M., Sadock, B.J. *Comprehensive Textbook of Psychiatry/III.* Baltimore: Williams & Wilkins, 1980.

Zetzel, E.R. A developmental approach to the borderline patient. *Am. J. Psychiatry* 128:867–871, 1971.

14

Eating Disorders
ELIOT SOREL, M.D.

Severe dysfunctions in eating behavior, or eating disorders, include a cluster of signs and symptoms defined by Urte: frequent body weight changes, fluctuations in kind and quantity of food intake, vomiting, and an accompanying mood disturbance. Transactions between the identified patient and his or her family play a prominent role in the dysfunction. Eating disorders occur in childhood, adolescence, and young adulthood. These disorders include anorexia nervosa, bulimia, pica, rumination disorder of infancy, and atypical eating disorder. Anorexia nervosa is the clinically best-documented dysfunction among the eating disorders and thus constitutes the major part of this chapter. Both anorexia nervosa and bulimia occur in females at a rate that is 10 to 20 times greater than in males. Pica and rumination disorder seem to affect both sexes equally. Atypical eating disorder refers to all other eating disorders that cannot be classified under any of the other categories.

Anorexia Nervosa

DIAGNOSTIC CRITERIA AND CLINICAL FEATURES

Anorexia nervosa, a disorder of uncertain etiology that usually begins in childhood or adolescence, is characterized by an unrealistic fear of becoming obese, distortion of body image, refusal to maintain a minimal normal body weight, and often amenorrhea. Physical illness must be ruled out as a factor causing the weight disturbance. Individuals with this disorder think of themselves as fat even when they are quite emaciated. Bulimia, use of laxatives, and compulsive exercising may accompany the clinical picture of starvation. There is a preference shown for low-calorie foods as well. Psychological denial of the illness is always a prominent feature. Sexual development is generally delayed or lost.

The current diagnostic criteria in the *Diagnostic and Statistical Manual of Mental Disorders*, Third Edition (DSM-III) emphasize an individual focus even though family pathology is usually quite evident (see Table 14-1 for these criteria). Until it was recently surpassed by bulimia, anorexia nervosa was the most prevalent of all eating disorders. Despite the even greater progression of bulimia, anorexia has become increasingly prevalent, and it has been recently stated, "One might speak of an epidemic illness, only there is no contagious agent" (Bruch, 1978).

The first recorded case of an eating disorder dates back to the eleventh century, when Avicenna, the Persian physician, treated a young prince for anorexia nervosa (Sours, 1980).

In the English medical literature, a case reported by Morton in 1689 clearly illustrates essential features of anorexia nervosa (see Case 1). In the nineteenth century, the renowned English surgeon William W. Gull and a Parisian internist Professor Ernest C. Laségue independently presented to their colleagues cases of *apepsia hysteria* and *l'anorexia hysterique* respectively. Initially, Gull thought that apep-

Table 14-1. Diagnostic Criteria for Anorexia Nervosa

A. Intense fear of becoming obese, which does not diminish as weight loss progresses.
B. Disturbance of body image, e.g., claiming to "feel fat" even when emaciated.
C. Weight loss of at least 25% of original body weight or, if under 18 years of age, weight loss from original body weight plus projected weight gain expected from growth charts may be combined to make the 25%.
D. Refusal to maintain body weight over a minimal normal weight for age and height.
E. No known physical illness that would account for the weight loss.

Reproduced with permission from *Diagnostic and Statistical Manual of Mental Disorders*, 3rd ed. Washington, D.C.: American Psychiatric Association, 1980, p. 69.

sia hysteria was an illness of psychogenic origin with the absence of pepsin as its biologic marker.

Clinical data indicating the presence of pepsin led Gull to reconsider both the etiology and the nomenclature of the disturbance, and he introduced the term *anorexia nervosa*.

Laségue's description of the illness integrated biologic, psychological, and social dimensions in a three-stage progression. The first stage was characterized by decreased food intake and increased activity; the second stage was defined by the family's increased anxiety and the patient's decreased weight (relating to each other in a feedback loop); and the third stage was characterized by amenorrhea, constipation, severe depression, and markedly depressed activity. He described the illness as follows:

> ... hypochondriacal ideas or delusions often intervened. The physician has lost his authority; medicaments have no effect except laxatives, which counteract the constipation. The patients claim that they have never felt better; they complain of nothing, do not realize that they are ill and have no wish to be cured. This description would, however, be incomplete without reference to their home life. Both the patient and her family form a tightly knit whole and we obtain a false picture of disease if we limit observations to the patient alone (Laségue, 1873).

Laségue's observations, which were revolutionary for his time, descriptively integrated biologic, psychological, and social dimensions. Therapeutically his interventions, nevertheless, remained circumscribed to the identified patient and increasingly met with resistance, particularly in the middle and late stages of the illness. The primary underpinning of the disturbance was thought to be psychological.

A period deemphasizing the psychological basis of anorexia ensued after Simmonds in 1914 postulated that anorexia nervosa was due to pituitary insufficiency. His observations were based on data that later proved to be erroneous.

Today, a century after the observations of Gull and Laségue, the interconnections between biology, psychology, and social context are still relevant. Until very recently, however, the emphasis has been primarily on the identified patient. Alexander in 1950 (see Case 2) highlighted individual, family, and professional dynamics that are frequently brought to bear on the outcome of anorexia nervosa. Although Alexander's emphasis was on the individual, his family tasks assignment, which promotes positive parent-child transactions, uses Laségue's original phenomenologic observations in an effective therapeutic intervention. Alexander's concept of multicausality extends, albeit linearly, from the individual to the dyadic and family dimensions of an eating disorder.

Bruch (1973), based on her several decades of clinical work with patients with eating disorders, conceptualizes anorexia nervosa as a disturbance of delusional proportions characterized by distortion of the body image, impaired perception and interpretation of stimuli arising from the body, and a feeling of ineffectiveness in the struggle to gain control of one's life.

Bliss and Branch (1960), defining anorexia nervosa, emphasize the predominant factors:

> What is common to all patients with anorexia nervosa is not the "anorexia" but the "nervosa" that causes the loss of weight. The appetite may be absent but also may be present, increased or perverted. Some have a true anorexia and genuinely have no desire for food. Others crave food but refuse to eat. Some eat and then vomit; whereas, others, surreptitiously hide or dispose of their meals so as not to arouse the suspicion and disapproval of their families and physician. There are those who fear to eat because digestion may cause fearful somatic distress or lead to obesity; and there are a few who eat docilely and then purge themselves of the offensive nutriments by cathartics and enemas. But, in every case, although the reasons and stratagems will vary, the final result is a reduction in the intake of calories, a loss of weight and semi-starvation.

Clinicians and clinical researchers have, in the last 10 to 15 years increasingly focused on the family involvement in anorexic dysfunction. This change of emphasis may be in response to the increasing incidence of anorexia nervosa (Crisp et al., 1977); in England, among girls 12 to 18 years of age, the disorder affects one of every 100 in private schools and one of every 550 in public schools. The growth of family systems theory and therapy has brought about a theoretical and therapeutic shift in the assessment and treatment of anorexia nervosa.

ETIOLOGY

The etiology of anorexia nervosa is unknown. In 63 percent of the patients a disturbed relationship with their families existed before the diagnosis and treatment of anorexia nervosa (Hsu et al., 1979), while 70 percent of the patients were from upper and upper-middle social classes.

INDIVIDUAL AND FAMILY FACTORS IN ANOREXIA NERVOSA

Crisp (1977) and Kalucy and associates (1977) focused on the diagnosis, treatment, and outcome of anorexia nervosa; in their view, weight phobia is central in the diagnostic process, and they believe that etiology involves both the individual and the family. Regarding the role of the identified patients, Crisp emphasizes their investment in maintaining a subpubertal body weight and the belief that their body size and form determine their fortunes in life. A second important dimension refers to the patients' need to maintain a vigilant control over their impulses to eat. On this second level there is usually a very intense commitment to school work and secretiveness. A third level of understanding involves the struggle with developmental, maturational issues as one of the contexts of the dysfunction, particularly regarding relationships with peers and differentiation from the nuclear family. A fourth level of assessment might reveal that the identified patient has a close relationship with the father and that there is some brief history of impulsive behavior causing panic in the family. The patient may have previously been a compliant high achiever. The family would share or mask dysfunction in one or both of the parents, and the family system is probably isolated.

Kalucy and his colleagues (1977) identified several variables that were found in 44 families that had one member hospitalized for treatment of anorexia nervosa. The family system variables include weight pathology, sexual maladjustment, illness in parents, and disruptions of family equilibrium, among others. In the weight pathology category they found a history of overweight in 20 percent of both mothers and fathers, and a low adolescent weight had been present in 16 percent of the mothers and 23 percent of the fathers. Age phobia was present in 23 percent of the mothers. In 43 percent of the parents, sexual activity was rare or nonexistent. Migraine and phobic avoidance were present in 30 percent of the mothers. Among the fathers, 19 percent presented with alcohol abuse, 29 percent with marked obsessional thinking, and 40 percent with manic-depressive psychosis.

Assessment of family equilibrium found some revealing data as well. This evaluation focused on the family status before the onset of anorexia in the identified patient; 20 percent of the families had experienced one death in their network, usually the death of a grandparent. Departures or separations were also significantly present—in 34 percent of the families, the patient was leaving home, and in 32 percent of the families, a sibling was leaving. Illness in the father was present in 21 percent of the families, and parental separation threatened in 34 percent of the cases.

The families in the group presented with what Kalucy and colleagues (1977) described as "narrow, inflexible and concrete range of coping mechanisms," and their coping mechanisms were minimally applicable to transactions outside the family system. In these families, with identified dysfunction in one or both spouses, as well as losses or threatened loss such as death, departures, and separations, the adolescents constitute a group at risk.

PHYSICAL AND LABORATORY FINDINGS IN ANOREXIA NERVOSA

The physical and laboratory findings in anorexia nervosa are of uncertain etiologic significance; most of the findings are likely to be results, not causes, of anorexia. In severe cases involving a weight loss of 25 to 30 percent, physical examination reveals muscle atrophy, disappearance of the fatty layers of the tissues, and the presence of lanugo. The patient's extremities appear cyanotic, and nails are unusually brittle. Bradycardia, hypotension, and hypothermia are present. In severely emaciated patients, loss of teeth and multiple dental caries are also present. Use of cathartics and diuretics may enhance dehydration.

Laboratory findings revealed fasting blood sugar in the range of 60 to 80 mg/100 ml. Basal metabolic rate is reduced 20 to 40 percent (Sours, 1980). Oliguria is usually present, but renal functions are responsive to increased water intake. Urinary ketones are usually found with cachexia. Hepatic functions are usually normal, and there is slowing down of the gastrointestinal tract. The electrocardiogram shows with bradycardia, inverted or flattened T wave, and ST-segment depression (Sours, 1980).

The use of cathartics and diuretics in many of these patients enhances dehydration and electrolyte imbalance, with hypokalemia a frequent finding. Endocrine assessments revealed the previously mentioned decreased basal metabolic rate and the presence of amenorrhea, the latter due to gonadotropic insufficiency. The metabolic imbalance precipitated by the use of cathartics and diuretics is reversible with free feeding.

TREATMENT OF ANOREXIA NERVOSA

The treatment of anorexia nervosa, an illness that has a mortality of 5 to 15 percent, presents a challenging proposition for the clinician since he has to focus on the family systems. Models for treatment of family systems were developed by Palazzoli (1978) in Philadelphia; in these models, family functioning and dysfunctioning are considered a crucial underpinning in anorexia nervosa. They postulate that psychosomatic dysfunction such as anorexia nervosa in children and young adults is predicated on at least three conditions, namely: (1) a certain type of family organization that encourages somatization; (2) involvement of the child in parental conflict; and (3) physiologic vulnerability. The family organization that emerges is one characterized by enmeshment, overprotectiveness, rigidity and lack of conflict resolution.

Evaluation of Family Systems

Enmeshment refers to fused boundaries between the parental subsystem and the sibling subsystem, with confused hierarchies and frequently ineffective parental leadership. Enmeshment is further characterized by a high degree of intrusiveness in communications, thoughts, and feelings—often one family member finishes another's sentence. In effect, the family system is dysfunctional in the five markers identified by Fleck (1980) in assessing family systems—that is, leadership, boundaries, communication, affectivity, and task goals.

Usually in such a system, individuals have a lower level of differentiation of the self, or a higher degree of fusion. Individuals with lower levels of differentiation are stressed into dysfunction by weaker stimuli and require longer periods to recover than is true of people with higher levels of differentiation. Having a lower level of differentiation also involves a lesser degree of flexibility (higher rigidity) and a greater dependency on others (Bowen, 1978).

The symptomatic child in such families is overprotected by the parents. In turn, the attention to the symptom maintains conflict-avoidance patterns. One frequently encountered pattern in conflicted parental subsystems involves the triangulation of the child; a stable coalition is formed with one parent while the other parent becomes the outsider.

Overprotectiveness interferes with children's ability to learn to compete, cooperate, and negotiate with their peers, thus retarding their development of autonomy and competence. This process, of course, interferes with their differentiation of self.

Overprotecting or blaming the symptomatic child is also a major way used by the parents to avoid conflict resolution and maintain symptoms. The dysfunctional family system will probably enact this pattern repeatedly, maintaining conflict, while a family that functions successfully will usually confront their problems, negotiate, and resolve the conflicts.

The treatment in anorexia nervosa frequently has two phases—an inpatient phase and an outpatient phase; at times treatment can be conducted wholly on an outpatient basis if the case is identified early enough. Hospitalization becomes essential when weight loss reaches a threatening degree.

The psychiatric clinician must work closely with the family physician or the pediatrician to make a decision as to how to proceed in treatment. Ideally, the family physician or the pediatrician carries out a thorough medical evaluation including a complete battery of laboratory tests to rule out any organic conditions such as metabolic abnormalities, central nervous system tumors, or gastrointestinal disease. After this evaluation, the decision to hospitalize, if necessary, should be made jointly by the psychiatric clinician and the referring physician. It is desirable for the family physician or pediatrician to follow through on a complete medical evaluation even if hospitalization is necessary. A supportive nutritional regimen should also be started as soon as possible.

Inpatient Treatment
The inpatient phase, which has as its chief emphasis the critical issue of weight gain, has two stages: a medical-behavioral stage and a psychotherapeutic family systems stage, as postulated by Crisp (1967), Blinder (1970), and Minuchin (1978) and their respective associates. At times the degree of nutritional deterioration of the patient might require nasogastric feeding. The patient's weight should begin to increase before the start of the psychotherapeutic intervention since successful psychological treatment is greatly impeded by a deteriorating physical condition.

The success of the medical-behavioral stage is facilitated by a competent nursing staff and by the use of a protocol that is clear, concise, and consistent with specific target weight gains per day and per week. The diet should be nutritionally balanced, and the patient should be allowed reasonable time to complete the task of eating. There should be clear reinforcement schedules involving rewards for meeting targets and negative reinforcement for failures. The model varies somewhat according to the developmental stage of the patient. For an older adolescent and young adult there should be firm guidelines with some room for negotiation to foster autonomy, while younger children would be given less flexibility.

In addition to nutritional status, other factors that enter into the decision to hospitalize include the need to engage the family in a family-oriented treatment approach and the need to assess the impact of prior outpatient therapy. Some therapists prefer to work as a team with the pediatrician or family physician (Minuchin, 1978), until the completion of the first segment of the inpatient phase—the evaluation. After the family session at which the results of the evaluation are presented, the psychiatrist is fully in charge, and family therapy formally begins. Other psychiatrists prefer being in charge from the first day of the hospitalization. There are as yet no solid comparative data to differentiate the two approaches.

Goals to allow discharge vary. The pediatrician-psychiatrist team may set as a goal the point at which the patient has regained half of the difference between the actual weight at hospitalization and the ideal weight for the specific developmental stage. In this approach, the team also sets a target of a two-pound weight gain per week in the outpatient follow-up until the weight is appropriate for height and age. Some other practitioners, including Crisp (1977), are willing to discharge the patient only after the full restoration of body weight to match population mean levels.

Outpatient Treatment
Most of the patients who require hospitalization involve cases that are referred or diagnosed after the acute onset of the illness. Hos-

pitalization may be required in such patients as a life-saving initial intervention, allowing close monitoring of intake and output to correct the nutritional and metabolic imbalance. Case 3 at the end of the chapter represents a patient who was referred early in the course of the disorder; hospitalization was not needed and she therefore started directly in outpatient therapy. The case of D.S. exhibits the hallmarks of anorexia nervosa—(1) the fear of weight gain even while body weight is diminishing; (2) decreased food intake, alternating with bouts of binge eating and vomiting, and (3) a loss of 25 percent of combined body weight plus the projected weight gain expected from growth charts for her age. At the time of referral she was clearly below the minimum normal weight for age and height. There was no physical illness that accounted for her weight loss.

Working in family therapy with D. and her family, it also became evident that D.'s older sister, a very important member of the family system, was planning her departure from the household for a job in another town. The sister had been the *parent surrogate;* that is, she was frequently entrusted with the care of her two younger siblings; this was particularly true in recent years as the mother had increasingly disengaged from the system. The family system presented with a history of depression in the mother, who was overprotective and intrusive of D., and of alcohol abuse in the father. As D. started dating and receiving letters from friends, for example, her mother frequently read D.'s letters without her permission.

Therapy sessions involved the system as a whole as well as meetings with subsystemic components. At the outset the sessions were held weekly and then gradually, as progress ensued, were changed to alternating weeks and finally to monthly sessions for approximately a year. The work with the family system as a whole initially redefined the problem from one of *sickness* to that of *control.* Further, the work helped to rearrange hierarchies and promote parental leadership, with clear definition of tasks and goals in the household. The parental subsystem was taught to delegate age-appropriate responsibilities to D. and to respect her privacy, thus facilitating differentiation and autonomy. Bringing the parental subsystem together sharply defined the subsystemic boundaries and enhanced parental leadership; it also further facilitated differentiation of the adolescent.

Task assignments between sessions provided a major avenue for systemic intervention, correcting hierarchies, establishing clear subsystemic boundaries, enhancing leadership, and promoting differentiation. The choice of tasks usually derived from the family's actual needs. One among many tasks that was assigned involved responsibility for the family meal. Meal times for the family as a whole were regularly scheduled with all members participating in the tasks related to it. Parental leadership, which had been previously abandoned, became a renewed function of the system. Each assigned task was carried out with some regularity, providing opportunities for cooperation and sharing that had been absent or relegated to one member, namely the parental child. The initial stages of the task created therapeutically induced crises that mobilized the parents to help their daughter and further brought into focus the previously descibed corrections in the system.

Activating the parental executive into an effective leader of the system redefined the subsystemic boundaries from the sibling subsystem. D. began gaining weight. The increasingly effective confident parental executive became more open to exploring existing conflicts between the spouses, between spouses and children, and among siblings. They began identifying solutions, with a diminished focus on D. and with enhanced self-assurance about the family's ability to identify, negotiate, and solve problems.

At the time of termination D.'s weight was stable and within normal limits for her height and age, and her eating patterns were normal. She was now age-appropriate in her relationship with her peers and her family and was well on the way to her self-differentiation.

TREATMENT OUTCOME
AND FOLLOW-UP

Outcome and follow-up studies to date have been difficult to compare because treatment approaches have varied, particularly in psychotherapeutic models. Outcome studies done by Crisp (1977), Kalucy, and Minuchin (1978) reveal varying rates of therapeutic success and raise a number of issues warranting further investigation.

Crisp's (1977) follow-up studies after two years revealed a 50-percent recovery rate, while his four- to seven-year follow-up revealed a 60-percent recovery rate and a 5-percent death rate. Crisp's follow-up data indicated that males do less well and that patients in social classes IV and V present with a more severe and chronic illness. Furthermore, family nutritional disorders concerned with weight, premorbid obesity, and long duration of illness before treatment all worsen prognosis.

Kalucy (1979) reviewed the outcome in 44 families with anorexia and found a rate of 45-percent improvement in patients from social classes I and II, a 50-percent improvement in patients from social class II, and only a 20-percent improvement in patients from social class IV and V.

To date, the most promising outcome and follow-up data come from Minuchin (1978) and his group in Philadelphia; they have followed 80 percent of their 53 anorexic patients treated in structured family therapy of a minimum of 3 to a maximum of 16 months. Follow-up, which began 6 months from start of treatment and ranged from 18 months to 7 years, revealed an 86-percent recovery rate based on both medical and psychological assessment.

In all of the outcome and follow-up studies that have been cited, treatment intervention early in the illness (preferably within the first six months) is a major predictor of positive outcome.

Bulimia

DIAGNOSTIC CRITERIA
AND CLINICAL FEATURES

Bulimia, another eating disorder, usually begins in adolescence or young adult life. It is frequently encountered on a continuum with anorexia nervosa, although in bulimia the weight loss is never in the 25- to 30-percent range. It is rarely, if ever, life-threatening but often presents with a chronic, fluctuating course. As stated previously in this chapter, bouts of binge eating can occur in anorexia nervosa. Like anorexia, bulimia is found predominantly in females, and a family history of weight problems is frequently present.

Clinical research data on bulimia have been reported less in the medical literature, although current estimates refer to a 90-percent prevalence of binge eating in the female college population in the United States. It is unlikely that this group would meet the strict diagnostic criteria for bulimia as presented in Table 14-2. In most patients with bulimia the weight fluctuation is usually around the normal range; cases present during the course of

Table 14-2. Diagnostic Criteria for Bulimia

A. Recurrent episodes of binge eating (rapid consumption of a large amount of food in a discrete period of time, usually less than two hours).
B. At least three of the following:
   1. consumption of high-caloric, easily ingested food during a binge
   2. inconspicuous eating during a binge
   3. termination of such eating episodes by abdominal pain, sleep, social interruption, or self-induced vomiting
   4. repeated attempts to lose weight by severely restrictive diets, self-induced vomiting, or use of cathartics or diuretics.
   5. frequent weight fluctuations greater than ten pounds due to alternating binges and fasts
C. Awareness that the eating pattern is abnormal and fear of not being able to stop eating voluntarily.
D. Depressed mood and self-deprecating thoughts following eating binges.
E. The bulimic episodes are not due to anorexia nervosa or any known physical disorder.

Reproduced with permission from DSM-III, pp. 70–71.

the illness at weights above or below ideal for height and age. Many of the individuals in this group also present with a history of substance abuse.

Case 4 exemplifies the salient clinical features of bulimia. Reviewing the case we notice that the onset was in adolescence, shortly after her separation from family of origin. The young woman's weight had a 35-pound variation, but at times it was within the normal range for her height and age. She presented with a history of substance abuse, including marijuana and amphetamines.

The clinical data meet the diagnostic criteria for bulimia, including the recurrent episodes of binge eating; consumption of high-calorie, easily ingested foods during the binge; termination of such eating by social interruption; and frequent weight fluctuations of more than 10 pounds between alternating binges and fasts.

The patient was also aware that her eating patterns were abnormal and was constantly in fear of not being able to stop eating voluntarily. She often felt depressed and had self-deprecatory thoughts after the eating binges. No anorexia nervosa episodes could be identified. Her family history revealed a conflictual system with an ineffective parental executive, a blurring of boundaries between the parental and sibling subsystems, and coalitions across generational boundaries, with one parent as the outsider.

TREATMENT
Clinical work with such patients is extremely challenging, particularly since many go undetected or untreated for months and frequently for years. Rigid transactional patterns are deeply embedded in the family system, and the role of the identified patient in detouring conflict has been long established. Furthermore, in such cases the "patient role" frequently becomes an "identity card" for the symptomatic family member. Work with this adult patient must focus primarily on the current life situation, helping the patient develop appropriate skills that would make her competent. The work usually proceeds with the individual alone as well as with the family. Many of the therapeutic strategies applied to family systems in the treatment of anorexia nervosa are applicable to these family systems as well, particularly when the patient is an adolescent.

Early detection and treatment are by far the best predictors of outcome, particularly when the approach to treatment is a problem-solving one that involves the family system.

Community support and self-help groups are developing in many areas and seem likely to be of considerable assistance to affected individuals, at least in the area of personal and social adjustment. New studies have suggested that some cases of bulimia may be related to primary affective disorders, and there may be a treatment role for antidepressant medication in these patients.

Pica
Pica, a rare disorder, is encountered in the first three years of life and is present equally in males and females. The illness involves the ingestion of nonnutritive substances such as paint, plaster, hair, cloth, pebbles, leaves, and dirt. The illness usually remits in childhood but may continue through adolescence and adult life. In planning therapeutic intervention, one must assess the family system, paying particular attention to the care (or lack of care, or possible neglect) of the infant or child, as well as any nutritional or mental deficiency.

Rumination Disorder of Infancy
Rumination disorder of infancy is a rare disorder that is present equally in males and females. It usually starts in the first year of life although it may begin later in mentally retarded children. Rumination disorder involves repeated regurgitation without nausea or associated gastrointestinal illness for at least one month after a period of normal functioning. There is accompanying weight loss or failure to achieve expected weight gain.

The difficulties that may develop as the result of the disorder involve particularly the relationship between mother and infant. There is a potential for bonding impairment because the mother might be repulsed by the infant's behavior. Intervention obviously requires work with both the infant and the mother.

Case 1. "In the month of July she fell into a total suppression of her Monthly Courses from a multitude of Cares and Passions of her Mind, but without any Symptom of the Green-Sickness following upon it. From which time her Appetite began to abate, and her Digestion to be bad; her flesh also began to be flaccid and loose, and her looks pale.... She was wont by her studying at Night, and continual pouring upon Books, to expose herself both Day and Night to the injuries of the Air.... I do not remember that I did ever in all my practice see one, that was conversant with the Living so much wasted with the greatest degree of a consumption (like a Skeleton only clad with skin) yet there was no Fever, but on the contrary a coldness of the whole Body.... Only her Appetite was diminished, and her Digestion uneasie, with Fainting Fits, which did frequently return upon her." (Morton, 1689)

Case 2. "In an 8 year old girl, a severe anorexia developed during the Summer vacation. The child refused practically all food, and every meal was the occasion for violent scenes in which she was forced to swallow a few bites. She lost weight and soon showed clinical evidences of undernourishment. The pediatrician prescribed the usual roborants and completely overlooked emotional factors. After the psychiatrist had won the child's confidence, it was not difficult to uncover the emotional background of the condition. She had a younger sister, at that time 2 years old, who was fed by a nurse usually in the presence of the mother, at the same time that the patient ate. The psychiatric interview revealed that the older girl had experienced strong jealousy of her younger sister. This little intruder absorbed all the parent's attention. It became evident that the child's refusal to eat was motivated first by her wish to capture both the nurse and the mother's attention and to direct it away from the little sister. By means of her stubborn symptoms she succeeded in doing so. The second motive was a guilt reaction. She wanted to receive all the love, to take away everything from her little sister, and she had to do penance for this envy by not eating. The third factor in her anorexia was spite towards the parents, getting revenge for all their attention being given to her younger sister. At the psychiatric interviews in which all these emotions poured out dramatically and the change in the management of their routine, promptly eliminated this dangerous symptom. The patient was taken along by the parents to a restaurant for her meals which she consumed with her parents and in this way she was being given a premium for being the older one, and this helped her tolerate the attention given to her younger sister. Enjoying the advantages of being the older child, she could more readily renounce the privilege of the baby." (Alexander, 1950)

Case 3. D.S., a 16-year-old high school student, the second of three daughters of an executive family, was referred for consultation following bouts of self-induced vomiting of three-months duration, decreased appetite, diminished food intake and a weight loss of 25 pounds (25 percent of the combined total body weight and projected weight gain). D. told the examiner that she had been inducing vomiting, usually after meals, by inserting the knife handle of a table knife in her mouth. D. stated that she had been "feeling fat" particularly since her schoolmates and parents had been teasing her about her weight.

She has for a long time been worried about her grades although generally she has been maintaining an A minus to A average. Concern about her weight, her grades, and more recently, changes in the relationship with her father would make her feel worried and depressed and she would not eat or at times secretly eat more; she would then "regret it, and would run to the bathroom, throw up, and then feel better." The relationship with her father has been changing only in the last year. She had previously felt close to her father, and she would side with him in fights involving her mother, particularly as they related to her freedom. D. stated that now her father only "yells" at her. When he found out that she was "throwing up," he told her to stop because it was not good for her health.

Although D.'s weight progressively diminished, she continued to feel fat and be afraid that she would gain further weight. She also said she had school problems with her classmates; she felt older than they were, avoided them, and thought that they were avoiding her.

Exploration of the family system revealed high parental expectations regarding the children's school performance. Furthermore, the father described the identified D. as "my buddy," engaged in sports activities with her, and said, "She has been taken from me by her growth...[and] my overconcern with her becoming sexually active." He acknowledged that there was a distancing in his relationship with his wife; he had a history of alcohol abuse, and his wife had disengaged herself from the household.

Case 4. S.T., a 24-year-old single female architectural designer sought a consultation after three years of psychoanalysis and "feeling trapped." S. lived with a roommate; frequently when she was alone in the apartment after work, she would "eat until full, spoonfuls of peanut butter, ice cream, nuts, jelly," and she stopped only if interrupted by the arrival of her roommate. Then she would hate herself for doing it, and at night, while thinking about her hatred of being fat, she would vow not to do it again. The following day, however, the same binge eating would happen again, and S. then spent hours at night "thinking about how to be thin...how to control it."

One approach that S. took to control her food urges was to avoid having any food at home; she had been unable to maintain that method for longer than a week. Her inability to control her urges made her feel "fat, stupid, and angry." She had been "fighting with food" for the previous six years since shortly after leaving home. S. stated that her body repulsed her and that she was not interested in having a sex life. She described her periods as being irregular. In order to be able to sleep she had been using diazepam (Valium), 10 to 20 mg, which had been prescribed for her for the past five to six years. Her weight had been varying between 125 pounds and 160 pounds, and S. had also abused marijuana and amphetamines.

Family history revealed that S. was the third of four siblings with an alcoholic father and a critical, distant mother. S. described her parents as spending their time fighting each other, and the children were usually "on the father's side." She "hated him for being so passive, never fighting back."

References and Further Reading

Alexander, F. *Psychosomatic Medicine*. New York: Norton, 1950.
Bowen, M. *Family Therapy in Clinical Practice*. New York, London: Jason Aronson, 1978.
Bruch, H. *The Golden Cage*. Cambridge: Harvard University Press, 1978.
Crisp, R.H. Diagnosis and outcome in anorexia nervosa. *Proc. R. Soc. Med.* 70:464–470, 1977.
Fleck, S. Family functioning and family pathology. *Psych. Ann.* 10(2):17–35, 1980.
Hailey, J. *Problem Solving Therapy*. San Francisco: Jossey Bass, 1977.
Hudson, J., Laffer, P.S., Pope, H.G. Bulimia related to affective disorders by family history and the dexamethasone suppression test. *Am. J. Psychiatry* 139:685–687, 1982.
Kalucy, R.S., et al. A study of 56 families with anorexia nervosa. *Br. J. Med. Psychol.* 50: 381–395, 1977.
Minuchin, S. *Psychosomatic Families*. Cambridge: Harvard University Press, 1978.
Morton, R. *Phthisiologies: or Treatise of Consumptions*. London, 1689.
Palazzoli, M.S., *Self Starvation*. New York, London: Jason Aronson, 1978.
Sours, J.A., *Starving in a Sea of Objects*. New York, London: Jason Aronson, 1980.

15

The Psychiatric Disorders of Adolescence
JOHN E. MEEKS, M.D.

It is important to remember that adolescents do not have some magic immunity to the psychiatric disorders of adulthood. A few years ago seriously disturbed adolescents were often viewed as merely showing phase-specific *growing pains*. Seriously antisocial young people were misdiagnosed as if they were only demonstrating the natural rebelliousness of the adolescent period. Psychotic adolescents were thought to be showing a temporary disorganization designated as *adolescent turmoil*. Careful follow-up studies have long since clarified the reality of adolescent psychiatric disability.

The true prognostic outlook for adolescents with serious behavioral or psychiatric symptoms is extremely guarded unless they receive active and effective treatment. Mental health professionals were reluctant to recognize this because of their hesitancy to label unhappy adolescents out of a fear that they might thus acquire a more-or-less permanent negative image or identity. As will be discussed later, there are very good reasons why diagnosis in adolescents can be a confusing process. People in that age group may actually present their psychiatric symptoms in somewhat different forms from those seen in adult patients. In addition, the nature of their relationship with the adult mental health professional may lead to difficulties in obtaining the necessary diagnostic information.

This disparity between adolescents and adult psychiatric patients needs to be recognized but should not be exaggerated. Although it is probably true that some practitioners will find themselves unable to work effectively with adolescents, there is no need for physicians and other members of the helping professions to consider the adolescent as, in some basic way, different from the adults they are accustomed to. Although the developmental thrust of this age group accentuates certain human behavioral patterns and tends to obscure others, the adolescent—in or out of psychiatric difficulty—is still more like a human being than anything else! Though this comment is made jokingly, it is surprising that many adults find it difficult to empathize with adolescents and assume that youngsters in that age group are in some basic emotional way deviant from the remainder of the population. For example, they will insist that adolescents are insensitive to criticism, show no remorse, or are lacking in empathy. In fact, one is most likely to have a correct understanding of an adolescent's emotional state by imagining how you would feel if you were in similar circumstances. In short, the basic interviewing skills and capacity for empathy that are used in any doctor-patient relationship serve very well in relating to the adolescent with psychiatric disability.

Special Characteristics of the Adolescent Phase
Having noted that adolescents are very similar to other human beings of any age, it is important, nevertheless, to look at some of the areas where apparent differences exist and where particular needs of the developmental period lead to confusing self-presentation. It might be best to begin with the area of dependency.

Blos has referred to adolescence as the second individuation, comparing it to Mahler's earlier developmental formulations. Other writers have emphasized the adolescent's striving toward emancipation and independence. Often this desire for self-direction is offered as the explanation for the fabled rebelliousness of adolescence. Certainly there is some truth in these ideas.

It is important to recognize, however, that adolescents' attitudes toward dependency are by no means so simple and straightforward. Faced with the incipient tasks of adulthood and struggling with the pressures of sexual and aggressive arousal, identity confusion, and rapid changes in body image, adolescents tend to be shaken in their sense of mastery. Their world seems to be crumbling around them and they are struggling to build a new one. In this type of life situation, which is characterized by high stress, the human mind tends to return to earlier and simpler approaches to life and its problems. For this reason, adolescents show great unevenness in functioning. As parents often say, "One day she acts as though she's 30 and the next day as though she's three."

During these episodes of childlike feeling and behavior, adolescents are in fact, hungry for dependency support. This desire, however, is in sharp conflict with the recognized need to move toward independent development. In other words, adolescents are not in single-minded pursuit of independence but they are in desperate need of maintaining the *appearance* of independent functioning both in the eyes of others and in their own estimation.

This extraordinarily complex attitude toward dependency shows up in many aspects of adolescent behavior. For example, while declaring themselves free spirits, adolescents are often slavishly conforming to the norms of their peer group and are, therefore, extremely susceptible to peer pressure. Adolescents can also tolerate dependent relationships when these are justified by a face-saving purpose. For example, adolescents are often able to form warm and friendly dependent relationships with adults who help them achieve specific tasks and goals—for example, coaches or music teachers. Relationships of this kind permit the adolescent to focus on the skill-mastery while covertly enjoying an almost touchingly dependent relationship with the adult instructor.

Unfortunately the adolescent's initial perception of an adult who is offering psychiatric assistance has no such comfortable place to hide. It is apparently humiliating that the adolescent is the weak, supplicant member of the relationship. In addition, the very behaviors that may be identified by others as "the problem" may be emergency defensive operations that the adolescent perceives as essential to survival.

These interactions involving dependency help to explain why many adolescents adamantly refuse to admit their need for help and why the therapeutic relationships that they do develop are often tenuous and easily broken. However, there is a bright side to these characteristics of adolescence. Since the developmental phase is a fluid one, the potential for change is great. If appropriately managed, adolescent patients can show much more rapid positive progress than adults with comparable degrees of psychopathology. The treatment of the adolescent patient can be difficult but it can be also extremely rewarding.

NARCISSISTIC AND OMNIPOTENT DEFENSES IN THE ADOLESCENT

The approval of parenting figures is the primary source of self-esteem in younger children. Elementary school youngsters feel proud of themselves when their parents praise them. It is also important in the development of self-regard that youngsters feel they are competent people who are able to deal with most of the surrounding world successfully. Youngsters who are seven to 11 years old expend great efforts to learn about the world and to organize it carefully in their own minds. Because they think of themselves as competent and intelligent, they feel safe.

In early adolescence both of these gyroscopes of worthiness begin to spin wildly off course. Because of their compelling need to emancipate themselves and move toward independence, as well as the need to modify the inward rules of conscience to fit the realities of adult living, adolescents must gain psychological distance from parenting figures. Because of their secret yearning for dependency, as already described, this distancing is often accompanied by a subtle or overt denigration of important adults. After all, if your dad is a jerk, who would want his help anyway? Certainly you would not want his praise; in fact if he should offer it, you might well feel worse. At the same time that adolescents are deprived of praise as a nurturing dew to the flower of their self-esteem, their sense of competence is also shaken. With the maturation of their intellectual and cognitive capacities they begin to recognize that the world is larger and much more complex than the one that they had previously felt able to control. Education, the media, and contact with a wider world forces adolescents to recognize that life is much more complex than they imagined and that success in the adult world is not the simple matter of "playing house" and mimicking adults that they had once believed. To some extent, interpersonal relationships with peers may worsen the problem. Since most adolescents are extremely frightened about their worth, they often use age-mates to bolster self-confidence and to prove their capacity for conquest. This can create a very fickle pattern of relating in which there is little security. At the same time, each rejection increases the adolescent's need for reassurance, and an escalating intrigue of cliques, scapegoats, and social climbing can result.

With many of the previous underpinnings of self-esteem pulled away, it is not surprising that emergency measures have to be taken. If one can no longer feel competent, it is not hard to understand why there would be a return to earlier fantasies of omnipotence to reduce anxiety and restore value in the self. This method of addressing the world is also reinforced through the flowering of formal process cognition. Adolescents use this new capacity to construct brilliant and fanciful world systems, thereby rising above all practical difficulties, and equalizing or even defeating adult competitors. As a result, they feel much better about the world and their place in it. Unfortunately, omnipotence is a difficult state of mind to maintain because there is a pernicious tendency of other people and situations to produce challenges and defeats.

The impact of this pattern on the practitioner can be extremely confusing. If the adolescent is seen at one particular time—when his or her omnipotence defenses are working—he or she may appear almost bizarrely unconcerned about problems that seem serious and pressing to the physician. At these times the adolescent is comforted by a buoyant sense of being able to handle all difficulties without any need to be bothered with silly details. On the other hand the adolescent who is encountered at the time of collapse is more approachable but may be so helpless and despondent that he or she can bring little enthusiasm to the job of evaluation or treatment.

In view of these multiple forces acting to lower self-esteem it is little wonder that adolescents are preoccupied with the effort to build themselves up. As a result, they seem very self-centered. In addition, the rapid changes in body image and body sensations also focus self-interest and magnify the tendency toward self-absorption. For most adolescents it is not a pleasant process. Their efforts at self-love are thwarted by real and imagined defects in their perfection, which often lead to open or secret self-loathing. This is particularly true of the adolescent girl who regards herself as "ugly" because she compares herself with an imagined ideal of female beauty.

The adolescent boy does not fare much better and is plagued by vague or specific worries regarding his adequacy, strength, sexual prowess, and potential competency as an adult male. These painful defects in self-esteem, prodded by the absence of external sources of narcissistic support, lead to a variety of behaviors that may be viewed critically by adults. For example, adolescent girls may spend inordinate amounts of time primping, may speak for hours on the telephone with friends who can bolster self-esteem, or may show fickle behavior toward boyfriends and girlfriends alike. Adolescents must consider seriously the narcissistic implications of any friendship that they choose, particularly in the early stages of adolescent development. Relatively healthy adolescents may be able to tolerate a friendship with a youngster who is regarded as unpopular but many cannot. To belong to the "right" group is an important balm to the adolescent's aching ego.

Adolescents often find it difficult to accept criticism either from friends or from adults. This may lead to difficulties in school, where taking chances and making mistakes are required in order to progress educationally. It is obvious that referral for psychiatric treatment would be extremely difficult to accept. People who must admit that they need professional assistance to handle their emotional affairs suffer a blow to their pride, but such an admission is particularly excruciating to already anxious adolescents.

ACTING OUT
Another characteristic of the adolescent period that differs quantitatively although not qualitatively from people of different ages is the use of action. Most adolescents have a tendency to act first and think later. This is developmentally appropriate since adolescents do need to expand their life experience, encounter the wider world, and challenge old frames of reference. This cannot be done without actually trying out behaviors; just thinking is not enough. Physiologically this push to action is related to hormonal changes and to an apparent increase in aggressive drive that may be related to the accelerated growth process characteristic of the period.

Many psychotherapists find this proclivity toward "acting out" a negative aspect of the treatment effort with the adolescent. Many of us have come to value—if not overvalue—reflection, introspection, and thought. There is also a great need to support healthy defense mechanisms and self-control in the adolescent patient. This makes vigorous interpretation and exploration of the unconscious less desirable than in treatment efforts with the older individuals.

PSYCHOTHERAPY AND ADOLESCENTS
All of these characteristics definitely affect the way in which adolescents tend to approach their adult psychotherapist and in addition affects the way adolescents view the presence of "illness" in their personality. However, it is important to realize that all of these issues, while they require some technical adjustments, can be managed effectively if they are understood. Remember, adolescents are primarily more similar to than different from all other human beings. The therapist who has good basic skills in empathy and basic interviewing and a solid foundation in theoretical understanding of the process of psychotherapy can easily adapt these capabilities to the psychotherapy of the adolescent patient. The section on treatment will discuss some of the adjustments suggested by various practitioners in this field.

Diagnostic Evaluation of the Adolescent Patient

A medical student on his first psychiatry rotation was interviewing a 15-year-old adolescent boy in a group setting. The adolescent and the medical student talked for 15 or 20 minutes about the youngster's problems. The adolescent explained that he had family difficulties, particularly because his parents disapproved of his smoking marijuana, staying out late, and running around with a "a bad crowd." The medical student had been told that friendship patterns among adolescents could reveal valuable diagnostic information and decided to pursue the issue of friends and peer relationship.

Medical student	You have a lot of friends, then?
Patient	Yeah, lots of friends.
Medical student	Who would you say is your best friend?
Patient	I would say God is my best friend.
Medical student (smiling and nodding)	I understand that but I meant human friends like those you can talk to.
Patient	God and I talk.

The medical student was obviously flustered but recovered after a few moments and elicited an elaborate delusional system accompanied by hallucinations in this schizophrenic adolescent.

The point of this vignette is that all adolescents try to present themselves in some sort of conformity to the social stereotype—that is, they emphasize conflict with parents, good relationships with friends, and some capacity for acting out. However, although they wear the same uniform, their marching orders can vary widely. Careful diagnostic evaluation without prior assumptions is extremely important in order to discover the basic pathologic process, which may be obscured to some extent by the external accoutrements of the developmental period. It is particularly important with adolescents to resist the temptation to make a one-to-one connection between the presenting symptoms and their basic difficulty. For example, many delinquent youngsters in fact suffer from severe cases of traditional psychiatric disorders.

In planning the diagnostic evaluation of the adolescent, there are some practical issues that do not arise in regard to adult evaluations. For example, should one interview the adolescent's parents prior to meeting for the first diagnostic interview with the adolescent? Should one utilize a family conjoint interview as part of the diagnostic process? There are no definite answers to these questions; in fact the situation is to some extent unresolvable. If one sees the adolescent first, there are risks that he or she will leave out significant information, present facts in a distorted way, or manipulate the evaluator, who may be somewhat more vulnerable because of a lack of data. For example, delinquent adolescents may present a very one-sided view of family circumstances and events, challenging the therapist to defend the appropriateness of psychiatric intervention. This can be dealt with if the therapist is comfortable saying, "I would be glad to respond to that question, but only after collecting all available information from a variety of sources." The real danger, however, is that the adolescents may, in the process, "paint themselves into a corner" by solidifying a resistant position that might not have developed if the therapist had been better informed regarding the overall situation. On the other hand, if the parents are seen first, there is always the danger that the adolescents will see the evaluator as only an agent of the parents and may adopt a passive-aggressive position of, "Why are you asking me? My parents have probably told you all about that." Again, all of these attitudes can be successfully managed if they are anticipated and if their subtle forms are recognized quickly.

As a rule of thumb some have recommended that adolescents age 15 and older be seen first before their parents, while those younger than 15 should be seen after the parents have been interviewed for background history. This dividing line is related as much to cognitive development as to psychological issues. In other words, it is usually only at around age 15 that an adolescent is able to conceptualize an overall situation and report it in a somewhat "adult" fashion. In addition, it may be wise to see the parents first if there is reason to believe that the adolescent is going to be strongly resistant to the evaluation process; in this case, in spite of the dangers that have been described, the need to ensure total parental cooperation and to plan appropriate strategies that allow completion of the evaluation becomes the most important factor.

INTERVIEWING THE PARENTS

Regardless of whether they are interviewed before or after the adolescent is seen, it is imperative that interviews with the parents be included as part of a diagnostic evaluation. A great deal of information is needed that can be obtained only from that source. Each parent should be asked separately if there is a history of mental illness on either side of the family. This question should be gentle but probing, searching for "peculiar aunts" who on closer inspection may appear to be schizophrenic or to suffer from a major affective illness.

A careful social history is a basic requirement for understanding psychological development. This history includes a history of the marital adjustment or any separations and remarriages that affected this youngster's history; the family structure, including siblings and other relatives who have lived within the home; important separations from parenting figures; geographic moves; and all of the other events that shape external experience. In addition, one should seek as much detail as possible regarding the youngster's intellectual and psychosocial developmental progress. Although parental reports of dates and events may be factually inaccurate, the overall picture may indicate certain clusters of difficulties in the development process. In addition, reviewing this early history of the child often allows the parents an opportunity to reveal important emotional attitudes toward the youngster that predate the current difficulty. Temperament is an important aspect of early development to pursue. Was he or she extremely active, very intense, accepting of novelty, or inclined to settle into a natural and predictable habit pattern? In addition to this background material concerning development, a social history should carefully focus on possible precipitating events that may help to shed light on the adolescent's current illness. These events have important diagnostic and prognostic implications since the presence of clear-cut major external stress is often associated with a stronger premorbid personality and therefore a more positive outlook for cure.

In deriving both a family history and information regarding recent precipitants, one should ask about external sources of information that may be useful. These may include family photographs, baby books, school records, and other more objective information sources.

Finally, it is important to assess the parental motivation for therapy and the degree of alienation that may exist because of the adolescent's difficulties. It is also important to determine the degree to which parents are able to support independence and emancipation, as opposed to the degree to which there may be pathologic needs to maintain the adolescent in a dependent posture with the family.

DIRECT INTERVIEW WITH THE ADOLESCENT

A careful diagnostic interview of the adolescent patient may reveal a surprising amount of usable information. Some adolescents, after a brief period of testing, are able to relate with a fair degree of honesty and openness. In these cases the overall interview experience is not materially different from that involving an adult psychiatic patient.

Direct information may be much more difficult to obtain from other adolescents. Because of their discomfort with adults, as described earlier, these adolescents tend to be extremely wary of the evaluator. There are a number of ways they may use to test the diagnostician. They may present in an argumentative or uncooperative manner that is motivated both by a desire to divert attention from their difficulties and by an unrecognized wish that the diagnostician will recognize and respond to this indirect indication of discomfort. It may be informative to observe the assumptions that the adolescent seems to make regarding the diagnostician. For example, some adolescents seem to approach the examiner as though they anticipated harsh criticism; others may behave in such a way as to suggest that they expect to be able to intimidate and overwhelm adults; while still others may approach in a subservient and obsequious manner, flattering the adult. All of these approaches are likely to occur more blatantly with adolescents because they are somewhat more naive about the conventional behavior expected in an interview situation with a physician. This is actually fortunate in that it allows a more direct view of some of their images of adults and their relationships to them. Of course, from a practical viewpoint it is necessary for the diagnostician to correct any extreme distortions of perception—whether these derive from the adolescent patient or from misinformation provided by the parents. The examiner needs to explain the real purpose of the interview accurately and briefly.

In any case it is important to proceed patiently in the collection of both the direct verbal information and the inferred and nonverbal data while providing the adolescent with some appropriately chosen immediate feedback. Adolescents are very frightened of adult evaluation of them and will be extremely apprehensive about the impression and attitudes they may be making on the examiner. For this reason it is important not to remain silent and noncommittal but to offer some verbal reaction as the interview progresses. Naturally, this does not include detailed speculations; instead, brief comments that are truthful and informative are appropriate. For example, when interviewing adolescents who describe a variety of situations in which they have become angry even if they regard themselves as victimized, one could say, "It sounds as though you feel a lot of people are treating you unfairly, and under those circumstances you have a pretty hot temper." This is important not only to convey your dispassionate, neutral, and understanding attitude toward the material presented but also in order to begin to offer the adolescents a conceptual framework within which they can view his difficulties and begin to reflect on their problems in living.

It needs to be reemphasized that the basic diagnostic interview needs to be completed with the adolescent even if this requires a longer period of time and a greater amount of tact than might be necessary with the adult patient. The mental status examination involves the same basic framework that one uses in evaluating adult psychiatric disorders; one must analyse solid data regarding state of consciousness, memory functions, evaluation of affect, and presence of pathologic thought processes, even if the adolescent patient has trouble cooperating. Some adolescents may be offended when asked, for example, if they have heard voices speaking to them when no one was there. When this reaction occurs it is because of the concreteness, narcissism, omnipotence, and self-centeredness of those individual adolescents. They are offended because they feel that the question reveals an opinion of them—namely, that they are crazy. When the examiner makes clear that the question is routine and is part of an effort at completeness, the problem is usually solved. In fact, it is useful with anxious or suspicious adolescents to forestall such a response by explaining, "I will ask many routine questions that may not apply to you."

ANCILLARY STUDIES

After interviewing the adolescent and his or her family it may be necessary to obtain additional information. Psychological testing may be desired in order to assess treatment strengths or to continue probing for a suspected underlying psychotic disorder. Educational testing may be necessary in order to determine the presence or absence of a learning disability and to assess the current capacity for dealing with school demands. Other youngsters may require neurologic evaluation, electroencephalography, special endocrine studies, or other data to complete the diagnostic process.

With the adolescent patient it is important to give a careful explanation of each test and its purpose while firmly insisting on the necessity that the tests be completed. Even if the adolescent is frightened and distrustful, medical responsibility requires insistance that necessary procedures eventually be performed. It is not essential, of course, to have an instant showdown and a battle for control. In fact, some adolescents will resist necessary procedures in order to learn something about how the diagnostician responds to rebellion and disobedience. This is important diagnostic information since many of these youngsters have long utilized defiance of adults as a means of avoiding anxiety-producing information about themselves and their personalities.

FAMILY INTERVIEW

Many diagnosticians prefer to have at least one conjoint family interview as part of the diagnostic process. At times family alliances and interactions become much more obvious when the entire family meets together in a single room. Family interviews can be particularly useful in determining the role that peers may play in the adolescent's difficulties. This interview is also useful in clarifying the neutral diagnostic attitude of the evaluator. The adolescent has the opportunity to see the interviewer respond to parental complaints and accusations as data to be understood rather than as divinely revealed truth. For example, the parents say, "Johnny is totally hopeless; I'm sure he'll end up in a reform school." This gives the interviewer a chance to say, "At this point the problem is even worse because *you're* feeling frustrated and discouraged. It sounds as though you have lost some of your faith in Johnny and in yourself as parents. We'll have to try to understand how things got to this point."

This family interview is a model that many practitioners also use as a vehicle to convey their diagnostic findings and recommendations. Although it may take some experience to learn how to discuss the adolescent's difficulties in a family setting, there is a great deal to be said for the process. Needless to say, it is important to avoid blame, taking sides, or overstatements of certainty regarding diagnosis or prognosis. At the same time, it is important to be informative and to avoid a bland, noncommittal position that may leave the family totally in the dark regarding your findings. For example, in discussing a schizophrenic youngster it is important to describe the confusion, disorganization of feelings, and other aspects of the illness in human terms but in ways that do not artificially diminish their importance and seriousness. If questions are raised about the chronicity of the illness or its prognosis, or if one of the family members asks directly about the presence of schizophrenia, an approach of modest honesty is probably best. Often it will be necessary to say that the illness does resemble some types of schizophrenia, while adding that there are many varieties of the illness and that it is too early to predict the probable long-term course of the problem. Obviously, it will be important to ask for perceptions of the implications of such a diagnosis. None of this is meant to imply a suspension of clinical judgment. For example, if a family has a pattern of making the youngster the scapegoat, one should avoid falling into that trap by holding back from applying the label. In those instances it might be more appropriate to say, "I think the family's desire to have a simple explanation for Johnny's difficulties, although understandable, may be making things worse. Merely assigning a name to the problems your son is having will not help."

In short, although these reporting interviews need to be handled with delicacy, there may be advantages to doing them in the family format in order to establish a generalized understanding of the nature of the problem, the planned treatment interventions, and the contributions each family member needs to make to the success of that effort.

In other cases it may be wise to hold separate reporting interviews. Examples of this kind of case include those families in which the interaction is so malignant that one can be virtually assured of a negative result on any effort at joint discussion. As a rule, patients with problems this severe would be those who probably require hospitalization or other separation from the family at any rate. The decision should be based on the goal of the completed diagnostic evaluation. This goal is to derive a clinical and dynamic diagnosis, to devise a rational treatment plan, and to provide the groundwork for cooperation with the treatment effort. Since with almost all adolescent patients this involves at least some passive cooperation from the family, it is wise to include them in some form.

Pediatric Treatment of the Adolescent

OUTPATIENT TREATMENT

As already mentioned, the goal of the diagnostic evaluation is to determine a treatment plan that addresses the psychiatric disability of the adolescent. For most patients evaluated the needed intervention will involve some form of outpatient treatment. There are certain basic requirements for successful outpatient therapy. The adolescents treated in this way must have some capacity to contain themselves short of dangerous or self-destructive behavior, and there must be some provision for reasonably accurate presentation of on-going life experiences in the interview situation. If individual psychotherapy is contemplated, this implies a capacity on the part of the patients to bring a significant portion of their personal experience to the therapist for discussion. In family psychotherapy this ability may be less crucial, since other family members may be able to provide the factual information and observations required to intervene. Group psychotherapy may also require less overt cooperativeness and verbalization since one can depend on the peer pressure in an adequately functioning group to push individual adolescents toward a more expressive stance.

In order to consider outpatient psychotherapy in any form, it is necessary to ensure a reasonable degree of family cooperativeness. Many families of disturbed adolescents have ambivalent feelings about permitting their youngsters to mature. One can anticipate certain resistances and unconscious efforts to sabotage therapy under the best of circumstances. However, it is essential that the basic thrust of the family be toward permitting if not encouraging maturation. For example, the family that genuinely desires independence for their adolescent may still continue to infantilize or intrude but are prepared to recognize and accept the impact of this behavior on the adolescent's efforts to become emancipated; the family members are willing to open this behavior to therapeutic scrutiny in the interest of the mental health of their child.

There are no diagnoses that absolutely rule out the possibility of outpatient therapy, although many serious cases of drug abuse, disorganized psychotic youngsters, habitual runaways, and adolescents with other dangerous symptom presentations are difficult to treat successfully on an outpatient basis. Even more crucial is the patient's ability to become involved in a relationship with the therapist. Youngsters with relatively severe acting out may be rapidly able to control this behavior when provided with the support and assistance of a therapist.

Outpatient psychotherapy with the adolescent is in many respects not substantially different from individual, group, or family psychotherapy with adult patients. Adolescents become involved in transference relationships, demonstrate resistance behaviors, and respond to confrontations, clarifications, and interpretations in much the same way as do psychiatric patients of any age. As mentioned earlier, the initial period of therapy is often somewhat more tumultuous than with adult patients because adolescents have difficulty in comfortably accepting responsibility for their own lives and because of their tendency to be anxious regarding dependency relationships with adults. If the therapist is patient and empathic, yet clear and firm during the early phases of therapy, these testing behaviors are often answered to the patients' satisfaction so that therapy can proceed in a relatively routine manner. (The discussion of the details of outpatient psychotherapy with the adolescent is beyond the scope of this chapter.)

PHARMACOTHERAPY

Surprisingly little is known about the use of psychoactive medication in adolescents. Research in this area does not even approach the depth of studies of medication effects in older patients. This lack of information is partly because of a general reluctance to use medications with younger patients, but perhaps there may be a tendency to deny the intensity of severe psychiatric disorders when they appear in the young.

It does seem clear that schizophrenic adolescents require and respond to antipsychotic medication in much the same way that older schizophrenics do. There are dosage variations that are difficult to explain. These variations in response may be related to the rapid physiologic changes of adolescents but may also result partially from the developmental turbulence of the period and perhaps from the adolescent's reluctance to accept ther dependent position implied by accepting medication. Appropriate dosage is often achieved only by trial and error, and medication acceptance may be encouraged by the use of a single dose administrated at bedtime. Many severely disturbed adolescents may require a brief period of hospitalization in order to stabilize them on the appropriate medication and dosage. Compliance may be a greater problem than among adult patients but can be obtained if a good therapeutic relationship exists with the prescribing physician.

Antidepressant medications seem to benefit some depressed adolescents, but the indications for the use of these medications is not entirely clear. Therapeutic trials with very depressed adolescents are probably wise since some of these youngsters show considerable amelioration of symptoms through this approach. It may be that medication is especially effective with those patients who have a family history of unipolar or bipolar depression, but this is by no means proved at present. Occasional adolescents show clear-cut bipolar illness, and they may respond to lithium for treatment of the manic phase and prevention of depressed episodes.

Minor tranquilizers are of dubious assistance during the adolescent phase of life, as are stimulants such as dextroamphetamine (Dexedrine) and methylphenidate (Ritalin); however, they may be useful in specific cases. The potential for drug abuse and self-medication is extremely high in adolescents because of the endemic dissatisfaction with the self and the difficulty in maintaining and regulating a positive mood and positive self-esteem. Many of the minor tranquilizers are in fact, utilized "on the street" as drugs of abuse and should be prescribed with extreme caution to adolescent patients.

It should be noted that many adolescents and their families are somewhat negative toward the use of any kind of medication, particularly in youngsters who have a history of drug abuse. The philosophical issues that are often raised in this age group might be summed up as, "Why are your drugs any better than mine, Doc?" Although there is superficial cogency to this question, the major tranquilizers and the antidepressant drugs are rarely used as drugs of abuse. They provide little in the way of pleasurable altered states of consciousness and carry with them unpleasant side effects that make them unattractive for recreational use. It should be noted that in this stage of our understanding, all use of pharmacologic agents in adolescents should be viewed as ancillary to the primary psychological approaches to them and their families. If drugs can add constructively to the youngsters' ability to benefit from these treatment approaches, the aid should not be withheld. In all likelihood over the next decade we will understand a great deal more about the appropriate use of this type of treatment in younger age groups.

HOSPITAL TREATMENT

The decision to hospitalize an adolescent is always reached reluctantly. There are obvious disadvantages in that hospitalization may encourage a self-identity as a "mental patient," because of separation from the community and because of the potential infantilizing effects of the hospital experience. In spite of all of these concerns, many adolescents do require inpatient treatment. Some of them have to be hospitalized because they are dangerous to themselves or to others in their environment. Many depressed and suicidal adolescents fall into this group, as do a large number of psychotic youngsters and those in panic states. Other adolescents have to be hospitalized not so much because of acute emergencies related to their immediate behavior but because they are totally immobilized in their capacity to continue psychological development. These impasses in the developmental process may be related to chronic family psychopathology that cannot be treated without separating the youngster from the family setting; the problems may also result from crippling defenses that the adolescent has erected, effectively removing him or her from adolescent life. Youngsters who have developed such defenses of constriction and avoidance that they cannot attend school or leave their home can only be reached by placing them in an atmosphere where they will have human contact within the limits of their anxiety.

The goals of hospital treatment need to be carefully considered in each clinical situation. For most adolescents the hospital involvement is only a phase in an overall treatment plan, which may require a period of partial hospitalization or outpatient treatment for an extended period after the inpatient care. The current pressure for brief hospitalization can be carried to extremes, however, if the problems that required the inpatient placement are not resolved before attempting a continuation in a less restrictive environment.

Effective hospital treatment of the adolescent is a complex topic that cannot be adequately treated in a general text. Effective programs seem to combine peer interaction, family intervention, psychotherapy, appropriate medication, and construction of a corrective and healing milieu. Follow-up studies suggest that appropriate hospital treatment is an effective intervention for many psychiatrically disturbed adolescents.

RESIDENTIAL TREATMENT

Residential treatment centers as a rule provide a level of care somewhere between the supportive boarding school and the intense inpatient hospital setting. The residential treatment centers that exist vary greatly; some specialize in particular types of youngsters, such as those with learning disabilities, while others serve a wide variety of youngsters from a geographic region. Many residential treatment centers not only serve as sources of therapy but are seen as long-term substitute family placement for youngsters who have no viable family support system. For this reason many residential treatment centers require placement of at least a year, and they often try to provide corrective living experiences for a youngster over an extended part of their adolescent years.

FAMILY PARTICIPATION
IN ONGOING THERAPY

In all treatment approaches except for long-term residential placement, the family remains actively involved in the adolescent's life. Recognizing the truth of this situation, most therapists provide for active family treatment and contact.

It has to be recognized that many families of disturbed adolescents are ambivalent about being involved in the treatment process. Although many are quite cooperative, others may be so angry or frightened that they find it extremely difficult to accept any responsibility for the adolescent's difficulties. In other cases, the parents are so overwhelmed with guilt and self-blame that they find it difficult to support a treatment effort that asks their youngster to assume some responsibility for helping himself or herself. These parents often identify with the adolescent in a regressive manner; in addition, they find fault with the treatment attempts of the therapist in a way as dependent and unrealistic as the attitude of the adolescent toward the parents. The parents anticipate the same kind of guilty capitulation and are often reassured and supported when the therapist maintains self-respect and firmly indicates the expectation for the adolescent's support and assistance in the treatment effort.

Many other parents are in fact to some extent emotionally neglectful of their adolescents. This neglect may be because of inherent psychopathology in the parent or it may be the result of an extended period of interaction so negative that emotional withdrawal was the only feasible solution that allowed the parents to maintain some sanity and self-esteem. At any rate these parents need to be given some opportunity to ventilate their negative and rejecting feelings; they should not be burdened with excessive guilt-inducing comments. Often, provided with some evidence of the adolescent's improvement and approachability and offered some support and understanding, these parents become excellent collaborators in the treatment effort and are gradually able to look at some of their own responsibility for inducing the original difficulties.

Most parents are neither overly involved nor neglectful. They are understandably perplexed about the nature of their adolescent's problems and need support and direction in becoming helpful in the treatment effort. Mental health professionals need to recall that most parents have had no training in the style of thinking or the technical approaches of psychotherapeutic intervention. Parents deserve an explanation of the treatment plans and some assistance in understanding how "just talking" could possibly be beneficial in a problem that they regard as so catastrophic and puzzling. A therapeutic alliance with the parents is a crucial part of the treatment effort directed to any adolescent patient.

Case 1. T.L. was a 15-year-old male brought to the emergency room because of fear, agitation, and strange thoughts. History revealed that T. had always been a quiet and compliant youngster, mildly fearful of authority. His parents were divorced and T. lived with his mother and maternal grandmother until two weeks prior to admission, when T.'s mother abruptly left the grandmother's home and T. She had not contacted T. during the following two weeks. T. went to live with his father and immediately threw himself into vigorous efforts to improve his life. He learned to drive and got a job at whirlwind speed.

While at work the night before admission, T. began to think everyone suspected him of drug use (he had never used drugs). He began to fear his father and his siblings, suspecting that they planned to kill him. He felt automobiles were passing his house to observe him. He was frightened of the examiner, thinking he could be part of the conspiracy. T. felt he had been brought to the hospital for execution.

Mental status revealed a frightened, agitated youngster with flushing, tachycardia, and dilated pupils. Affect was flattened and associations were loosened. Blocking was noted. T. was guarded and suspicious. Sensorium was clear and memory was intact.

Diagnosis was of acute schizophrenic reaction. T. was treated with phenothiazines, and the symptoms cleared rapidly. After four weeks in the hospital he was discharged to outpatient therapy.

Case 2. M.C., a 16-year-old male, was admitted to a psychiatric hospital because of extreme seclusiveness. M. had always been shy but had gradually isolated himself to a degree that his family could not accept. He stopped attending school, almost never left the home unless accompanied by parents, and became very quiet even in the household. M.'s parents were interested in him but had very different perceptions of his problems. His mother felt sorry for the boy and felt that her husband "pushed" M. too much. The father, on the other hand, felt that his wife was overly indulgent with her son and complained that she and M. were "too close."

Mental status evaluation revealed no evidence of psychosis or brain damage in M. He was shy but warm and socially aware. He said he did not go to school or out into the neighborhood because "the kids are too tough." A diagnosis of avoidant disorder of adolescence was established. Treatment with family, group, and individual psychotherapy was begun in the hospital, along with active efforts to encourage M. to socialize. After some months the therapy was continued on an outpatient basis, with continuing success.

Case 3. B.R. was admitted to a psychiatric hospital after several efforts at outpatient treatment over a three-year period had failed to influence her antisocial behavior. B. was in complete rebellion against her family's rules and, in fact, basically ignored them. She attended school sporadically and, as a result, was failing the tenth grade. The parents had reason to believe B. was active sexually, used drugs of all kinds extensively, and stole from stores and from her brother.

On examination B. was belligerent, challenging, and uncooperative. She denied problems and suggested her parents should be hospitalized instead of her. A mental status evaluation, which was completed with great difficulty, showed no evidence of psychosis or organic brain disease.

On the unit B. broke rules, taunted staff, and organized the other patients in rebellious groups. She required extensive supervision yet complained bitterly that "no one trusts me." The parents were clearly both angry with her and intimidated by her. They felt very guilty and ashamed because of her problems.

The patient gradually responded to the firm rules of the unit and began to behave more appropriately. The parents also began to be more effective, although the mother sometimes expressed concerns that the hospital's expectations were perhaps too "conventional" for a "free spirit" like B. Progress was very slow over an extended period of inpatient, day-hospital, and outpatient treatment.

Betty was diagnosed as suffering from a conduct disorder and as being undersocialized and nonaggressive.

APPENDIX A
The Psychiatric Disorders of Adolescence
I. Major psychotic disorders
   A. Affective psychoses. Both unipolar depressive disorders and bipolar depressive disorders occur during the adolescent years. They may be somewhat atypical in comparison with the comparable syndromes in adulthood but the basic patterns of diagnosis including family history, severity of mood disturbance, and response to organic therapies still obtain.
   B. Schizophrenic disorders. The schizophrenic disorders were at one time referred to as dementia praecox because of their common onset during adolescence. Symptom pictures are those described in other portions of the text pertaining to adults.
II. Neurotic disorders
   A. Depressive neurosis.
   B. Anxiety neurosis.
   C. Phobic disorders. These include school avoidance or school phobia, as described elsewhere.
   D. Neurotic inhibitions. These include school failure, social withdrawal, and other patterns of personality constriction.
III. Primary disorders of behavior
   A. Disorders of socialization (see diagnostic criteria in Appendix B).
   B. Exaggerated behavioral patterns. This includes excessive shyness, extreme patterns of social avoidance, oppositional behavior, and passive aggressive behavior when these are so pervasive and repetitive that they impair flexibility and adaptive management of life problems.
   C. Substance abuse. Alcoholism or excessive intake of other drugs may be a major component of antisocial behavior or may begin in an atmosphere of anxiety or depression as an effort at self-treatment. Eventually the drug addiction may become the primary difficulty.

IV. Psychological maladjustments secondary to physical illness, organic brain damage, or primary learning disabilities. Any illness, brain damage, mental retardation, or learning disability that interferes with the capacity to learn adaptive skills and rules of socialization may result in secondary symptoms of emotional maladjustment. Youngsters with problems of this kind are often less sure of themselves, more suspicious of adults, and frequently mildly depressed. Their chronic difficulties in achieving the success comparable to their age-mates and the negative reaction that they elicit in many adults may cause severe adjustment problems, particularly when the real nature of their difficulties are unrecognized.

Appendix B
DSM-III Categories Related to Adolescence

MENTAL RETARDATION
Mental retardation is divided into four subtypes:

317.0, mild retardation, IQ 50–70
318.0, moderate retardation, IQ 35–49
318.1, severe retardation, IQ 20–34
318.2, profound retardation, IQ below 20

Although it is unusual to encounter adolescents who are being diagnosed as mentally retarded for the first time, there are adolescents whose emotional difficulties are primarily secondary to mental retardation. One should be particularly alert to this possibility in youngsters with behavior disorders since some delinquent behavior is a result of chronic frustration and is based on a need to gain positive recognition and a sense of mastery after years of continued academic failure.

Appropriate educational intervention is indicated for adolescents with mental retardation. It is important to recognize the adolescent's sensitivity to appearing childish. For this reason, educational materials have to be carefully constructed so that they are simple enough for the retarded youngster while avoiding content and style more appropriate for younger children.

ATTENTION DEFICIT DISORDERS
The attention deficit disorders are divided into three subgroups.

314.01: attention deficit disorder with hyperactivity
314.00: attention deficit disorder without hyperactivity
314.80: attention deficit disorder, residual type

In adolescents one most commonly encounters the residual type of attention deficit disorder. Most adolescents who were hyperactive or had severe attention deficit problems as younger children have dropped the most flagrant symptoms as they mature. However, restlessness, impulsivity, and general disorganization may still be apparent. These problems may result in poor school performance, difficulty in relating with family members, and problems with gaining appropriate independence.

CONDUCT DISORDERS
The conduct disorders are divided into five types:

312.00, conduct disorder, undersocialized, aggressive
312.10, conduct disorder, undersocialized, nonaggressive
312.23, conduct disorder, socialized, aggressive
312.21, conduct disorder, socialized, nonaggressive
312.90, atypical conduct disorder

The first four conduct disorders are self-explanatory. The atypical conduct disorder diagnosis is used when a youngster regularly transgresses societal norms without a clear pattern that would allow classification in the four primary diagnostic categories.

Conduct disorders are common during the adolescent years. While a certain amount of rebelliousness is normal for this phase of life; thus it is necessary to differentiate the conduct disorders from nonpathologic behavior. It is also important to rule out mental retardation, learning disorders, severe temperamental deviations, and other constitutional and organic predisposing conditions. If these are present, remediation for the basic problems must accompany the psychological approach to the family and youngster in the treatment process.

ANXIETY DISORDERS
OF CHILDHOOD OR ADOLESCENCE
There are three specific anxiety disorders of childhood or adolescence:

309.21, separation anxiety disorder
313.21, avoidant disorder of childhood or adolescence
313.00, overanxious disorder

The diagnosis of separation anxiety disorder is used particularly in youngsters with a pattern of school avoidance. When separation anxiety appears first during adolescence it should be investigated carefully since it may indicate a more severe basic psychopathology. For example, some adolescents with school avoidance are in fact schizophrenic or manic depressive.

Youngsters with avoidant disorder of childhood or adolescence are often pathologically shy and yet do not show the severe personality distortion associated with schizoid disorders. They usually relate well to family members and people they have known for a long time but are extremely reluctant to interact with strangers. This behavior in its less severe forms is one variant of normality; in fact the problem should be diagnosed only if there is genuine interference with appropriate development—for example, if the condition is so severe that it precludes appropriate friendships.

OTHER DISORDERS OF ADOLESCENCE
The specific disorders related to adolescents included in this DSM-III category are as follows:

313.22, schizoid disorder of adolescence
313.23, elective mutism
313.81, oppositional disorder
313.82, identity disorder

Schizoid disorder of adolescence, as mentioned earlier, is a more damaging and severe reason for shyness and withdrawal. The problem is typically quite chronic and the youngster often has unusual or even bizarre secret interests without, however, clear evidence of psychosis.

Youngsters with elective mutism seem warm and affectionate but simply refuse to speak in most situations outside of their home.

Youngsters with oppositional disorder do not show clear conduct disturbance in that they do not break major rules or seriously violate the rights of others. They are primarily "troublemakers" who violate minor rules, argue chronically, and provoke others. They are notable for their extreme stubbornness.

Identity disorder is a common diagnosis in middle to late adolescence, when issues of identity are quite central to development. It is important, however, to be sure that more serious illnesses such as schizophrenia are not dismissed as "adolescent turmoil" or identity disorder.

EATING DISORDERS
The following are the specific eating disorders that affect adolescents (they are fully discussed in Chapter 14):

Anorexia nervosa
Bulimia
Pica

STEREOTYPED MOVEMENT DISORDERS
AND OTHER DISORDERS
WITH PHYSICAL MANIFESTATIONS
Transient tic disorder
Chronic motor tic disorder
Tourette's disorder

Stuttering
Sleepwalking disorder
Sleep terror disorder

PERVASIVE DEVELOPMENTAL DISORDERS
The diagnosis of childhood-onset pervasive development disorder, residual state (299.91) fits some youngsters whose early development was not so distorted as to justify a diagnosis of infantile autism but who do show severe enough symptoms of extreme anxiety, peculiarities of movement, and resistance to change that they seem quite atypical in their peer group.

SPECIFIC DEVELOPMENTAL DISORDERS
The specific developmental disorders, which are coded on axis II, are as follows:

315.00, developmental reading disorder
315.10, developmental arithmetic disorder
315.31, developmental language disorder
315.39, developmental articulation disorder
315.50, mixed specific developmental disorder

These diagnoses are based on the demonstration of a significant defect in learning capacity in one or more cognitive areas, when the defect is not due to mental retardation or organic brain damage. The negative impact of development and the likelihood of secondary psychological symptomatology developing during adolescence have been mentioned earlier in this chapter (p. 230).

References and Further Reading

Blos, P. *On Adolescense*. New York: Free Press of Glencoe, 1963.
Blos, P. The second individuation process of adolescence. *Psychoanal. Stud. Child* 22: 162–186, 1967.
Blos, P. Character formation in adolescence. *Psychoanal. Stud. Child* 23:245–263, 1968.
Freud, A. Adolescence. *Psychoanal. Stud. Child* 13:255–278, 1958.
Gitelson, M. Character synthesis: the psychotherapeutic problem of adolescence. *Am. J. Orthopsychiatry* 18:422–431, 1948.
Josselyn, I.M. The ego in adolescence. *Am. J. Orthopsychiatry* 24:223–237, 1954.
Josselyn, I.M. Psychotherapy of adolescents at the level of private practice. In Balser, B.H. (ed.), *Psychotherapy of the Adolescent*. New York: International Universities Press, 1957.
Kett, J.F. *Rites of Passage: Adolescence in America 1970 to the Present*. New York: Basic Books, 1977.
Lewis, J.W., Beavers, W.R., Gossett, J.T., Phillips, V.A. *No Single Thread: Psychological Health in Family Systems*. New York: Brunner/Mazel, 1976.
Masterson, J.F. Psychiatric treatment of adolescents. In Freedman, A., and Kaplan, H. (eds.), *Comprehensive Textbook of Psychiatry*. Baltimore: Williams & Wilkins, 1967.
Meeks, J.E. *The Fragile Alliance*. Malabar, Fla.: Robert E. Krieger, 1980.
Novello, J.R. (ed.). *The Short Course in Adolescent Psychiatry*. New York: Brunner/Mazel, 1979.
Robins, L.N. *Deviant Children Grown Up*. Baltimore: Williams & Wilkins, 1966.
Thomas, A., Chess, S., Birch, H.G. *Temperament and Behavior Disorders in Children*. New York: New York University Press, 1968.

16

Geriatric Disorders
DAVID H. FRAM, M.D.

Aging is a physiologic and psychological process that affects us all. For those of us fortunate enough to reach the older years, aging becomes a reminder of the finite time each of us has to live. Although we have devised numerous ways—religious, cultural, and psychological—to attempt to come to terms with our eventual deaths, the passage of time affects us all, no matter how we attempt to cope.

In the course of growing older, people encounter certain problems that need special focus. The elderly are likely to encounter repeated losses and are, therefore, especially vulnerable to depression. Older people are subject to a gradual physical deterioration that may manifest itself in the nervous system through organic mental signs from extremely subtle to marked degrees. While most psychiatric disorders may continue into older life, there are several that are characteristic of old age.

The latter years of life have the potential for being the creative climax of life, but far too often they are years of misery and decline. This period of life should be a time for enjoying the ripened fruits of one's life experience. The older person needs to continue to view each day as holding the possibility for new experience, new learning, and new beginnings. It is the creative integration of new experience with the wealth of previously accumulated experience that enables the older person to remain vibrant and vital. Health professionals must try to minimize the effects of disabling processes and to foster continued growth and development through the final phases of life.

The Aging Process
The definition of old age is certainly not clearcut. Age 65 is commonly considered the boundary between middle age and old age, and age 75 can be said to be the boundary between early and late old age. It is evident that there is much variability among individuals, rendering chronologic age only a rough estimate of the status of a given person's aging process. Emotionally healthy older people, then, are those who integrate the losses and changes that inevitably occur with time into their previous experience so that life continues to have meaning. The developmental struggles and crises of the earlier phases have ideally resulted in the achievement of wisdom and maturity not possible in earlier years. The perspective of time may give older people a deeper understanding that may enhance the quality of their lives. It is important that the older person see this period of life as a final developmental stage in which a flexible approach to life is maintained, and life can be contemplated as a nearly completed whole.

Individuals, as conceptualized by Erikson (see also the discussion of the etiology of personality disorders in Chapter 13), arrive at late adulthood having faced certain developmental milestones. Building on childhood development, they have struggled for identity during adolescent years, have attempted intimate relationships with other autonomous individuals beginning in early adulthood, and have given of themselves in later adulthood by their unique contributions and by inspiration to others.

Arriving at old age, much of what previously had been meaningful may have disappeared. Children may have grown up and established their own lives. Career goals may have been achieved, but retirement transfers the responsibilities to others. Life may not have had all the satisfying achievements sought after, and older people may come to realize that these goals may never be achieved. The work of old age is partly to take stock of the past and to find a purpose for leading the rest of life.

Some of the reminiscing that elderly people do is, to a significant degree, an attempt to find purpose. The maintenance of ego integrity includes the creative recollection of the important aspects of the past with preservation of the meaningful aspects of the present in the person's identity. Coupled with this must be an active search for new meaning. New activities and interests must emerge for true personal development to continue.

BIOLOGIC FEATURES OF AGING

The elderly are frequently seen as rigid, forgetful, cantankerous, suspicious, and weak. They are often seen as sickly and dependent on others. Intellectual functions are thought to be in decline. The elderly are often considered to be nonsexual, and they may be thought of as deviant if sexual interests persist. While it is true that some of the above characteristics may be present to a degree in elderly people, there is great variability in appearance as people grow older. Some individuals seem to age very rapidly while others retain youthful characteristics despite advanced age. Sexual activity in both sexes has been shown in various studies to continue into advanced age in healthy individuals. Negative attitudes about sexuality in the elderly appear to contribute to premature demise of sexuality. It is important to distinguish between aging and disease. Quite apart from the multitude of diseases that can afflict people, especially the elderly, the aging process itself is a distinct entity to be considered. Research into the biologic aging process has proceeded into a number of interesting areas, which are discussed in the references. The future will undoubtedly bring greater understanding of the biologic aging process.

PSYCHOSOCIAL FEATURES OF AGING

Coping with loss is a dominant theme for the elderly. As individuals grow older, people around them die and must be mourned. Moreover, other losses may occur due to events increasingly beyond the control of individuals as they get older. For example, lost relationships and activities of work need to be mourned at the time of retirement. Commonly people discontinue what has been their major vocational thrust somewhere between the ages of 65 and 70. This change may be voluntary or involuntary. Historically, since males have dominated the work force, retirement loss has affected chiefly men. With the marked increase of women in the work force, however, the losses of retirement should increasingly affect both sexes. Women have, of course, traditionally suffered an analogous loss in the "empty nest syndrome," as children have grown up and left home. Retirement, rather than being the sought-after leisure that was fantasized, may be a time of stress, anxiety, and depression. The loss of a major focus for life, one's vocation, must be worked through in some effective manner. The loss needs to be mourned and a modified self-concept evolved. When such mourning has been inadequate, the retired individual remains vulnerable to depression and to a pervasive sense of meaninglessness. The much higher incidence of suicide among elderly men compared with that in women attests to the special problem of the elderly retired men.

It is of utmost importance for elderly people to maintain an interest in the world around them and to participate as much as possible in social activities. If social withdrawal appears, it is important to prevent it from becoming an ingrained pattern. Older people may be reluctant to try new things. They may consider themselves incapable of change, or they may consider such new activity as unsuitable to their senior role.

A problem that contributes to the loneliness and isolation of the elderly is the preponderance of women among that population. Since the life expectancy of women is seven years longer than that of men, we find that women overwhelmingly outnumber men in the older population. The result of this fact is that elderly widows are very unlikely to remarry, and eligible unattached elderly men are rare. With the organization of society based on the nuclear family at the core, single elderly woman are frequently left out of the social network.

Economic difficulties of the elderly also need consideration. There is a clear-cut correlation between poverty and old age. The elderly are overrepresented among the poor, especially among the black population. Older people commonly have fixed incomes, with limited ability to earn additional money. Previously self-sufficient persons may become economically dependent on children or others. The loss of economic well-being is another loss to be faced by the older person.

The loss of health and the awareness of the proximity of death is another stress of aging. Chronic health problems affect 86 percent of the older population; only 5 percent, however, have health problems severe enough that they require institutionalization. The awareness of one's mortality, so often ignored during youth, becomes unavoidable in the face of increasing health problems and loss of physical vigor.

Psychiatric Disorders of the Elderly
The elderly are subject to the full range of psychiatric disorders that afflict people of other age groups. Disorders that commence in younger years may continue into old age, manifested by similar or modified characteristics. Disorders may also develop in old age in individuals previously free of psychiatric disturbance. Although there are no diagnostic categories in the *Diagnostic and Statistical Manual of Mental Disorders,* Third Edition (DSM-III) limited to the elderly as there are for other age groups, there are several that are more characteristic of the elderly and will be discussed here in some detail (see Table 16-1). Mention will also be made of special characteristics of other psychiatric disorders as they appear in the elderly.

Table 16-1. Common Psychiatric Disorders in the Elderly

I. Organic disorders
  A. Delirium
  B. Dementia
    1. Primary Degenerative
      a. Senile onset
      b. With delirium
      c. With delusions
      d. With depression
      e. Uncomplicated
    2. Multi-infarct dementia
    3. Dementia associated with Physical Disorder(s)
II. Functional (nonorganic) disorders
  A. Affective Disorders
    1. Depression (pseudodementia)
    2. Bipolar Disorder
  B. Paranoid Disorder
  C. Hypochondriasis

ORGANIC MENTAL DISORDERS
Some degree of organic brain impairment is commonly found among elderly people. For many, of course, organic changes are minimal and do not greatly affect life functions. For others, there are major, often disabling organic deficits present. Among the elderly population in psychiatric hospitals or other residential care facilities, severe organic impairment is frequent.

Organic impairment may be reversible or irreversible, stable or progressive. The rate of development may be very slow or there may be very rapid progression to dementia.

In order to understand the nature of organic impairment, we will describe the extreme case, dementia, and discuss the situations with lesser manifestations.

Dementia (as presented in detail in Chapter 4) is characterized by a pervasive loss of intellectual abilities sufficient to impair social or occupational functioning. There are deficits not only in memory and abstract thinking but also in social skills, subtle personality features, and judgment. Decline in areas that influence interpersonal adjustment may in fact be more problematic than are the obvious intellectual losses.

Senile-onset primary degenerative dementia is the most common dementia and, by definition, has onset at age 65 or older. The onset is insidious and the course progressive. Death, which typically results from infection or general organismic failure, usually occurs four or five years after the condition is diagnosed. Aside from the age of onset there do not appear to be consistent distinguishing characteristics between senile and presenile dementia. There are pathologically demonstrable subtypes of primary degenerative dementia—Alzheimer's disease and Pick's disease. There does not, however, seem to be much clinical usefulness at present to these pathologic distinctions, which are usually made at autopsy.

Elderly people with lesser degrees of organic impairment will manifest some of these characteristics, but not to an extent that warrants the diagnosis of dementia. Some people will have significant atrophic brain changes demonstrable by computerized axial tomographic (CAT) scan with only mild loss of function. Others show little brain atrophy on CAT scan but have marked impairment. Minor memory disturbances, especially of short-term memory, are common among the elderly. The disturbance is compensated for in many by an increased preoccupation with the past and a tendency to reminisce. The elderly may also be subject to decreased concentration, decreased ability to think cognitively, decreased motor performance, and slowness of problem-solving. Furthermore, mild organic impairment may be manifested in ways characteristic for the elderly, such as incontinence (of both bladder and bowel) and regressive personality changes. Physical, psychological, and social stresses in an elderly person may exacerbate organic mental symptoms, and relief of stress results in marked improvement.

Differential Diagnosis

Differential diagnosis of the elderly is most important, since treatable conditions may be discovered. A good history, physical examination, and laboratory examination must be performed. It is crucial to seek out treatable causes of dementia and to identify the presence of a delirium (an acute disorder) when it is present, either alone or superimposed on a dementia. While Chapter 4 reviews the treatable dementias associated with physical disorders and the causes of delirium, it is worth emphasizing how vulnerable the elderly are to all types of interference with normal brain function. With the loss of reserve capacity, the brain function is much more easily disrupted by internal and external factors. Relatively mild medical illnesses (for example, urinary tract infections) can produce a delirium with serious consequences. When brain changes are combined with the decrease in the body water compartment that occurs with aging, prescription medications in typical doses can suddenly become quite toxic. The polypharmacy that so often occurs in older people is virtually ideal for producing an iatrogenic delirium or worsening of a dementing process.

Pseudodementia is another phenomenon that is most important to understand and consider in the differential diagnosis. Individuals with major depression may show evidence of moderate to severe organic changes on mental status examination and psychological testing. In these individuals, however, it is the disturbance of mood that is the primary difficulty, not an organic cognitive deficit. The time course of the disorder tends to differ from that of true dementia. The onset of symptoms, when accurate history can be obtained, is more abrupt and the course fluctuating. There is also inconsistency in the presence of the organic manifestations, while in patients with dementia repeated examinations show consistent presence of signs. When the diagnosis is unclear, treatment with appropriate antidepressant measures may be a diagnostic procedure in itself by *producing* a marked remission of symptoms. Often marked organic features may be superimposed on milder organic problems when the patient also has a major depression; in such patients, treatment may result in significant improvement but the residual organic deficit will remain (Case 1 represents an example of this phenomenon).

Functional Psychiatric Disorders of the Elderly

DEPRESSION

Older people are particularly vulnerable to depression. As discussed earlier, they are subject to multiple losses as the years progress. These losses are significant stresses to cope with and often precipitate depression. People who previously had no psychiatric difficulties may develop depression of major proportions, with or without psychosis. Moreover, the depression of the older person may manifest itself with symptoms and signs different from those in the younger person and thus go undetected. In addition to typical manifestations (such as a persistent sense of helplessness, hopelessness, or worthlessness; anorexia; weight loss; early-morning insomnia; psychomotor agitation or retardation; decreased energy; suicidal thoughts; and difficulty concentrating), depressed elderly people may exhibit marked memory problems, confusion, incontinence, and regressed behavior. In the extreme case the depression may be completely masked by the features of pseudodementia picture that resemble organic disorders, as discussed earlier. The recognition of the depression syndrome in such patients is of utmost importance; otherwise one might mistake a dementia with poor prognosis for a depression with a much better prognosis. (See Chapter 8 for the diagnostic features of major depressive disorders, including psychotic features.) Somatic symptoms are very often more prominent in the elderly than in those with typical depressive illness. This somatization can complicate the diagnosis of the primary depression and result in unnecessary and ineffective treatment of assumed physical illness.

Differential Diagnosis

Differential diagnosis of major depression in the elderly is the same as in other age groups, with the addition of organic affective syndrome (see Chapter 4).

Major depression with psychosis may have features similar to the paranoid disorders (described in the next section). Awareness of the primary mood difficulty, however, makes the distinction possible.

Treatment

Treatment of depression in the elderly should include appropriate psychological and biologic measures. A therapeutic relationship with these patients must be formed early in order to help them overcome contributing psychodynamic issues and to modify contributing environmental conditions. Optimal management of medical disorders needs to be instituted. If a pharmacologic approach is indicated, the tricyclic antidepressants in small initial doses should be started. Of those currently available, doxepin is considered safest because it is the least cardiotoxicity. Desipramine is probably the second choice because of its low anticholinergic effect. If the diagnosis is major depression with psychosis, an antipsychotic drug such as fluphenazine or trifluoperazine should be prescribed as well. Electroconvulsive therapy (ECT) should be considered and is recommended when less intensive measures have failed. This treatment can be especially crucial in treating the elderly since it is rapid and avoids the side effects of pharmacologic interventions.

PARANOID DISORDERS

Paranoia is considered an uncommon condition in the population as a whole. Paranoid symptoms are more commonly a feature of other disorders in which paranoid thinking is a part. Such disorders to be included in the differential diagnosis are organic delusional syndromes; the bizarre thoughts, loose associations, and prominent hallucinations of schizophrenia; the marked pressure of thought and speech in mania; the presence at some point of depressed mood in psychotic depression; and the absence of delusions in paranoid personality.

In the elderly, paranoid disorders are much more common than in the younger populations. Indeed, the typical age of onset of a paranoid disorder is considered to be middle to late adult life. Moreover, suspiciousness is a characteristic that frequently develops in the elderly in the absence of other manifestations of mental disorder. (The DSM-III diagnostic criteria for paranoid disorder are presented in Chapter 6.)

The varieties of paranoid disorder reflect the time period and social context of the disorder rather than any fundamental differences.

Diagnosis

Paranoia is defined as a chronic and stable persecutory delusional system of at least six-months' duration. Acute paranoid disorder has the same features, but the duration is less than six months. Shared paranoid disorder refers to the condition in which the delusional system develops as a result of a close relationship with another person or persons who have an established disorder with persecutory delusions; this disorder has been called *folie à deux* in the past. In all paranoid disorders stressful events in the person's life, deafness, or pre-existing paranoid or schizoid personality disorders may predispose the person to develop a paranoid disorder. *Paraphrenia* is a term formerly used in the attempt to distinguish late-onset paranoid disorder from schizophrenia. In DSM-III this term has been deleted from use. Either a diagnosis of paranoia or one of schizophrenia with late onset should be made in these cases.

Treatment

As with other psychiatric disorders of the elderly, paranoid disorders can be effectively treated. Symptoms may fluctuate markedly depending on the effectiveness of clinical management. An elderly person may remain significantly paranoid despite treatment but become delusion-free and much more functional.

It is most important to form a good therapeutic relationship and to use appropriate pharmacologic measures. When symptoms are florid, neuroleptic medication can be effective in lessening the intensity of the delusional belief. It is best to begin at a low dose and to titrate upward to an effective dose. Response is often quite gradual (over weeks) and incomplete.

HYPOCHONDRIASIS

Hypochondriasis is another disorder particularly common in the elderly. The diagnostic criteria are presented in Table 16-2.

While this disorder may occur at any age, it occurs with greater frequency among the elderly, who may become excessively preoccupied with their physical functioning. Fairly minor difficulties may be blown out of proportion and become the central concern of the person's life. Such disorders are most difficult to treat. Polypharmacy, multiple physicians, and lack of clarity must be avoided. It is important for the physician to form a warm and caring rela-

Table 16-2. Diagnostic Criteria for Hypochondriasis

The predominant disturbance is an unrealistic interpretation of physical signs or sensations as abnormal, leading to preoccupation with the fear or belief of having a serious disease.

Thorough physical evaluation does not support the diagnosis of any physical disorder that can account for the physical signs or sensations or for the individual's unrealistic interpretation of them.

The unrealistic fear or belief of having a disease persists despite medical reassurance and causes impairment in social or occupational functioning.

Not due to any other mental disorder such as schizophrenia, affective disorder, or somatization disorder.

Reproduced with permission from *Diagnostic and Statistical Manual of Mental Disorders*, 3rd ed. Washington, D.C.: American Psychiatric Association, 1980, p. 251.

tionship with these patients and to be as reassuring as possible about the extent of the illness and the meaning of symptoms. If referral to a psychotherapist becomes necessary, a close collaboration between physician and therapist is important. It is also quite important to appreciate that somatic symptoms and concerns are common features of depressive disorders in the elderly.

Other psychiatric disorders that commence in earlier years may continue into the geriatric period of life. Schizophrenia may continue unabated into a person's older years with continued acute episodes or continued chronic psychosis. Similarly, bipolar affective disorder may continue into the latter years of life, and there are occasional cases of late-life onset of manic disorder.

Assessment of the Elderly

The assessment of the elderly person must take into account many of the factors involved in assessment of a person of any age. In addition, the special needs and difficulties of older people require focus in areas that may need little attention in people of other age groups. A mental health team of specialists can often most effectively investigate the various important factors.

PSYCHIATRIC ASSESSMENT

The psychiatric assessment should describe the development of any psychiatric disorder that is suspected, particularly focusing on the development of symptoms or behavorial manifestations of the disorder. A careful mental status examination should be performed. Personal and family history should be taken. Care must be taken to get as reliable data as possible by providing a comfortable and reassuring setting for the interview and by getting data from other individuals who may have knowledge of the patient. Psychological testing may be useful to the clinical psychiatric examination in providing data regarding the patient's mental functioning.

ASSESSMENT OF LEVEL OF INDEPENDENT FUNCTION

An evaluation of the level of independent function is an important feature of the assessment of the elderly. While this should be included in the psychiatric evaluation, it is often the assessment of other members of the mental health team with closer, more consistent contact with the patient that will provide the information. The detailed assessment of the nurse, who is often the closest and most consistent observer, will frequently be the most knowledgeable about personal hygiene; sleep patterns; amount of care required; need for assistance in feeding, bathing, and toileting; ability to interact with others to get needs met; and so on.

SOCIOCULTURAL ASSESSMENT

A sociocultural assessment should be made. When a mental health team is functioning it is often the social worker who provides this part of the evaluation. The patient's living arrangement needs to be understood. Elderly people may live in their own housing; board with family or others; live in a retirement home, nursing home, or foster home; or live in some other setting. It is important for older people to retain as much autonomy in living as possible, but this goal must be weighed against their ability to care for themselves adequately, as well as the amount of social interaction that is possible. Living alone helps to maintain autonomy and should be reinforced when possible. On the other hand, some individuals are unable to care for their daily needs and may not have involvement with friends or family. An assessment of the transportation available to these patients, or their mobility, ought to be done. If an automobile, good public transportation, or a helpful friend or relative is available, their quality of life may be enhanced. One must evaluate the family constellation and friendship pattern, as well as the availability of family members and friends. An assessment of educational and vocational functioning, past and current, should be prepared.

A particular focus on issues related to retirement is important. The patient's economic status must be considered, especially since it affects planning for optimal living arrangements. Interests, activities, and community involvements of the patient should be documented.

MEDICAL EVALUATION

A medical evaluation should be conducted on an elderly person presenting with a suspected psychiatric disorder. Although it will commonly be the internist or family medicine specialist who will conduct this part of the examination, it is important for the psychiatrist to understand the nature of any significant medical disorder and what treatments are being instituted.

The medical assessment should involve a complete medical history and physical examination with a laboratory examination including complete blood chemistries, chest x-ray, and electrocardiogram. Skull x-rays, electroencephalogram, and (CAT) scan should be done if organic brain pathology is suspected. Audiometry and a visual examination will often produce important data if disorder in these areas is suspected. Further diagnostic studies may be indicated to evaluate positive findings on the initial tests.

Psychiatric Treatment of the Elderly Patient

It is important to devote considerable time and effort into formulating an appropriate, integrated treatment plan when working with the elderly patient. This plan should include all aspects of the assessment—medical, psychiatric, sociocultural, and functional. Responsibility for carrying out specific aspects of the plan should be established, and periodic conferences should be held to monitor progress and to make modifications of the treatment plan. Although use of the mental health team of professionals is often the most effective treatment approach, whatever resources are available should be employed.

USE OF PSYCHOPHARMACOLOGIC AGENTS

It is important to prescribe appropriate medication without increasing the patient's difficulty through overmedication or polypharmacy. As noted previously, older people are more sensitive to drugs commonly used in psychopharmacology, and lower doses than would be used in younger people should be prescribed initially. Also, as the elderly person is more likely to be taking other medications for physical illnesses, it is important to monitor him or her for possible drug interactions.

Drugs should not be used without undertaking concomitant psychotherapeutic and social measures; they should be part of the treatment plan. The problem of self-medication or possible substance abuse should be considered. While elderly patients are not likely to obtain drugs nonmedically, the misuse of prescribed hypnotics and sedatives by these patients is too frequent an occurrence. The practitioner should be alert for side effects and toxic effects of drugs that have been prescribed.

Treatment of Depression in the Elderly

Antidepressant drugs are as useful in the treatment of major depression in elderly patients as they are in other age groups. These drugs are also important in the treatment of the patient considered demented or senile, because positive response to the drugs will demonstrate the presence of a treatable pseudodementia. In dysthymic disorder, psychotherapeutic measures and minor tranquilizers are likely to be more effective. When antidepressant medications are to be used, the tricyclic antidepressants are more effective and less risky to use and should be tried initially. The various tricyclic agents available are imipramine, desipramine, nortriptyline, and protriptyline (which tend to be nonsedating) and amitriptyline and doxepin (which tend to be more sedating). The sedative effects usually diminish in a few days, however. Differences among this group of drugs, in addition, are that doxepin has less of a tendency to produce cardiac arrhythmias than do other agents—an advantage in the elderly patient with heart disease—and nortriptyline and desipramine may have a more rapid action. Side effects of the tricyclic antidepressants include excitement, exacerbation of psychosis, anticholinergic effects, cardiac arrhythmias, urinary retention, delayed ejaculation, and worsening of glaucoma.

Patients should be started on an initial low dose of antidepressant; the dose can be increased gradually with careful monitoring for toxicity and therapeutic effect. A full therapeutic dosage may prove necessary. Antidepressant blood levels may be helpful in monitoring the patients' progress. A course of six to eight weeks should be attempted for maximum therapeutic effect. A gradual tapering of the dose is also suggested when discontinuing antidepressant medication.

For elderly patients who do not respond to tricyclic antidepressants, the monoamine oxidase inhibitor (MAOI) drugs such as phenelzine and tranylcypromine may be tried. Those drugs should be used in the elderly only with caution and preferably in a hospital setting. It is generally considered appropriate to wait two weeks after discontinuing tricyclic antidepressants before instituting MAOI treatment because of the toxic interaction. While there has been some recent indication that the two classes of antidepressant drugs can be safely used in combination, in the elderly population it is best to use the more conservative approach. Side effects of the MAOI drugs include hypertensive crises from consuming tyramine-containing foods and sympathomimetic drugs, orthostatic hypotension, excess weight gain, and insomnia. Stimulant drugs such as the amphetamines and methylphenidate have been used in the past as antidepressants. They do indeed intend to be mood elevating and stimulating, and some authorities contend that there is still a role for amphetamines in mobilizing withdrawn, depressed patients. The drug effects, however, tend to be short lived and may be followed by a rebound worsening of depressive symptomatology. Their use is not recommended.

Treatment of Bipolar Affective Disorder and Mania

Lithium carbonate is a useful substance in the treatment of bipolar affective disorders and mania in the elderly. It is especially useful in the prevention of recurrent episodes of bipolar and manic illness, but is also useful along with antipsychotic drugs in treatment of the episodes themselves. Antidepressant drugs are useful in the treatment of depressive episodes, as already discussed. Because elderly people are more sensitive to lithium than are younger groups, a lower dose is indicated. An effective starting dose is 300 mg per day. An effective maintenance dose that produces a therapeutic serum level of lithium may be 600 to 900 mg per day in an elderly patient. In addition, a lower serum lithium level may be sufficient for older patients.

Side effects to lithium carbonate may appear more readily in the elderly and need careful monitoring. These side effects include gastrointestinal symptoms, fine tremors, ataxia, polydipsia, polyuria, weakness, and confusion. Serum levels of lithium should be monitored every few days as therapy is initiated and at less frequent intervals thereafter. As in the younger person, elderly patients with bipolar affective disorders may be very effectively controlled by the use of maintenance doses of lithium.

Treatment of Psychotic Conditions of the Elderly

For the elderly with schizophrenia, paranoid states, agitated depression, mania, and dementia with psychotic manifestations, the antipsychotic drugs may be very effective forms of treatment. There are a large number of antipsychotic drugs available. Although patients differ in their responses to the various drugs, there is as yet no systematic rationale for selecting one drug over another. It is best to become familiar with how to use a select few of the different types. Effective doses of all of the antipsychotic agents may be lower than those for younger populations. After starting with an initial low dose, one should titrate upward the amoung of drug prescribed until the desired antipsychotic effect is achieved, while monitoring closely for side effects. Needless to say, the beneficial effects of these drugs need to be weighed against their considerable toxicity.

Treatment of Dementia
Other drugs have been advocated for use in treatment of dementia. Some of these, the vasodilators, are thought to act by increasing cerebral blood flow; others, such as vitamins, ergoloid (Hydergine), procaine, and hyperbaric oxygen, act by beneficially affecting cerebral metabolism. Unfortunately none of these have been clearly determined as yet to have beneficial effects in dementia. Vitamins are, of course, effective in the presence of vitamin deficiency.

Treatment of Anxiety States,
Sleep Disturbances, Dysthymic Disorder,
and Adjustment Disorders
Minor tranquilizers are often helpful as an adjunct in the treatment of anxiety states, sleep disturbances, dysthymic disorder, and adjustment disorders. Although these medications should be prescribed for specific conditions for limited periods of time, there is little doubt that they are being used for chronic conditions for long periods of time in the elderly as well as in other age groups. Although there has been evidence of significant abuse of these drugs in the population as a whole and although adverse withdrawal effects have been reported, the minor tranquilizers are relatively safe in comparison to drugs of other categories. The most popular of these drugs are the benzodiazepines, such as diazepam, chlordiazepoxide, oxazepam, flurazepam, temazepam, and clorazepate. The short duration of action of oxazepam can be especially useful in the elderly. Flurazepam and temazepam are often used to treat insomnia. Accumulation of flurazepam over several days can cause major delayed toxic effects. Drugs to be avoided if possible for use as minor tranquilizers, sedatives, or antiinsomnia agents include the barbiturates, meprobamate, glutethimide, ethchlorvynol, and methaqualone because of their addictive potential and because they are lethal when used in suicide attempts.

ELECTROCONVULSIVE THERAPY
Electroconvulsive therapy (ECT) has a useful place in the treatment of major depression in the elderly. Usually a trial of antidepressant medication is given first before ECT is tried. In situations of severe suicidal risk, however, ECT may be appropriately given as the initial treatment. When organic changes are prominent, ECT should be avoided. A course of five to 10 treatments given over several weeks is usually adequate. The beneficial effects of ECT are often startling. It is unfortunate that there is such fear and popular negativism toward this treatment. (See Chapter 22 for further discussion.)

PSYCHOSOCIAL APPROACHES

Psychotherapy with the Elderly
Psychotherapy with the elderly involves many of the same issues that apply to such treatment in any person; in addition, some special considerations also apply. As with all patients, the elderly psychotherapy patient needs a formulation to be made of the psychodynamic issues involved, and a treatment approach needs to be devised. As the problems of the elderly are multicausal, as already discussed, this formulation and treatment plan needs to take into account sociocultural, interpersonal, medical, and environmental factors as well as strictly intrapsychic psychological ones. The assessment and treatment are best performed by a team of mental health professionals. In order to make an accurate assessment and to form a trusting therapeutic alliance with the elderly patient, a warm, comfortable, optimistic environment needs to be created. The elderly patient needs to feel that the therapist under-

stands his or her special problems and requirements and has helpful ideas for their solution.

It is traditionally thought that the rigidity of elderly patients renders them untreatable by psychotherapy. Indeed, extensive uncovering therapy for the purpose of major personality change, according to the psychoanalytic model, is not appropriate. The proper approach involves a therapy that is much more reality oriented and problem solving, and that is based on as deep an understanding of the person as possible. Treatment should attempt to help the patient solve practical problems such as financial or housing difficulties as well as focus on traditionally psychological problems. Hospital-based therapy is indicated for the crisis situation. It is most important that inpatient stays be minimized to prevent regression and hospitalism, to which the impaired elderly person is so vulnerable. Therapy should be oriented toward resolving conflictual interpersonal difficulties, coping with the recurrent losses of living, maximizing autonomous function, and maintaining active interest in old and new activities. The subject of death should not be avoided but rather should be discussed as the unfortunate but unavoidable end for us all.

Both individual and group therapies are useful, as is family therapy. The elderly person may be very responsive to various expressive therapies and to activity-oriented groups. Group therapy with a peer group of elderly patients is often a very rewarding experience.

It is important for the therapist to be aware of the countertransference issues that arise in working with the elderly. There is the tendency in general to avoid the elderly person, partly from a reluctance by many people to face their own inevitable aging and mortality. Working closely with the elderly person makes such denial much more difficult and may result in uncomfortable reactions on the part of the therapist. Recognizing these problems and coping with them will make the clinician more effective in working with an older person. When these concepts are kept in mind, the therapist will frequently find the elderly patient a responsive person to work with and the treatment involvement very rewarding.

Other Psychosocial Interventions

As discussed in the section on assessment, it is important to work with the elderly people in a manner that maximizes autonomy while at the same time ensuring that dependency needs are met appropriately. In some situations older people may attempt to live alone when it is not possible to care for themselves adequately. The professional team needs to aid the patients and their families to get appropriate assistance, which may take the form of help with meal preparation, housework, or a live-in companion if a significant degree of autonomy is possible. Intervention to enhance the quality of life for the elderly person should be focused on. It is important to suggest and help arrange daytime activities. Day care centers or social centers may be effectively used to add interest and variety to the elderly person's existence. It is important to work closely with families to encourage meaningful activities together that will lessen the isolation that can be prominent in this age group.

At some point one may need to acknowledge that the elderly individual is not capable of living on his or her own. It may be necessary to select some form of group, residential, or institutional living arrangement. A careful assessment of the degree of autonomy possible is important because the least restrictive type of setting should be chosen. The healthy individual, fairly autonomous but in need of a moderate amount of assistance, may do very well in a residential home for the elderly. Those in need of continued active nursing care because of medical conditions or because of major loss of self-care functions may need nursing home placement. Some individuals may remain sufficiently behaviorally disturbed or incapable of self-care despite all therapeutic and humane care possible. Even in such unfortunate patients, it is important to focus on the least restrictive setting so that they have as much autonomy as possible.

Case 1. A.L., a 75-year-old-woman, was admitted to the gerontologic psychiatric service in a markedly withdrawn, regressed state. A.'s ability to attend to the environment was greatly impaired. A. was disoriented and at times incoherent, had impaired memory, did not care for her personal hygiene, had to be fed, and was incontinent. Her affect was shallow and silly. A. denied sadness and depression. A. gave a history of having lived independently without disabling symptoms until three months before admission when she was persuaded to move to a retirement home from the farm where she had lived for 25 years. A's decompensation took place in the context of planning and arranging for the move, which was completed by her children.

In retrospect, A's children could recall episodes of memory loss and illogical thinking over the past few years in their mother, but no major symptoms, including at the time of the death of her husband two years earlier.

Medical work-up revealed only mild atrophic brain changes on CAT scan. A. was treated in a supportive therapeutic milieu, was seen daily in a supportive group therapy attended by other gerontologic patients and staff, and was treated pharmacologically with doxepin. Over a period of several weeks, the organic signs diminished markedly and it was possible to discharge the patient to the semi-independent setting of a retirement home. She has continued to have residual memory difficulty.

References and Further Reading

Amaducci, L., Davis, A.N., Antuono, P. *Aging of the Brain and Dementia.* New York: Raven Press, 1980.

Brocklehurst, J.C. *Textbook of Geriatric Medicine and Gerontology.* Edinburgh, London: Churchill Livingstone, 1973.

Busse, E.W., Blazer, D.C. *Handbook of Geriatric Psychiatry.* New York: Van Nostrand Reinhold, 1980.

Butler, R.N., Lewis, M.I. *Aging and Mental Health: Positive Psychosocial and Biomedical Approaches.* St. Louis: C.V. Mosby, 1982.

Cole, J.O., Barrett, J.E. *Psychopathology in the Aged.* New York: Raven Press, 1980.

Ennar, S.J., Samorajski, R. Beer, F. *Brain Neurotransmitters and Receptors in Aging and Age-Related Disorders.* New York: Raven Press, 1981.

Erikson, E. Growth and crisis of the healthy personality. *Psychol. Issues* 1:50–100, 1959.

Hendrick, J., Hendrick, D.C. *Aging in Mass Society.* Cambridge, Mass.: Winthrop, 1977.

Jarvik, L.F., Greenblatt, D.J., Harman, D. *Clinical Pharmacology in the Aged Patient.* New York: Raven Press, 1981.

Kalish, R.A. *The Later Years: Social Applications of Gerontology.* Monterey, Calif.: Brooks/Cole, 1977.

Kaplan, O.J. *Mental Disorders in Later Life.* Stanford, Calif.: Stanford University Press, 1956.

Kaplan, O.J. *Psychopathology of Aging.* New York: Academic Press, 1979.

Kart, C.S., Manard, B.B. *Aging in America: Readings in Social Gerontology.* Port Washington, N.Y.: Alfred Publishings, 1976.

Kelly, J.T., Weir, J.H. *Perspective on Human Aging.* Minneapolis: Craftman Press, 1976.

Levenson, A.J., Hall. R.C.W. *Neuropsychiatric Manifestations of Physical Disease in the Elderly.* New York: Raven Press, 1981.

Verwoerdt, A. *Clinical Geropsychiatry.* Baltimore: Williams & Wilkins, 1981.

Psychiatric Manifestations of Medical Disorders and Therapies
RALPH W. WADESON, Jr., M.D.

The greatest challenge in the practice of medicine is to establish for each patient a correct diagnosis and subsequent treatment plan. This chapter is intended for the student seeking greater understanding of the psychiatric signs and symptoms associated with a broad array of medical illnesses and therapies. By becoming more familiar with the mental manifestations of physical disorders, the student should also become more able to establish the fundamentally correct diagnosis rather then being misled by apparently functional psychiatric signs and symptoms.

One problem that continues to plague the practice of medicine is the imagined gulf between psychiatry and physical medicine. Studies have shown that as many as one-third of patients referred by other physicians to psychiatrists were suffering from an unrecognized medical disease. The multiaxial diagnostic structure of the *Diagnostic and Statistical Manual of Mental Disorders,* Third Edition (DSM-III), provides the opportunity for specificity in psychiatric and physical diagnosis in the best tradition of medical care. Axis III, which is specifically designated for recording physical disorders relevant to the clinical management of the patient, emphasizes that there may occur a complex interaction between physical and psychiatric disorders. It is also essential to remember that these physical disorders may include the effects of specific medical therapies, many of which are quite capable of producing psychiatric symptomatology. An awareness of which medications and surgical interventions are capable of producing mental manifestations can be extremely important.

The specific message of this chapter is intended to communicate (1) the many different types of physical illness that can manifest as diverse psychiatric syndromes and (2) the more important manifestations that are commonly encountered. The brain is vulnerable to insults that occur anywhere in the body. It is a valuable clinical learning experience to observe the confusional states that occur in a high percentage of patients on medical units. It is also quite instructional to visit a neurosurgical unit and observe the behavorial and mental aberrations that result from direct manipulations and trauma to the brain.

Major mental changes can result from medical disorders and treatments involving any organ system. Changes in organ function can also mimic a broad array of specific psychiatric syndromes. These diagnostic problems will be approached from two directions:(1) with emphasis on the specific organ system involved and (2) by the psychiatric syndrome imitated (see Table 17-1).

Medical Disorders Known to Cause Mental Changes

CARDIOVASCULAR SYSTEM

Cardiovascular disease is a common although often overlooked cause of numerous psychiatric symptoms. Hypertension, congestive heart failure, arteriosclerotic cardiovascular disease, cerebral insufficiency, aortic stenosis, mitral stenosis, paroxysmal atrial tachycardia, conduction defects, and rheumatic heart disease have all been known to present initially as psychiatric illnesses. The most common presentations include signs and symptoms of anxiety or depressive disorders. In advanced cases, a delirium with prominent psychotic features may be produced that only later is appreciated to have an organic component. The precise etiologies of these psychiatric symptoms vary. Certainly many cardiovascular diseases can create tension and fear of death or loss of function. Decreased profusion and oxygenation of the blood can

Table 17-1. Specific Psychiatric Signs and Symptoms with the Recognized Medical Causes

Signs and Symptons	Medical Causes	Signs and Symptons	Medical Causes
Depressive Symptoms of Low Severity, Chronic Presentation	Arteriosclerotic cardiovascular disease, diabetes mellitus, essential hypertension, hepatic insufficiency, hyperparathyroidism, hypochromic anemia, hypothyroidism, infectious mononucleosis, infectious viral hepatitis, metastatic carcinoma of the uterus, myasthenia gravis, peptic ulcer, pneumonia, pulmonary embolism, and pulmonary infarction	Impaired Sensorium (Delirious or Dementiform Presentation)	Bronchogenic carcinoma, chronic bronchitis, cirrhosis, congestive heart failure, diabetes mellitus, emphysema, hepatoma, hypertension, hypochromic microcytic anemia, infectious hepatitis, metastatic carcinoma of the uterus, neurosyphilis, other hepatic insufficiency, pancreatitis, pneumonia, and pyelonephritis
Acute and More Severe Depressive Symptomatology	Aortic stenosis, black lung, central nervous system stimulant withdrawal, cerebral anoxia, chronic bronchitis, congestive heart failure, emphysema, erythremia, hypertension, hypothyroidism, hyperthyroidism, pernicious anemia, pulmonary emboli, pulmonary infarction, pulmonary insufficiency, and viral pneumonia	Altered Personality Features	Cerebral vascular accident, congestive heart failure, hypertension, iron deficiency anemia, mitral stenosis, rheumatic heart disease, sickle-cell anemia, viral pneumonia, and rheumatoid arthritis.
Generalized Anxiety Symptoms	Arterioscleotic cardiovascular disease, bundle branch block, hyperparathyroidism, hyperthyroidism, hypochromic anemia, hypothyroidism, paroxysmal atrial tachycardia, pneumonia, scabes, and ulcerative colitis		
Disordered Thinking or Perception (Schizophreniform or Atypical Psychotic Symptoms)	Acute intermittent porphyria, brain neoplasms, central nervous system depressant withdrawal status, congestive heart failure, diabetes mellitus, encephalitic processes, hepatic insufficiency, hypoglycemia, infectious hepatitis, neurosyphilis, renal insufficiency, systematic lupus erythematosus, temporal lobe epilepsy, thyrotoxicosis, vitamin deficiencies, Wilson's disease		

also contribute by either creating subjective fear or causing altered neuronal dysfunction. In specific abnormalities such as paroxysmal atrial tachycardia or conduction defects, the physical sensation of the altered cardiac rhythm may first mimic anxiety and then produce a secondary anxiety state.

PULMONARY SYSTEM
Pulmonary disorders frequently produce psychiatric symptoms. Acute pulmonary disorders, such as pneumonitis of any origin, may generate hypoxemia followed by lessened mental acuity and a reactive anxiety state. Asthmatic conditions are also well known to be closely linked with anxiety. In this group of illnesses there is often anticipatory fear of the onset of breathing difficulties. There may also be major distortions in personality development and an adaptation as a result of the need to cope with a chronic illness. Chronic obstructive pulmonary disease, such as emphysema, black lung disease, and other forms of pulmo-

nary insufficiency, may produce hypoxia or carbon dioxide intoxication. Commonly resulting psychiatric symptoms include lethargy, fatigue, hypersomnia, depression, and disorientation.

GASTROINTESTIMAL SYSTEM

Numerous gastrointestinal disorders have presented initially with psychiatric symptomatology before the underlying medical diagnosis was established. Cirrhosis, infectious hepatitis, hepatic insufficiency, malabsorption-induced vitamin deficiencies, ulcerative colitis, and peptic ulcer are among the disorders that are recognized as capable of causing diverse psychiatric effects. Decreased cognitive function, anxiety, and depression are the most common manifestations. Once again, in more severe cases, an organic psychotic state, often of a paranoid nature, may ensue.

ENDOCRINE SYSTEM

Diseases of the endocrine system are probably most widely recognized as causing psychiatric difficulties. Increased or decreased function of any endocrine gland can lead to mental changes. Hyperthyroidism, hypoglycemia, hyperadrenalism, and Cushing's disease more commonly produce anxiety states or agitated psychotic disorders mimicking schizophrenia, mania, or an agitated delirious state. Exogenous sources of steroids and thyroid hormone may also produce similar psychiatric changes. Corticosteroids, either endogenous or exogenous, are especially provocative of underlying tendencies toward any psychiatric illness. Major depression, mania, and paranoid psychoses have long been recognized as resulting from excesses of these hormones. If there is a previous pyschiatric history, a physician prescribing steroid or adrenocorticotropic hormone (ACTH) therapy will be especially alert to the development of psychiatric symptoms. Disturbances of parathyroid function can produce diffuse psychiatric symptomatology of mild to severe degree, although psychiatric manifestations are uncommon. Sexual dysfunction is a frequent result of many of the endocrinopathies, and an endocrine disorder should always be investigated when there is a presenting complaint of sexual difficulties.

METABOLIC REGULATION

Metabolic abnormalities are easily missed in patients who seem to be suffering from psychiatric syndromes. Renal insufficiency and electrolyte disturbances can produce a diffuse encephalopathy but the patient may also present primarily with depressive symptoms. Anxiety, depression, and personality changes as well as dementia have often been reported in association with renal dialysis. Wide electrolyte swings, accumulating toxic substances as well as a rather helpless dependence on the dialysis program can contribute to psychiatric difficulties.

Disorders of hepatic function of any origin—such as chronic infectious hepatitis, chemical damage, or alcoholic cirrhosis—may produce restlessness, tremulousness, agitation, and even psychosis. This is presumed to result from excessive blood ammonia, although the correlation is imperfect. Delirium and dementia can also result.

Diabetes mellitus can produce acute or chronic mental changes through either hyperglycemia or hypoglycemia. The specific adjustment difficulties that may occur in child and adolescent diabetics are probably the result of an interaction of physical, individual psychological, and family factors.

Two specific, but uncommon, metabolic disorders that produce striking psychiatric changes are Wilson's disease and porphyria. Wilson's disease is known to present as a major mood disorder or schizophreniform psychosis. Eventually a dementing process will become evident, but this may be relatively late in the patient's involvement with psychiatric treatment. Physical evidence such as parkinsonian tremors, rigidity, cirrhosis, portal hypertension, and Kayser-Fleischer rings should be sought. A deficiency in serum ceruloplasmin and increased urinary copper excretion are characteristic. Porphyria, especially of the acute intermittent type, is a recognized cause of an acute paranoid or schizophreniform psychotic state, which may be difficult to differentiate from the functional disorders. Urinary porphyrin excretion will probably be increased during this phase.

Vitamin deficiencies, such as pellagra resulting from an insufficiency of nicotinic acid, may present as depression or atypical psychosis. A thiamine deficiency syndrome, Wernicke's encephalopathy, typically presents with an agitated confusional state often associated with a partial ocular palsy. Pernicious anemia, vitamin B_{12} deficiency resulting from lack of intrinsic factor, may produce an atypical psychotic state as well as symptoms of depression.

INFECTIOUS PROCESSES
Infectious and parasitic diseases once commonly caused patients to seek psychiatric treatment. Neurosyphilis was long known to be a condition that masqueraded as various psychiatric or medical disorders. Before the introduction of antibiotics, as many as one-third of psychiatric hospital admissions resulted from neurosyphilis. This disorder is a relatively uncommon cause of psychiatric symptoms today but should always be considered because of the ease of diagnosis and the availability of treatment. Today infectious hepatitis and mononucleosis are more commonly encountered, with psychiatric symptoms of depression being most typical. Other unrecognized acute or chronic infections, of course, may produce a general feeling of disease including vague anxiety reactions. Infectious processes involving the brain directly, such as herpes encephalitis, may produce a delirium or organic or schizophreniform psychosis.

CENTRAL NERVOUS SYSTEM DISORDERS
Central nervous system diseases, as one might expect, are common causes of diverse psychiatric symptoms. Epilepsy, especially when it involves the temporal lobe, may produce personality changes, anxiety, depersonalization, or a schizophreniform psychosis. Irritability, impulsivity, and even violent behavior have been reported during the ictal or paraictal phase of temporal lobe seizure disorders. Encephalitis, particularly herpes encephalitis, may cause symptoms appearing to be of a nonorganic nature. While dementia may eventually result from herpes encephalitis, a paranoid psychosis difficult to distinguish from paranoid schizophrenia may present much earlier in the course of the disease. Brain neoplasms, of course, almost invariably produce psychiatric symptoms as well as eventual major cognitive changes. Tumors located in the frontal region most often produce mood changes, loss of social inhibition, thought disorder, and psychomotor retardation. Temporal lobe tumors, like ictal disorders in this region, may produce illusions, hallucinations, affective changes, religious or paranoid delusions, and emotional lability. Parietal lobe lesions will characteristically be associated with specific agnosias, apraxias, and aphasias with distortion of body image and spatial disorientation. These may be interpreted as being of hysterical or even psychotic origin. Tumors in the occipital region may produce visual hallucinations and illusions that may be interpreted as functional hallucinations. Diencephalic tumors, on the other hand, produce emotional liability or manic symptoms. Finally, posterior diencephalic lesions are associated with hypersomia and akinetic mutism, which can be misdiagnosed as functional catatonic psychoses.

NONCEREBRAL MALIGNANCIES
Noncerebral malignancies may also generate psychiatric symptoms through distant effects. Carcinoma of the pancreas is classically known to produce a depressive syndrome often assumed to be primary. Insulinomas, by producing hypoglycemia, may cause irritability, personality changes, anxiety, and depressive symptoms. Bronchogenic tumors, carcinoid syndrome, hepatoma, and endometrioma have also been reported to cause diffuse emotional symptomatology. The ability of such tumors to cause psychiatric changes is not completely understood. In certain instances the distant effects appear to result from vasoactive substances produced by the tumor.

CONNECTIVE TISSUE DISEASES

Collagen diseases seem particularly able to affect mental processes. Systemic lupus erythematosus, of course, has received great attention for its ability to generate an atypical psychotic disorder potentially misdiagnosable as schizophrenia. In addition to lupus, however, rheumatoid arthritis, inflammatory angiopathies (such as periarteritis nodosa and cranial arteritis), and other pathologic collagen conditions that impair cerebral blood flow may produce psychiatric changes including depression, irritability, mood swings, and psychosis. Depression is often reported in association with rheumatoid arthritis; however, the nature of the interrelationship of the two disorders is not well established. Certainly chronic disability and sleep disturbances associated with painful arthritis can generate depression, and that depression in turn can aggravate the primary physical disorder.

EXOGENOUS TOXINS

It is especially timely today to emphasize the possible role of toxic exogenous substances in the production of psychiatric symptoms. Depression, anxiety, and atypical psychosis can result from poisoning by heavy metals, (such as mercury or lead), aliphatic hydrocarbons, aromatic hydrocarbons, ketones, and industrial alcohols. These substances appear to be increasingly prevalent in the environment, and a careful work history for toxic exposure should be taken from any patient presenting with these psychiatric symptoms.

IATROGENIC DISORDERS

Certain iatrogenic psychiatric disorders should be noted. The roles of exogenous thyroid and corticosteroid medications have already been mentioned. In addition, adrenergic-depleting and adrenergic-blocking agents, such as reserpine and beta-blockers, are well known to cause depressive disorders, potentially of severe and even suicidal intensity. Numerous anti-inflammatory agents have been recognized to cause symptoms of anxiety or depression. An acute delirium can, of course, result from excessive doses of medication or from injudicious polypharmacy. Withdrawal from addictive central nervous system depressants (that is, tranquilizers or hypnotics) may produce anxiety and sleep disturbances with nightmares. More severe withdrawal states can also result in delirium with psychotic features. Sudden cessation of central nervous system stimulants such as dextroamphetamine may produce a severe depression. This list is by no means exhaustive, and physicians should be familiar with the potential psychiatric complications of any medication they prescribe.

SURGICAL EFFECTS

Psychiatric reactions are also known to occur postoperatively. Surgical intervention, especially open heart surgery with pump support, may result in an agitated, paranoid psychotic state. Some correlation has been suggested between preoperative fear on the part of the patient and the potential for postoperative psychosis. This psychotic state usually involves a delirious clouding of consciousness and is resolved with relatively standard antipsychotic therapy.

Psychiatric Presentations of Medical Disorders

The second approach to the interrelationship of medical and psychiatric disorders is shown in Table 17-1, which lists the medical causes of mental changes according to the specific psychiatric symptomatology produced. An understanding in both directions—that is, medical problems that involve psychiatric manifestations and psychiatric disorders that present with medical symptoms—will increase the clinician's index of suspicion and probable recognition of a covert medical illness presenting as a psychiatric syndrome.

Treatment

Having once reached a diagnostic conclusion, one then proceeds to treat the primary medical illness according to basic therapeutic principles. If the psychiatric symptoms disappear after appropriate treatment of the underlying physical illness, then one can assume that the correct physical diagnosis was made. At times, however, psychiatric symptoms may be so severe as to require acute intervention, or there may be a psychiatric illness concomitant with the physical illness. In such a case, skilled management, possibly including psychotropic medication, as well as other medication or therapy procedures, must be used. For those purposes one should consult the other chapters in this book relevant to the psychiatric disorder manifested. Needless to say, if the correct diagnosis is made, the physician will have the satisfaction of seeing the patient get the most efficient and effective treatment that is currently available.

References and Further Reading

Alexander, F.G., Selesnick, S.T. *The History of Psychiatry*. New York: Harper and Row, 1966.

American Psychiatric Association, APA Council on Research and Development. *A Report of the APA Task Force on Behavior Therapy*, 2nd ptg. Washington, D.C.: American Psychiatric Association, 1974.

American Psychiatric Association. *Psychiatric Glossary*, 4th rev. ed. New York: Basic Books, 1975.

Bion, W.R. *Experience in Groups and Other Papers*. New York: Basic Books, 1959.

Brenner, C. *An Elementary Textbook of Psychoanalysis,* revised and expanded. New York: International Universities Press, 1973.

Brill, A.A. (ed.). *The Basic Writings of Sigmund Freud,* New York: Random House, 1938.

Burns, David D. *Feeling Good: The New Mood Therapy*. New York: William Morrow, 1980.

Clark, D.H. *Administrative Therapy: The Role of the Doctor in the Therapeutic Community*. London: J.B. Lippincott, Tavistock Publications, 1964.

Cumming, J., Cumming, E. *Ego and Milieu. Theory and Practice of Environmental Therapy*. New York: Atnetan, 1962.

Green, E., Green, A. *Beyond Biofeedback*. New York: Dell, 1977.

Gunderson, J.G. Defining the therapeutic processes in psychiatric milieus. *Psychiatry* 41:327–335, 1978.

Hinsie, L.E., Cambell, R.J. *Psychiatric Dictionary,* 4th ed. New York: Oxford University Press, 1970

Jones, M. *The Therapeutic Community*. New York: Basic Books, 1953.

Steinberg, H., Torem, M., Saravay, S.M. An analysis of physician resistance to psychiatric consultations. *Arch. Gen. Psychiatry* 37:1007, 1980.

Webster's New International Dictionary of the English Language, 2nd. ed., unabridged. Springfield, Mass.: Merriam Webster, 1943.

Wolpe, J. *The Practice of Behavior Therapy*, 2nd ed. Pergamon General Psychology Series. New York: Pergamon Press, 1973.

Yalom, I.D. *The Theory and Practice of Group Psychotherapy,* 2nd ed. New York: Basic Books, 1965.

III

Treatment

Assessment and Management of the Suicidal Patient

C. TERRENCE CHASTEK, M.D.

The clinical assessment of suicidal behavior requires a careful examination of suicidal intentionality, the psychodynamic characteristics of the patient, and a comprehensive psychiatric history. Suicidal behavior is a final outcome of a psychosocial stressor, of conscious and unconscious psychodynamics, and of varying degrees of intentionality. Suicidal behavior is an *acute, time-limited crisis,* and skilled professional interventions reduce mortality and morbidity.

Epidemiology

RATE AND INCIDENCE

The United States Department of Health and Human Services estimates a reported suicide rate in the United States of 10 to 12 per 100,000 and a yearly incidence of approximately 25,000 deaths. The actual number of suicides may be in considerable excess of the reported rate. The rate of suicide attempts is much higher—an estimated 10 attempts for every completed suicide. Suicide attempts are a common clinical problem in hospital emergency services.

DEMOGRAPHIC FACTORS

Analysis of demographic data identifies patterns of suicide within the population. Although these factors are important in statistical population analysis, the acutal assessment of the patient's suicide risk must be made as part of an individual clinical evaluation.

Age

Although suicides may occur in the young, attempts appear uncommon until adolescence. Childhood suicide, which is rare, is generally impulsive, and is often the action of a child who feels unfairly punished and unloved and wants to punish those who would suffer and grieve because of his or her death. Children who attempt suicide are generally very disturbed and have pathologic family situations. Suicidal behavior in children may include attempted suffocation, hanging, jumping from heights, running in front of vehicles, or ingesting medications or toxic household substances. In preschool children, accidental injuries are the most frequent cause of death, and subintentional attempts at suicide may be suggested by lethal accidents or by the tendency to have repeated accidents in this age group.

Adolescent suicide occurs at a rate of approximately six per 100,000; as is true for adults, there is a ratio of about three male deaths for each female death. Suicide is a major cause of death in the adolescent population, and studies have shown that suicide is second only to automobile accidents as the most frequent cause of death. The precipitant of an adolescent suicide is frequently a feeling of rejection by a teenage peer group or by a partner in a teenage romance. Adolescents who attempt suicide are typically chronically unhappy and have long-standing problems in relating to their parents, difficulties in establishing an identification with their social peer group, and a history of behavior problems—often including rebelliousness, school dysfunction, legal problems, and drug and alcohol abuse and dependence.

Suicide in young adults and middle-age people is frequently related to a depressive episode that is often precipitated by severe feelings of rejection and social isolation. Increased social isolation also appears to be a significant factor in elderly suicides because older people may have lost a sense of meaningful purpose. The frequency of suicide increases with age in men until the seventh decade, with a decline beginning at 75 to 85 years of age. In women the peak frequency for suicide is between 45 and 65 years of age. The suicide rate appears to be increasing in young people, while the rate in persons older than 35 appears to be decreasing slightly.

Sex
Men commit suicide about three times as frequently as women. However, women attempt suicide more frequently; there are approximately three suicide attempts by women for each attempt by a man. Recent data suggest that the difference in the rate of suicide and attempted suicide between men and women is narrowing.

Marital Status
Suicide rates are higher among unmarried people, including those who never married as well as the divorced and widowed. Patients who have lost a spouse through death are at a significantly higher risk of suicide and suicide attempts.

Occupational Status
In general, people who are unemployed have higher suicide rates than those of skilled workers and other people with jobs. Suicide rates are distributed throughout socioeconomic levels. Higher suicide rates have been noted in specific occupations including policemen, musicians, dentists, insurance agents, physicians, and lawyers. Physicians as a group have one of the highest suicide rates among all occupations; suicide may be the leading cause of death among physicians under the age of 40.

Clinical Conditions Predisposing to Suicide

SCHIZOPHRENIC DISORDERS
Schizophrenic patients have a high risk of suicide; it has been estimated that up to 20 percent of them have made suicide attempts. Suicide is a danger in patients suffering from schizophrenic conditions in the acute, recovery, and chronic phases of the illness. Schizophrenic attempts may be related to delusional beliefs and auditory hallucinations during acute exacerbations of the illness. Patients with schizophrenia may suffer from a postpsychotic depression, or they may experience depression, anxiety, and impaired self-esteem as reality testing improves; recovery from an acute episode can place the patient at *greater* risk of suicidal behavior.

Chronic schizophrenic patients, who frequently have been estranged from family and community, have very impaired personal relationships and are frequently socially isolated. This isolation further increases the risk of suicide. Schizophrenic patients are generally unpredictable and impulsive, and suicidal behavior in this group of patients requires a particularly careful assessment and intensive intervention.

MAJOR DEPRESSIVE DISORDERS
Suicidal ideations and attempts are important symptoms of major depressive disorders, and suicide is a major cause of death in this group. Major depressive disorders can be recognized and diagnosed by careful evaluation of the fundamental characteristics of such symptoms as (1) dysphoric affects (sadness, irritability); (2) vegetative symptoms including changes in appetite, libido, and energy; (3) psychosomatic manifestations; (4) psychomotor changes including retardation or agitation; (5) cognitive changes including concentration problems; (6) feelings of hopelessness and helplessness; and (7) a sense of worthlessness and inappropriate guilt.

Mobilizing psychosocial resources is particularly important in patients suffering from major depressive disorders. Psychotherapeutic interventions can be of significant help in ameliorating acute symptoms and in reducing the risk of further suicide attempts. Psychopharmacologic interventions may also be helpful. Hospitalization is often warranted when the risk of suicidal behavior is significant.

BIPOLAR AFFECTIVE DISORDERS
Patients suffering from a manic-depressive illness need to be carefully assessed for suicide potential. The risk in this disorder is extremely high. Manic-depressive patients appear at

greatest risk during a change in the bipolar illness—the point at which a manic or depressive episode begins or ends. Brief hospitalizations to establish mood stabilization, psychopharmacologic interventions (especially the use of lithium), and long-term supportive psychotherapeutic relationships have been particularly helpful with this group of patients.

SUBSTANCE ABUSE DISORDERS

Substance abusers have a very high risk of suicide. Depressed mood is a common occurrence during substance abuse. Furthermore, people who abuse alcohol or drugs may have alienated their social supports, may have lost jobs, and are often in poor physical health. The chemical effects of alcohol and drugs also increase suicidal potential by releasing impulses and altering judgment. A particularly dangerous situation occurs for the recovered substance abuser who resumes drinking or using drugs. The guilt, shame, and emotional loss at such time can be enormous.

MEDICAL ILLNESS

Medical illnesses and therapeutic medical interventions can be significant psychosocial stressors that may result in suicidal behavior. Patients who undergo extensive medical or surgical treatment often experience loss of functioning, impairments in self-esteem, changes in interpersonal relationships, and psychological sequelae; these effects may occur as a result of the treatment or they may be related to the limitations of therapeutic interventions that are unable to cure the underlying disorder.

Patients who develop chronic debilitating illnesses appear at highest risk, and patients who suffer from chronic protracted diseases with intractable pain are in particular danger. Huntington's chorea has been extensively studied, and this progressively debilitating illness is not infrequently terminated by suicide.

ORGANIC CONDITIONS

Delirium of any etiology with impairment in reality testing, disorganized thinking, confusion, and memory impairments may result in suicidal behavior. A careful medical and psychiatric examination will be required to delineate the presence and cause of an acute organic condition and to initiate an appropriate intervention.

Evaluation of Suicide Risks

To evaluate the risk that a patient may successfully commit suicide, one should assess the degree of intentionality of the suicide attempt. The following characteristics of the suicidal tendency or act should be explored: (1) the severity of the suicidal wish including thoughts, impulses, and fantasies; (2) the lethality of the manner of implementation (overdose, hanging, fatal accident, shooting, cutting, or stabbing); (3) the availability of potential psychosocial resources for intervention and prevention. A *history* of previous suicide attempts is an indication of increased risk for future successful suicide, as is a positive family history of suicide.

PSYCHOLOGICAL RISK FACTORS

A number of psychological factors may increase the probability of a suicide attempt. Feelings of despair, sadness, hostility, anger, shame, guilt, hopelessness, or worthlessness contribute to a suicide attempt. Most suicide events are dyadic and represent an actual or fantasized threat of separation and loss of a loved object. Anger and hostility are frequent conflicts in suicide; patients repress the rage they feel about the loved object and turn that rage against themselves.

A *deterioration in self-esteem* is a frequent concomitant in the development of suicidal behavior. Diminution in self-esteem may be related to many factors other than the loss of a loved person. An assault to self-concept may result from physical trauma or medical illness. A loss of function basic to one's self-identity is an important correlate of suicidal behavior, and the loss of physical, sexual, or occupational functioning may contribute to a loss of self-esteem, shame, and guilt, thus increasing the risk of a suicide attempt. Another risk is a feeling of helplessness—the patient's perception that he or she is unable to modify the psychological experience of overwhelming forces in personal relationships or in the environment. Helplessness also implies the inability of the patient to be successful in having others help with the crisis. Hopelessness and despair frequently play a dominant role in the production of suicidal behavior.

The existence of any of the psychological and medical disorders previously identified is definitely a risk factor to be included in the evaluation of suicide potential.

In spite of the patient's feeling of helplessness and despair, the suicide event is generally an acute crisis of time-limited, often brief, duration. Although patients who attempt suicide frequently have histories of chronic emotional problems, the emergency represented by a suicide attempt is often capable of amelioration in hours or day. The crisis nature of suicide attempts mandates careful professional assessment and skillful medical and psychiatric interventions even in chronically unhappy and poorly adjusted patients.

Most patients in a suicidal crisis are *ambivalent*. Suicidal patients simultaneously struggle with conflictual wishes, impulses, fantasies, and ideas that include both (1) wishes of self-destruction and (2) wishes for rescue and intervention. The ambivalence of suicidal patients represents a critically important "cry for help" that must be utilized to assist in the recovery of a will to live.

Management of the Suicidal Patient

A suicidal patient represents a medical emergency and must be treated in a setting appropriate for crisis interventions. Patients who have made a suicide attempt require careful medical and psychiatric assessment and intervention. These patients require a safe environment to prevent further harm and a supportive, nonrejecting environment to help them reestablish an investment in relationships and a hope for the future. The attitude of the physician is particularly important, since such patient will probably continue to struggle with ambivalent feelings, including both suicidal wishes and wishes for rescue and help.

Suicidal patients frequently engender *countertransference* (unconscious emotional reactions) in medical and psychiatric professionals. Physicians should be particularly aware of the development of these feelings toward suicidal patients; the emotional reactions that constitute countertransference may include resentment, annoyance, indifference, denial, and rationalization. The physician's annoyance, hostility, or rejection may complicate the patient's anger, guilt, or shame and adversely effect not only the acute medical management but the outcome of the suicide event. The use of psychiatric consultation is frequently helpful in the assessment of suicide risk and the management of suicidal patients, and that consultation will frequently facilitate a thorough assessment, integrate medical and psychiatric management, and reduce countertransference problems.

Suicidal patients tend to have difficulty utilizing fantasy and imagination and to tend to polarize perception (everything is thought to be all good or all bad, all right or all wrong). Rigidity and constriction in the cognitive style of patients during a suicide event limit their ability to project and imagine themselves out of the crisis and into the future.

Crisis intervention techniques are particularly useful with suicidal patients. Because, as previously noted, the suicidal crisis is generally brief in duration and usually involves ambivalent wishes, the situation will frequently be ameliorated by crisis intervention. Given time and support, the great majority of suicidal patients will change their minds. The clinician's understanding, empathy, and concerned involvement with all threats of suicide fosters a sense of caring for the individual and may help the patient reestablish a sense of self-worth. Careful observation in a safe, protective, and supportive environment reduces the impulsive threat of these patients and helps them regain a sense of control over destructive impulses and opportunities.

Hospitalization may be required for patients with significant suicide risk; however, brief hospitalization may be all that is needed to reduce suicide risk and to initiate interventions in patients suffering from an emotional crisis. Interventions include mobilization of environmental resources, initiation of supportive psychotherapy, and establishment of a relationship with a therapist to prepare the patient for outpatient followup treatment. Patients suffering from psychiatric illness may benefit from a brief hospitalization to stabilize the illness and reduce suicide risk. Patients suffering from toxic reactions to alcohol overdose frequently require brief hospitalization until there is a full return of sensorium, cognition, memory, and judgment. Suicidal patients are in particular need of reestablishing psychosocial support in the environment. The reestablishment of crucial interpersonal relationships is of considerable value in the acute management of the patient and in the prevention of further suicidal behavior. Family and friends, who are viewed as potential support for the patient, can be extremely useful in assisting professional interventions and should be involved as much as possible.

Case 1. N.P., a 48-year-old woman, was brought to the hospital after an overdose of sleeping medications prescribed by her internist. N. had apparently been suffering for two to three months from an increasing sleep disorder including initial insomnia, frequent awakenings, and early morning awakening with an impending sense of doom and dread; she was then unable to return to sleep.

Psychiatric evaluation revealed a two- to three-month history of increasing sleep disorder, a loss of appetite and loss of weight, crying spells, and loss of energy. N. admitted to feelings of worthlessness and hopelessness about her future.

The patient was hospitalized for a few weeks, during which time psychotherapy and a course of antidepressants were initiated. After a period of stabilization following the alleviation of her severe symptomatology, N. was able to make the transition from the hospital to outpatient psychotherapy, assisted by antidepressant pharmacotherapy.

Case 2. R.B., a 20-year-old single woman, was brought to a crisis intervention service by a girlfriend because R. had expressed wishes to harm herself. She had apparently suffered a loss of romantic relationship, became increasingly preoccupied and tearful, and expressed impulses to hurt herself, although she had not made an actual attempt. R. voluntarily came to the crisis intervention service at the suggestion of her friend.

Psychiatric examination revealed a tearful young woman in acute distress. There was no evidence of a major depressive disorder or psychotic thinking. Premorbidly she had exhibited difficulty in romantic relationships but had no history of psychiatric problems. R. appeared very distraught over her romantic involvement, with a deterioration in her self-esteem and fearfulness of her impulsive self-destructive ideation.

R. was able to return home accompanied by her friend; she was scheduled to begin in outpatient psychotherapy the next day to allow a more comprehensive psychiatric evaluation.

Case 3. A.S., a 35-year-old recently separated man, threatened to shoot himself with a hunting rifle and was brought to the local emergency room by a family friend. A. appeared intoxicated and had apparently been drinking daily for the past two weeks and recently was threatening suicide during alcohol intoxication

A. was admitted to an alcohol treatment center for detoxification. Psychiatric consultation was requested after detoxification had been completed. A. had a chronic episodic problem with alcohol addiction and had become increasingly addicted to alcohol after a deterioration in his marriage.

He was able to be successfully detoxified and make a commitment to a supportive Alcoholics Anonymous group for continued alcoholism treatment. Outpatient psychotherapy was recommended but A. refused; however he did agree to episodic psychiatric consultation and consented to an exchange of information between the consultant and the alcoholism counselor.

References and Further Reading

Agee, V. L. *Treatment of Violent, Incorrigible Adolescents.* Lexington, Mass.: Lexington Books; 1979.

Barnhill, L.R. Clinical assessment of intrafamilial violence. *Hosp. Community Psychiatry* 31:543–547, 1980.

Basic intervention for violence in families. *Hosp. Comm. Psychiatry* 31:547–551, 1980.

Beck, A. *The Predictors of Suicide.* Bowie, Md.: Charles Press, 1974.

Child and Adolescent Suicide. Rockville, Md.: National Institute of Mental Health, 1981.

Farberow, N.L. *The Many Faces of Suicide, Indirect and Self-Destructive Behavior.* New York: McGraw-Hill, 1980.

Holinger, P.C. Violent deaths as a leading cause of mortality: an epidemiologic study of suicide, homicide, and accidents. *Am. J. Psychiatry* 137:472–476, 1980.

May, R. *Power and Innocence: A Search for the Sources of Violence.* New York: Norton, 1972.

Menuck, M., Voineskos, G. The etiology of violent behavior: an overview. *Gen. Hosp. Psychiatry* 3:37–47, 1981.

Perlin, S. *Handbook for Study of Suicide.* New York: Oxford University Press, 1975.

Pfeffer, C. R. Suicidal behavior of children: a review with implications for research and practice. *Am. J. Psychol.* 138:154–159, 1981.

Schneidman, E. *Suicidology: Contemporary Developments.* New York: Grune & Stratton, 1976.

Tardiff, K., et al. Assault, suicide and mental illness. *Arch. Gen. Psychiatry* 37:164–169, 1980.

Violent patient: rapid assessment and management. *Psychosomatics* 2:101–105, 1981.

Wekstein, L. *Handbook of Suicidology: Principles, Problems, and Practices.* New York: Brunner/Mazel, 1979.

Assessment and Management of the Violent Patient
C. TERRENCE CHASTEK, M.D.

A useful classification of the violent patient is difficult to achieve. Violence is here defined as behavior intended to produce physical harm or destruction. Although threats of violence are not uncommon among psychiatric patients, violent behavior itself is a relatively infrequent manifestation of mental illness. The subgroup of patients who exhibit violence as a direct product of mental illness appears to be relatively small. Patients exhibiting violent thoughts and impulses, on the other hand, are much more numerous than those who ever commit a violent act. Understanding and managing violent patients should begin with this larger, potentially violent group so as to prevent the more dangerous outcome.

Violence may occur in a number of settings and conditions, only a few of which are appropriate for medical and psychiatric intervention. Not all deviant behavior is a result of mental illness, and psychiatric intervention appears appropriate only when a diagnosable disorder can be identified.

Epidemiology

Violent behavior commonly includes a wide variety of physically harmful actions directed toward a person—for example, murder, sexual assault and rape, physical assault, spouse abuse, and child abuse. Social violence in the context of conflicting political and cultural ideologies, including mass violence, is broader than the content of this discussion and not appropriate for psychiatric intervention.

Statistical descriptions of violent behavior are available. In the United States the current homicide rate averages 10 deaths per 100,000 population. In the average year in America 20,000 people are murdered; 60,000 to 80,000 are victims of rape; 400,000 are threatened in armed robbery; and 500,000 are victims of significant physical assault. Data suggest that someone is admitted to an emergency room as a casualty of violence about once every minute in the United States.

Violence in the United States follows certain general patterns: high concentration in metropolitan centers, preponderance in socially and economically deprived areas, and an overrepresentation in young males. Half of rape arrests and a third of homicide arrests involve males under the age of 25. Additionally, young men are the most frequent homicide victims; for a black man in his twenties living in a socially deprived metropolitan area, murder is the most common cause of death.

Violence is clearly not only associated with criminal activity, and less than one-fourth of murders occur during the course of robbery or related crimes. Violent behavior is often related to alcohol, drug, and narcotic abuse. Alcoholics and drug abusers are overrepresented as both offenders and victims of violence.

Violence between family members accounts for approximately 20 percent of homicide victims; spouse murder accounts for the majority of family homicides. Lethal episodes represent a minority of familial violence, and spouse abuse is frequently unreported because of fear and shame.

Homicide rates vary depending on the day of the week; weekends and holidays represent statistical peaks, and there is a greater-than-average incidence in July and August and a peak at Christmas.

Child abuse is a significant form of violent behavior and may cause up to one-third of the fractures in children admitted to emergency rooms. Victims of child abuse appear to have an unfortunate potential for becoming child abusers themselves later in adolescence and adult life.

Classification

When violence is a manifestation of a mental illness, appropriate identification and assessment of the mental illness will assist in therapeutic interventions. *Psychological, neurologic,* and *toxic* factors may contribute to violent behavior. Cultural and sociological factors may influence the form of violent behavior.

Violence is not unique to specific diagnostic categories, and a diagnostic description does not enable one to predict violent behavior. The following is a description of some of the more common clinical situations in which violent behavior may be a manifestation of psychiatric, neurologic, or toxic conditions.

PSYCHIATRIC CONDITIONS LEADING TO VIOLENCE

Personality Disorders

Personality disorders are common in persons who exhibit violent behavior; numerous subtypes of personality disorders are represented. Patients with *antisocial personality disorders* represent a subgroup whose violence may also occur in association with criminal activity; these people typically have histories of early and excessive aggressive behaviors. The antisocial behavior and interpersonal impairments are typically chronic and persistent; psychiatric interventions generally have limited impact in modifying antisocial personality disorders.

Patients with *borderline personality disorders* reveal a chronic history of low frustration tolerance, impulsivity, unstable interpersonal relationships, and affective lability. These patients reveal limited ability to function under stress. Acute regressions of micropsychotic proportions may occur with impaired ability to integrate and control rage, anger, and aggression.

Additionally, the *overcontrolled, compulsive* person has been described as one who chronically suppresses frustration and rage. Overcontrolled individuals are externally cooperative, passive, and compliant, but occasionally under the influence of acute frustration they regress, and precipitous violence may occur.

Major Affective Disorder

Patients in a major depressive episode will occasionally attempt or commit homicide and follow it with their own suicide or suicide attempt. Violent behavior in depressed patients is generally precipitated by severe psychological stress (such as marital separation) with resultant symptoms of intense hopelessness and despair. These persons may act under the pessimistic belief that they are sparing others from a bleak and painful future.

Bipolar Affective Disorder

Bipolar affective disorders, particularly during manic or hypomanic phases, may cause very impaired control of aggression. Patients suffering from these disorders demonstrate mood lability, low frustration tolerance, and irritability, and they are often easily annoyed. These patients often exhibit pressured speech and behavior sometimes related to omnipotent and grandiose delusions; they may also become paranoid or abuse alcohol. Patients with bipolar affective disorders exhibiting violent behavior during a manic or hypomanic episode will generally require hospitalization and appropriate pharmacologic intervention until the illness can be stabilized.

Schizophrenia

Schizophrenic patients who are actively psychotic may exhibit violent behavior as a product of a delusional system. Such delusions may include the belief that a person (or some group) is attempting to control their mind or behavior, or that someone represents a serious threat to their safety and well-being (or the safety of others). Patients experiencing paranoid delusions or command hallucinations can be extremely unpredictable and dangerous.

Acutely ill schizophrenic patients who suffer from violent ideation or behavior generally require hospitalization and appropriate pharmacologic interventions. Patients exhibiting acute and bizarre destructive behavior may respond to aggressive pharmacotherapy with frequent administration of potent antipsychotic medications (for example, haloperidol) to achieve control of the violent behavior. Rapid antipsychotic titration is generally best performed in a hospital setting.

Conduct Disorders of Childhood and Adolescence

Aggressive behavior is frequently present in conduct disorders, which have their onset in childhood and adolescence. These children typically have impaired social attachments, egocentrism, and aggressive behaviors. The aggressive behavior of these children and adolescents generally includes defiance, negativism, verbal abusiveness, and bullying, although occasionally more severe aggressive behavior develops. Aggressive behavior in children and adolescents with conduct disorders may represent defensive acting out of psychodynamic conflicts.

NEUROLOGIC DISORDERS LEADING TO VIOLENCE

Episodic Dyscontrol Syndrome

The episodic dyscontrol syndrome has been described as a behavior pattern characterized by periodic violence. Aggressive behavior is presumed to represent an abnormality in the limbic system involving lesions of the temporal lobe, frontal lobe, amygdala, or hippocampus. Episodic dyscontrol appears related to an aura or postictal confusional state rather than directly to an ictal phenomenon. Episodic dyscontrol syndrome has been associated with pathologic intoxication, impulsive sexual behavior or assaults, and a history of serious traffic accidents.

The electroencephalogram will occasionally reveal subcortical dysrhythmias or epileptogenic discharges. Nasopharyngeal leads and sleep activation enhance the identification of anterior and medial temporal lobe abnormalities.

Controversy exists regarding the relationship of epilepsy to violence. Violence as a direct manifestation of seizure activity is very rare, and the vast majority of epileptics do not suffer from violent behavior.

Attention Deficit Disorders

Children, adolescents, and adults with a history of attention deficit disorder with hyperactivity (previously described as minimal brain dysfunction) will frequently reveal low frustration tolerance, mood lability, concentration deficits, impulsivity, and occasional aggressive outbursts. Attention deficit disorders always present in childhood but may persist into adolescence and adulthood. Psychostimulant medications such as dextroamphetamine and methylphenidate have been reported to reduce disruptive, impulsive, and aggressive behavior in some patients; in addition these medications improve concentration and attention impairments.

TOXIC AND ORGANIC CONDITIONS LEADING TO VIOLENCE

Alcohol Abuse

Alcohol appears to be a significant contributing factor to violent behavior in many individuals. Some patients appear sensitive to *pathologic intoxication*, a transient psychotic condition induced by even small quantities of alcohol. Disinhibition and impairment of judgment contribute to a release of violent behavior.

Drug Abuse

Studies have demonstrated violence associated with sedative-hypnotic drugs including barbiturates and benzodiazepines. Irritability is a common feature in withdrawal from drug and alcohol dependency.

Violent behavior appears particularly problematic in association with use of phencyclidine (PCP, "angel dust"). Phencyclidine may produce psychotic episodes with bizarre violent behavior that is often quite unpredictable in its timing or object.

In addition to the pharmacologic effects of a drug, other factors that significantly influence the final behavioral outcome are: the social setting in which the drug is used, the personality constellation of the individual abusing the drug, and the behavioral patterns of the social group in which the drug use is associated. These situational, personality, and social factors may either mitigate or augment the pharmacologic effects.

Other Medical Conditions
Premenstrual tension in women has been associated with increased irritability and occasionally aggressive behavior. Metabolic conditions such as hypoglycemia have been related to aggressiveness, but these appear to be rare causes. Medical and neurologic abnormalities should be investigated in patients whose violence or aggressiveness appears atypical for that individual.

Mental Retardation
Occasionally mental retardation may be associated with impulsive aggressive or sexual behavior.

Etiology

GENETIC FACTORS
An occasional genetic predisposition towards violence has been postulated to be associated with the XYY genotype in males. The condition is rare, and the relationship of this genetic condition to violence is controversial.

DEVELOPMENTAL CHARACTERISTICS
Family histories frequently reveal that violent patients come from homes with intrafamilial aggression, violence, or deprivation. Alcoholism and parental brutality are frequent in patient histories. The childhood history should be explored for hyperkinesis, cruelty to animals, enuresis, and temper tantrums. Although these traits are frequently seen in patients exhibiting violent behavior, their prognostic value is unclear. Patterns of frustration tolerance and impulse control should be explored for indications of the potential for violence and the etiology of the problem.

Impairments in the development of stable and caring object relations are frequent in aggressive patients who have inadequately developed basic, dependent, and trusting relationships. Aggressive patients are often described as infantile or immature, and they also frequently have limited ability to form close interpersonal relationships; they may reveal a schizoid intrapsychic development and defensive organization. A lack of trust appears related to an impaired sense of self and further augments their overreactivity to criticism.

Personality characteristics develop very early in life, and character structure and psychological defenses are generally unconscious. As a result these patients have difficulty learning from experience and tend to repeat maladaptive patterns of behavior. Intrapsychic change is difficult for violent offenders with personality disorders, and they also have difficulty generalizing from the therapeutic situation to other environmental situations.

PSYCHOLOGICAL FACTORS
An assessment of the violent patient should include a determination of the precipitant for the crisis, an evaluation of the intensity and the target of the anger or aggressiveness, and an assessment of internal psychological controls.

A common etiologic feature in violent patients is a narcissistic injury (that is, an injury to self-esteem) that threatens damage to the individual's self-concept and causes overwhelming and disruptive anxiety. Helplessness is a frequent underlying theme in such patients. Pseudohomosexual panic has been described as a condition in which violent behavior may occur in an effort to reestablish self-esteem and masculinity by using hyperaggressiveness to defend against passivity, dependency, and helplessness. (Child abuse frequently occurs as a defensive reaction formation against the parent's own helplessness and inadequacy. The parent distorts his or her anxiety into a perception that the child is "attacking" the parent's authority and caretaking.)

Morbid jealousy also can threaten the individual's self-esteem and result in rage and aggression to retaliate, damage, or destroy.

Management

PSYCHOTHERAPEUTIC APPROACHES

Individuals with personality disorders characteristically reveal limitations in tolerating and integrating dysphoric feelings such as anxiety, depression, and anger. This pathologic characterologic development appears to occur as individuals learn to protect themselves from dysphoric feelings with two major modes of defense. The first defense is *denial,* which involves denying both internal intrapsychic stress and interpersonal needs. Denial can be utilized so extensively as to cause reality distortion, which further impairs judgment and control of internal impulses. Psychotherapeutic interventions focus on helping the patient become more able to tolerate internal distress, reduce denial and reality distortion, and reestablish mastery over aggressive impulses. The second major defensive operation is *acting out,* which represents the attempt to relieve intrapsychic distress by behavior rather than by more mature defenses, such as fantasy and sublimation, which normally allow a person to postpone gratification. Psychotherapeutic and crisis intervention techniques frequently focus on reducing aggressive behavior by learning to talk about rather than act out conflicts. This not only helps patients to control aggressive violent impulses but also allows them to begin to form effective patient-therapist relationships.

ROLE OF THE PHYSICIAN AND TREATMENT PERSONNEL

Violent patients frequently provoke strong unconscious countertransference reactions in health professionals. The hostility of the patient can stimulate physicians' own anxiety, fear, and reactive hostility, thereby reducing their effectiveness in crisis and therapeutic intervention. It is most important that clinicians be aware of their own internal images and reactions to violence so that they can have better self-control in dealing with such patients.

The utilization of a professional team including psychiatric consultation is preferable to professional interventions by an individual because it decreases anxiety and misjudgment. The physician may function as the expert leader, but staff members from other disciplines such as nursing have a primary role in stabilizing the environment, communicating a sense of control and safety to these patients, and setting clear limits regarding behavior and threats. Above all, the team must present a consistent, uniform message to violent or potentially violent patients. This message usually includes a statement that the caretaking personnel recognize the difficulty the patients are having—especially their underlying fear. Furthermore, the caretakers are there to help the patients stay under control, not to hurt them. The expectations or plan is then presented in a clear, direct manner without overt fear, anger, or threats. The sense of calm control must be communicated and followed up. Adequate personnel to ensure control and safety should be immediately available and evident without prematurely surrounding the patients. The goal is to generate in these patients a feeling that encourages deescalation of violent impulses and reestablishment of self-control.

PHYSICAL INTERVENTIONS

Acute interventions, including physical restraint, may be required. When physical restraint is necessary, an adequate number of trained individuals is essential to prevent injury of either the staff or the patient. A combative patient must be controlled as quickly and effectively as possible to reduce the potential for injury to the professional team and to the patient. Efficient intervention further reduces anxiety and anger. A commonly utilized restraint procedure is to have one or more individuals assigned to each extremity and to the head, to enhance the smoothness and effectiveness of the physical intervention. A safe quiet room may be helpful by decreasing sensory stimulation, or limb and body restraint may be employed.

MEDICATIONS

Psychopharmacologic intervention depends on the conceptual and diagnostic understanding of the violent patient. Acutely violent patients may benefit from rapid tranquilization with antipsychotic medications. High-potency neuroleptics such as haloperidol (5 to 10 mg intramuscularly or orally) are generally preferable to avoid side effects of orthostatic hypotension or cardiac arrhythmias. The dosage may be repeated every 30 to 60 minutes until control is established.

Social and Professional Responsibilities

PREDICTION OF DANGEROUSNESS

A task force of the American Psychiatric Association has reviewed the prediction of violence and conceptualization of *dangerousness*. This task force report emphasizes the difficulty of predicting rare and infrequent events such as violence and suicide, and it stresses that the label of *dangerous* has been applied indiscriminately with far more false positives than true positives. Dangerousness is neither a psychiatric nor medical diagnosis. The single greatest useful predictor of future violent behavior of an individual is a history of previous violent behavior; severely recidivistic offenders are clearly more dangerous.

A continuing problem is that although the actual probability of violent behavior is small, the future occurrence of violent behavior may have considerable consequences. Since physicians, including psychiatrists, have limited ability to predict violence, the criteria for the prediction of dangerousness need to be based on societal and judicial determinations rather than solely on clinical judgment.

Courts in several jurisdictions have held that, in the interest of protecting society, the need for informing a potential victim (or notifying the police) of a serious threat of injury outweighs the protection of the patient's privilege of confidentiality in certain circumstances. This is always a difficult decision, and both medical and legal consultants can prove helpful.

Case 1. C.J., a 26-year-old single man, was brought to an emergency room by the police after threatening a female friend. During the altercation C. became increasingly excitable, verbally abusive, and then physically threatening.

On examination, C. appeared very agitated, with pressure of speech and tangential associations. He initially denied emotional problems. In discussing the precipitant, C. gradually admitted to a noticeable increase in sexual drive and acknowledged that the argument was precipitated by his suspicions that his girlfriend was refusing his sexual advances because of her presumed involvement with another man.

C. later acknowledged a previous two-month depression, approximately six months earlier, during which he felt very little energy, interest, and motivation, and was unable to continue his employment.

C. was hospitalized because of his mood lability, impulsiveness, and impaired judgment. Psychiatric evaluation suggested bipolar affective disorder. The patient was hospitalized and treated with neuroleptic medication and lithium carbonate.

Case 2. W.M. is a 24-year-old man referred (from detention) for forensic psychiatric evaluation pending a court hearing to determine competence to stand trial. W. had shot a patron of a local restaurant in the abdomen during a robbery attempt. He claimed to his attorney that he had been under the influence of phencyclidine (PCP, "angel dust") and was unaware of his actions.

Psychiatric examination of W. revealed a very guarded, withdrawn man who volunteered little information. Additional information from the family revealed a childhood, adolescent, and young adult history of antisocial activity with frequently aggressive behavior in the context of criminal activity. Psychological testing, which was ordered to complement the evaluation, revealed low-normal intelligence and personality impoverishment, but no active evidence of psychosis.

W. was determined to be free of overt psychiatric illness and was returned to detention for judicial proceedings. A diagnosis of antisocial personality could have been made but was considered to be no therapeutic or legal significance.

Case 3. P.C., a 14-year-old female, was brought to a crisis clinic by her parents after becoming verbally abusive and assaultive to her mother. P. had become involved in an altercation with her mother regarding a curfew and restriction for deteriorating school functioning and unmanageability at home, including severe defiance of parental authority.

Psychiatric evaluation of P. revealed a two- to three-year history of postpubertal acting out, including defiance of limits, deteriorating school performance, increasing drug and alcohol experimentation and abuse, sexual acting out, and episodes of running away. The parents had become increasingly concerned about their inability to control P.'s negative behavior, and they were worried that she was associating with a delinquent peer group. Family evaluation revealed chronic marital conflict; the parents had considerable differences in parenting styles and difficulty in supporting each other in parenting decisions.

Outpatient individual psychotherapy was arranged for P., who was initially resistant to therapeutic involvement but gradually became invested in treatment and began to work on her impaired self-esteem, developing anxiety and depression, and fears of social rejection.

The family was seen collaterally to improve familial communications and to help her mother and father with parenting techniques.

Case 4. E.N., a 17-year-old male, was admitted under commitment to a psychiatric hospital after destroying property in the home and threatening to kill his father.

A psychiatric examination revealed an extremely agitated young adult who appeared in very poor contact with reality. Parents described a two- to three-month history of increasing social isolation, mood lability, paranoia, and evidence of extensive drug experimentation. The patient appeared floridly psychotic and was hospitalized. A study of urine levels of drugs was performed on admission; it indicated recent ingestion of phencyclidine. The patient required extended hospitalization because of episodic, unpredictable, and violent outbursts. Antipsychotic medications in low doses helped the patient, but moderate doses of these medications appeared to result in deterioration and superimposed delirium. After six month of hospitalization, the patient gradually began to reveal improved reality testing and control of episodic regressive behavior. Cognitive testing showed considerable improvement over initial testing, and the patient appeared to have been suffering from a severe drug-induced psychotic brain syndrome.

References and Further Reading

Clinical Aspects of the Violent Individual. Washington, D.C.: American Psychiatric Association, 1974.

Madden, D.S., Lion, J.R. *Rage, Hate, Assault and Other Forms of Violence.* New York: Spectrum Publications, 1976.

Monroe, R.R. *Episodic Behavior Disorders.* Cambridge: Harvard University Press, 1970.

Pincus, J.H., Tucker, G.J. *Behavioral Neurology,* 2nd ed. New York: Oxford University Press, 1978.

The Psychological Therapies
JAMES T. QUATTLEBAUM, M.D.

For the purpose of this chapter, the term *psychological therapies* refers to all noninvasive systematic approaches to altering a patient's mood, thought processes, or behavior. This chapter will begin with an extensive discussion of the prototype of psychological therapy—psychoanalytically oriented individual psychotherapy—and then proceed to describe briefly various other current psychological therapies and the ways in which they relate to the prototype. In order to understand psychoanalytic psychotherapy (also loosely known as dynamic psychotherapy), some basic concepts must be presented.

Basic Concepts

THE UNCONSCIOUS

People do, say, feel, and think things without a conscious focus on these experiences and processes, and without understanding the reasons for them. The unconscious is defined in the American Psychiatric Association's *Psychiatric Glossary* (1975) as "That part of the mind or mental functioning of which the content is only rarely subject to awareness. It is a repository for data that have never been conscious (primary repression), or that may have become conscious briefly and later repressed (secondary repression)."

Anyone who is performing psychotherapy must confront the significance of the unconscious and recognize its role. The way in which unconscious processes are related to treatment techniques differs depending on the type of therapy and the philosophical assumptions of the therapist.

From one point of view, psychotherapy that is curative must include interpretation of unconscious resistances and must lead to a growing awareness by the patient of previously unconscious elements. At the other end of the spectrum, changes in conscious feelings and behavior alone (without any conscious changes in ideation or memory) are viewed as sufficient. Whatever unconscious changes take place do so unconsciously. Much psychodynamic psychotherapy includes a combination of these approaches.

There are many demonstrations of unconscious processes in everyday life. Dreams are among the most common, but perhaps the most dramatic examples of these processes, at least in terms of being reproducible, are those associated with hypnosis; denial and rationalization of unconscious behavior and feelings can be elicited in an objectively observable way in hypnotized persons.

Information about the unconscious is also obtained from (1) observations of the nature of the relationship of the patient with the therapist, (2) information about the patient's present relationships with other people and past relationships with family members, (3) slips of the tongue, and (4) other unconscious behavior.

FREE ASSOCIATION

In free association, a basic technique in a psychoanalytically influenced psychotherapy, the patient is instructed to say whatever comes to mind without any selection or exclusion whatever. The purpose is to permit the therapist (and the patient) to observe patterns in relationships among feelings, thoughts, and behavior that the patient previously could not see; at appropriate times, this material is used to provide the patient with a broader understanding of his or her own feelings and behavior.

TRANSFERENCE

Transference represents a patient's feelings about and behavior toward a therapist; these feelings are unconsciously influenced by earlier relationships with individuals in the patient's past. These responses must be distinguished from reactions to the "real" therapist. The patient's feelings and behavior may have been appropriate in the past situation but are not in the present; they may, therefore, be observed and their significance noted. The question that each therapist should have painted in red letters on the office ceiling is: "When have you felt this way before?"

Countertransference refers to the sometimes unconscious emotional reaction of the therapist to the patient as if he or she were someone from the therapist's own life experience. The dangers of countertransference do not negate the fact that therapists must have emotional reactions to their patients. Their emotional reactions constitute information about the patients (as well as, incidentally, about the therapists); there are many kinds of information they will never get unless their interaction with patients is to some extent emotional. It is the responsibility of therapists to see that their own feelings are used constructively, and that their behavior is circumspect.

RESISTANCE

Resistance is a tendency by the patient to avoid becoming aware of unconscious emotions. If people have remained unaware of feelings, behavior, or types of relationships that are important to them in their life, it may be assumed that there is some reason for this continued unawareness. Frequently, the reason is that they fear that this information will be so painful that it is actively kept out of consciousness. They will, then, naturally and unconsciously, in whatever ways present themselves, make efforts to *avoid* becoming aware of such feelings as a result of therapeutic techniques.

Because the ingenuity of patients in finding ways to evade potential awareness is infinite, it is important that the "rules" of psychoanalytic psychotherapy be observed. Tardiness must be noted, and missed appointments must be charged for; otherwise, what is actually an evasion of confrontation of unconscious emotions may be viewed by the patient as simply a series of practical coincidences. Family involvement (in this prototype), which is distracting, must be minimized. (The useful participation of families in evaluation and treatment planning must be distinguished from the intrusion of families into psychoanalytic psychotherapy.) Various ways the patient may use to make the therapeutic relationship a personal one, or to structure the discussions, in order to avoid free association, must all be dealt with in ways that sometimes seem arbitrary.

Types of Psychotherapeutic Approach

Psychoanalytically oriented psychotherapy can involve several approaches. Ideally, the therapist would make use of various perspectives simultaneously, but in actual practice it is probably necessary for the therapist to shift from one approach to another from time to time.

INTELLECTUAL OR
COGNITIVE APPROACH

The patient's own observations and those of the therapist lead to a new understanding of his or her feelings and behavior, and their relationship to past experiences. That is, the unconscious becomes conscious, casting illumination on mental and emotional operations. The patient acquires new information about himself or herself.

Current psychiatric thinking does not emphasize the importance of a single traumatic event or emotionally powerful moment, or the recalling of a single long-forgotten incident from a patient's childhood. Of more general significance are patterns and experiences that take place over a period of time. It must be remembered, however, that in traumatic neuroses, single incidents may be very powerful and long-lasting in their effects; for example combat fatigue may necessitate emotional reliving of a repressed memory. Similar processes are important in other psychiatric disorders.

RELATIONSHIP-ORIENTED APPROACH

A relationship with a therapist must be supportive to permit the patient to engage in the process. The therapist must be seen as a collaborative ally who merits a certain amount of trust. The relationship with the therapist is particularly important in fostering whatever "openness to learn" a patient may enter therapy with. It is important that the patient become increasingly willing to learn about himself or herself if therapy is to succeed.

The concept of the relationship with the therapist as a *corrective emotional experience* is a controversial one. But the meaning and impact of the therapist's total relationship with the patient must be considered, aside from specific events or techniques. This relationship can enhance the patient's self-understanding as well as help him or her feel better.

BEHAVIORAL APPROACH

Patients in therapy may be encouraged (positively reinforced) by the therapist, and may, as a result, behave in new, "experimental" ways in therapy sessions or in life outside the therapy sessions. As a result of these changes in behavior, patients may learn some things not only about themselves, but about the world. This may increase the frequency of the new behavior and lead to further experimental changes in behavior. A depressed divorced woman, for example, might feel enough better in a therapeutic relationship to attend business school; she succeeds, gains confidence, and then enters other socially challenging situations.

EMOTIONAL UNDERSTANDING

The understanding obtained in psychotherapy cannot be purely intellectual, but must make sense emotionally as well; successful treatment will not only lead to new thoughts, but also to new feelings. The influence of repressed emotions is referred to so often, and in circumstances where it is so difficult to demonstrate, that it sometimes seems that our awareness of such repressed emotions is useless. On some occasions, however, with suitable patients and suitable treatment, awareness of previously repressed emotions takes place so dramatically, with such overwhelmingly constructive consequences, that it is necessary at all times to take these into account. While anger is frequently repressed, other feelings—including love, sexual desire, fear, and sadness—must also be considered. Repressed anger was involved in both of the following cases.

Case 1. L.D., a sweet, redheaded 19-year-old woman, was hospitalized with intense headaches and weight loss (to a current weight of 85 pounds). She had received two complete neurologic evaluations in two separate university medical centers prior to psychiatric evaluation. In the second psychiatric session, L. began, for the first time, to express her rage (at her father, prosaically enough); within 72 hours she had no headaches and was eating and gaining weight.

Case 2. E.B., a man with undiagnosable gastrointestinal pain, was a half-owner of a corporation worth several million dollars, but he permitted the owner of the other half to run the company and to pay him a small salary (there were no dividends). In early psychotherapeutic sessions, E. was extremely sympathetic toward his boss and co-owner, pointing out to the therapist the many problems the boss dealt with and the reasons for his discourteous treatment of E. Within a year, E. was a millionaire, looking for new vocational challenges, without a stomach ache to bother him.

Variations of the Prototype

SUPPORTIVE PSYCHOTHERAPY

Supportive psychotherapy may be provided in once-a-week sessions or in sessions that are less frequent or of shorter duration. Rather than dealing with new awareness of unconscious patterns, patients treated with this approach to therapy benefit from the symptomatic helpfulness of the therapeutic relationship itself. The therapist may inform, advise, and clarify. Encouragement is provided for new adaptive forms of behavior, and for patients to use those strengths that they already have. Anxiety is reduced; the patients' defenses against distressing feelings are supported, and repression is not only permitted but may be assisted. Reassurance, suggestion, persuasion, inspiration and reeducation are used, and probing is avoided—or at least weighed carefully and used cautiously.

Psychotherapy that is initially supportive may continue over an extended period of time, however, and may become more analytic in its orientation. Some of the work of psychoanalytic psychotherapy may be done; the nature of the work being done may become confused—which can be either useful or destructive.

It is important that supportive psychotherapy not be considered the same as "having a friend to talk with." The therapist has a developed ability to support defenses, knows how to refrain from probing, can offer direct encouragement when effective, and uses supportive techniques sensitively; it is also important that the supportive therapist is paid a fee. The payment makes clear what obligations the patient does *not* have to the therapist; that is, the patient pays a fee and owes the therapist nothing else in return for his or her support. Nonprofessional friends are handicapped by having a vague limit on what they are to give the patient, but also they will tire, or be perceived as tiring, and may want something for themselves in return for the support they are giving. Professional support is, therefore, quite different from that of a friend, valuable though the latter may be.

Value of Medical Background
Some people may question the value of a medical education in this kind of therapy. It is true that much useful therapy can be provided by nonphysicians. It is also true, however, that medical background provides: (1) experience in bearing comprehensive responsibility in relationships with people in life-and-death situations—this responsibility is not provided by graduate school experience in a discipline with less breadth than medicine (airline pilots, but not flight engineers, and battlefield commanders, but not staff officers, have similar experiences); (2) a context in which decisions can be made taking into account both the biologic realm and the physical environment, and a holistic perspective in which individual patients and their management may be viewed; and (3) an ancient ethical heritage (of which most physicians are intuitively aware) that provides a structure of ethical conduct in situations where one person is professionally helping another. Nurses share this more clearly than do members of other nonmedical disciplines. These factors (and perhaps others) support a distinct and important role for physician participation in the development, use, and prescription of psychotherapeutic techniques.

Patient's Role in Psychotherapy
It should be made clear at this point that in psychotherapy, even more than in other types of treatment, patients have ultimate authority in their own treatment and the therapist is an instrument which patients may use to help themselves. A therapist may conscientiously do only what he or she has been commissioned to do—at least tacitly—by the patient, and must not impose his or her own values or goals. I explain to some types of patient that I am like an automobile's power steering—I never turn the wheel but try to make it easier for the driver.

The choice between supportive psychotherapy and analytically oriented psychotherapy is a difficult one that is ultimately based on the capability and goals of the patient. The patient's choice, however, may be an obscure and difficult one, and the actual therapy provided may remain an imprecisely defined mixture for an extended period of time.

PSYCHOANALYSIS
More intense and ambitious than psychoanalytically oriented psychotherapy, psychoanalysis involves four or five sessions weekly for several years. The definitive aspect of psychoanal-

ysis is the focus of attention on the transference and its analysis. The couch, rather than a chair, is used to allow full development of all possible transference manifestations as well as to facilitate free association. As in other types of psychotherapy, much of the work has to do with the interpretation of resistances.

Psychoanalysis has provided the theoretical foundation for most dynamically oriented psychotherapies. The discoveries of Freud have so much become a part of modern civilization that the grand hysterics who composed a significant part of Freud's practice are now rare except in isolated areas or undeveloped countries. This disorder has been successfully prevented by the influence of the culture on the individuals within it.

Psychoanalysis is the treatment of choice for the more integrated character disorders—those that are termed personality disorders in the *Diagnostic and Statistical Manual of Mental Disorders,* Third Edition (DSM-III); many think that this treatment is useful for some neuroses—the DSM-III categories of anxiety, somatoform, and dissociative disorders.

GROUP PSYCHOTHERAPY

The types of group psychotherapy vary in purpose, frequency, and technique; these variations are somewhat analogous to the types of individual psychotherapy. Sessions may be 60 to 90 minutes in duration, may meet one to four times weekly, and usually include seven to nine patients. The goals may be the same as in individual psychotherapy; however, the emphasis may also be on goals uniquely suitable for group settings. Psychodrama or other specialized techniques may be used.

Emphasis in group psychotherapy is more on the here-and-now relationships that a patient has with other members of the group and with the therapists, as distinct from relationships that existed in the past or those with people outside of the group. The primary instrumental task of a group member is to be increasingly open about his or her feelings toward people actually present during the sessions.

The relationships that may be looked at directly in group psychotherapy are, of course, more diverse. Issues of dependence are, in some cases, constructively diluted. Support and confrontive analysis may be given simultaneously, but the support that a group can provide is less finely varied in response to an individual member's changing situation than would be possible with an individual therapist. A group can provide observations and feedback to an individual patient given from a number of different viewpoints and with a kind of power that is quite different from, and sometimes greater than that provided by an individual therapist.

Some patients may require more stimulation than individual therapy can provide in order for emotional experiences of any richness and variety to be forthcoming, while others are so sensitive to group feedback that they are unable to tolerate it.

Patients who have a great deal of difficulty in verbal communication may learn more (although vicariously to start with) in group sessions. Those who are acutely anxious when called on to express themselves in unstructured settings, may, in a group, self-regulate the rate at which they become actively involved, to some extent. Those who are psychologically very unsophisticated may sometimes be oriented (that is, pick up the jargon) better in groups.

Many patients can accomplish the same goals in either individual or group psychotherapy. Group therapy usually costs less, but many patients resist groups because of a notion that they must expose themselves before strangers. The first step, of course, must be the conversion of strangers into colleagues.

Different Types of Group Therapy

A cotherapist is frequently used in group psychotherapy, to provide a second viewpoint, continuity during vacations and absences, opportunity for role-specialization (for example, confronter and supporter), and safer emotional responsiveness to patients (by either therapist, with the other remaining "cool").

Expressive therapies such as art, dance, and psychodrama groups, can foster awareness of subtle and long-hidden feelings that cannot emerge so clearly—or at all—in less global and symbolic ways. They may have both cathartic and insight value. *Gestalt therapy* involves specially developed techniques designed to help patients attend to holistic, here-and-now, biologic, perceptual, and social experiences, permitting growth through encountering themselves more intensely.

Groups with educational or other goals—among them assertiveness training, sensitivity training, training in group phenomena, and encounter groups—are important and may be useful; however, unless they are part of a treatment program, they should be distinguished from therapy groups. The former are usually not adapted for people in great pain or those who present powerful resistances, deal with dangerous unconscious forces, and use pathologic defenses.

In doing group psychotherapy, one must always pay attention to the qualities and behavior of the group as an entity. It is the therapist's responsibility to identify factors that interfere with the development of the group as an instrument that is potentially helpful to the individual members. In looking at a group therapy session, a number of different aspects may be observed: the theme of the group, as well as the content of its conversation; the mood of the group; the stage of the group along the course of its development as an organic entity; the communication pattern within it; the predominant defenses used against awareness of anxiety-producing unconscious emotions; the therapists' roles and the nature of the therapists' interventions; and the special roles of the group. Isolated patients must be noted as well as dominant patients.

Evaluation of Group Phenomena
The development of theory about group psychotherapy has been significantly influenced by the work of Bion (1959). He viewed the group as having, as its primary task, the *study of its own behavior* and internal tensions. The group is distracted from this task, however, to varying degrees, by emotional tendencies toward the acceptance of several basic assumptions:

1. Dependence: The assumption is that "success" will ensue if the therapist does what is required. The group feels and acts helpless.
2. Fight/flight: The group feels angry or afraid, and acts as if success depends on winning some battle or escaping some danger.
3. Pairing: The group feels optimistic, and this is related to an important relationship between two members of the group (the pair). There is anticipation that a new leader may emerge. The symbolic birth of a prince to a royal family (Bion is British), or the coming of a messiah, may be related. In any case, such a hope distracts from the task of group members taking the initiative for their own growth.

Yalom (1965) pays his respects to a number of curative factors in group psychotherapy other than those discussed for psychodynamic psychotherapy. He contends that groups instill hope; develop socializing techniques; and permit imitative behavior, interpersonal learning, universality (the alleviation of the sense of being utterly alone in one's misery), group cohesiveness; and altruism (the satisfaction derived from the act of giving), among other functions. He notes also the importance of the "corrective recapitulation of the primary family group" in the therapy setting.

FAMILY THERAPY
The general concept of family therapy includes treatment of an individual family, an individual couple, several families in a group, or several couples in a group. All of these types of therapy can be powerful treatment tools, and one or more of them may be necessary to treat an individual properly. They have in common

(along with group psychotherapy) the fact that they involve casting light on, and providing understanding for, individuals as members of a social system that must also be illuminated and dealt with as an entity. Many of the principles of psychotherapy that have already been reviewed can apply in these kinds of treatment, if it is understood that the social system, itself, is also a patient—and in many ways the preeminent patient. These approaches may be necessary if the observed pathology is in the system (the "fit" between the people involved) or in the social unit that maintains homeostasis in such a way as to prevent necessary change in an individual member.

Especially when a couple requires prolonged assistance in looking at and changing its relationship, a couples group can prove far superior to work with a single couple in reducing the intensity of the dialogue; the group permits the partners to look at themselves and their relationship in a broader perspective. Resistances, however, can be powerful even in a group setting.

MILIEU THERAPY

Milieu therapy will be discussed as a psychological therapy, although it might be called sociological or holistic therapy. The term *milieu* is from the French word that means environment or setting. In words engraved upon his tomb, Napoleon asked to be buried on the banks of the Seine in the "milieu" of the French people. Milieu therapy refers to the use of a patient's total social and physical environment, and every aspect of day-to-day life and human relationships, as part of a therapeutic process. It is an important and powerful therapeutic approach that is particularly relevant to hospital treatment of psychiatric patients.

Unfortunately, the term *milieu therapy* has been applied for years indiscriminately to programs that are, in many cases, essentially meaningless. As a result, milieu therapy is frequently thought of as trivial or incidental background therapy. But in a properly developed, serious milieu therapy program, three months in a psychiatric hospital should be about as meaningless in the life of an individual patient as, for example, three months in China, at Harvard, or in Marine boot camp.

A milieu approach is necessary when less-comprehensive approaches that involve smaller segments of the patient's life have failed, when the patient's own natural milieu has been powerfully pathogenic, or when the patient is so disorganized and desperate that he or she required the "splinting" by an external social group. Many patients requiring long-term hospital treatment are young adults, classified diagnostically as having borderline personality disorders, who require milieu therapy for effective personality change.

Therapeutic Processes

Milieu therapy was used, without the development of technical concepts, for thousands of years by people who were concerned about the helpful atmosphere in which patients were treated. Development of milieu therapy as a technical tool and body of knowledge was crystallized perhaps most notably by Maxwell Jones (1953), who wrote a book entitled *The Therapeutic Community*. The processes going on in such a therapeutic community have been defined and analyzed during the years since, and are reviewed and summarized by Gunderson (1978). Gunderson enumerated the following five processes and defined and discussed each in some depth.

Containment. It is important to maintain physical welfare and safety for the patient and others.

Support. The hospital unit must make an effort to reduce anguish and anxiety and increase feelings of self-esteem and security.

Structure. A stable and predictable social and administrative framework must be provided to reduce ambiguity and permit the patient to accept membership more confidently.

Involvement. Social interaction and emotional investment in the hospital community permit social learning and personal growth.

Validation. Hospital community processes can "affirm a patient's individuality" and, presumably, enable him to learn about it.

CRISIS INTERVENTION

Psychological therapy constitutes a part of a crisis intervention program, along with medication, hospitalization, and other types of treatment.

Crisis intervention refers to efforts made by a physician or other member of a mental health team to assist a patient in a period of emotional turmoil in which his or her usual defenses have broken down. Something has happened to weaken the individual, to disrupt old patterns of adaptation by making them unavailable or ineffective, or to increase the amount of situational stress he or she is subjected to.

The important point is that this highly emotional time of transition may end either in growth or in chronic illness. Patients have options that they do not have when less-than-optimal defenses are more rigidly fixed, and less adaptive techniques more firmly adhered to. Opportunities for growth present themselves, along with dangers of regression.

The crisis intervention process frequently begins in an emergency room or walk-in service, but it may well begin in a physician's office. Loss of a friend or family member, failure at school or work, physical illness, transfer to a new city, and many subtle variations and influences may serve as precipitants. Often a suicidal attempt or gesture leads to treatment. The most common mistake in managing such cases is to attempt to deal with the patients alone without recruiting for them a supportive social network, usually including the family. Very often patients will protest against involving the family while really yearning for its help, and professionals who do not press the issue will miss the point. As an example of this situation, a 25-year-old woman who was brought to a crisis center after an overdose gave absolute orders that her mother was not to be called; however, when the nurse asked for her mother's telephone number, the patient gave it immediately, along with another number where her mother could be found if she was not at home.

Other tasks of the crisis intervention team include: provision of support and reassurance; education and orientation of the patients as to the meaning of their symptoms and the nature of treatment; practical assistance (for example, vocational counseling) and environmental manipulation (for example, conferring with an employer or teacher); help in exploring the environment for new opportunities; help in reviewing of old goals, with examination of possible new ones; observation, definition, and encouragement of the use of the patient's strengths and special capacities; assistance in mobilizing internal personal and external environmental resources; and assistance in arranging long-term treatment.

BEHAVIOR THERAPY

Behavior therapy is the polar opposite of the prototype psychotherapy in that it is concerned primarily with evident manifestations (signs and symptoms) of a disorder and not unconscious origins. Behavior therapy is the "systematic application of experimentally derived behavior-analysis principles to affect observable and, at least in principle, measurable changes" interactions between person and environment. This definition implies a "detailed and objective description of the patient's problem behavior" in "observable and quantifiable" terms, a search for "particular situations in which the behavior typically occurs or fails to occur," "systematic manipulation of the environment and behavior variables thought to be functionally related to the disturbing performance," and "assessment of the treatment outcome in the same objective, quantifiable terms" (APA Task Force Report, July 1974).

This approach, in simplest terms, involves the rigid definition of stimulus and response, and the experimental observation of the relationship between them. It is the present psychiatric application of a long tradition of psychological and philosophical behaviorism.

One example of a behavior therapy is the token economy, which is an established system of rewards and punishments using some medium of exchange to alter behavior in a hospital setting or in some other social unit. Another example of a behavioral approach is the successful treatment of premature ejaculation by teaching the patient to anticipate the onset of ejaculatory inevitability, and to prevent it by the Semans "squeeze" technique, which lowers the threshold of penile excitability.

An important part of therapeutic work using a behavorial approach is that patients are instructed to observe, to count, and to record their own behavior in terms of instances and items. Usually they are asked to get a notebook and not only keep track of circumstances in which a given behavior occurs (for example, eating or smoking), but also estimate the degree of anxiety and to note who was present when the incident took place, so that a more or less objective record is available as a basis for observation and planning. There is also a great deal of interest in rating scales, questionnaires, and other measuring devices.

In order to give an overview of the field, several of the methods used in behavior therapy will be described in the following sections.

Systematic Desensitization

Systematic desensitization is the gradual, progressive exposure of patients to objects or situations that they fear to an excessive or disabling degree. The anxiety associated with such exposure is successfully counteracted by the use of relaxation techniques such as progressive deep muscle relaxation (associated with deep breathing and the imagining of calming scenes), which is taught to the patients and practiced by them until they become proficient.

A hierarchy is constructed—that is, a list is made of anxiety-producing situations associated with a specific fear, arranged in order of increasing or decreasing intensity of the associated anxiety. For example, if the fear is of flying in airplanes, the hierarchy might start with purchasing a ticket, proceed through arriving at the airport, and end, after 10 to 15 items, with the initial flight. Related to this is the use of a SUDS scale (that is, subjective units of distress). The patient is taught to estimate the level of anxiety experienced, in real or fantasy situations, on a scale from 0 (no anxiety) to 100 (maximum anxiety); the patients have initially established reference points from their own experience. The patient can use this scale to give estimates that will define the intensity of various experiences and the success of relaxation techniques. This is a tool for assessing and quantifying relative degrees of anxiety.

The patient will be asked to imagine (or later to confront in reality) the first (least intense) item in the hierarchy; then anxiety is reduced to zero by relaxation techniques. When the first item no longer produces anxiety, the next item on the hierarchy is used, and so on.

Some behavior therapists see many psychiatric disorders—including depression and conversion symptoms, as well as phobias and habit disorders—as capable of being formulated and treated in this or similar ways. Schizophrenia, however, is frequently viewed as organic.

Medications or other therapeutic interventions, such as diazepam (Valium) or carbon dioxide inhalation, may be used with patients whose anxiety is too intense to be dealt with by relaxation techniques alone. This intervention can reduce anxiety during therapy sessions so as to permit desensitization.

Biofeedback

Biofeedback, a behavorial application of modern electronic instrumentation, can provide patients with information about their physiologic processes and changes in functions so that these processes may be brought under control. Such physical measurements as heart rate, muscle tension, and skin temperature may be converted into auditory signals (varying tones) or visual signals (varying light intensity). The measurements may also be displayed by the deflection of a needle on a calibrated scale.

The autonomic nervous system and many physiologic processes, which were never thought to be subject to voluntary control, have been found to be responsive to the mental state of the person in such a way as to be experienced as volitional. Some examples of processes subject to instrumental measurement and feedback are (1) changes in temperature and vasomotor responses, (2) contractions of the intestine and uterus, (3) formation of urine by the kidney, (4) ejection of red blood cells from the spleen, and (5) electroencephalographic patterns.

Biofeedback has been used effectively in the treatment of cardiac arrhythmias, hypertension, migraine and tension headaches, epilepsy, asthma, and gastrointestinal disorders, among other problems. Penile and vaginal plethysmography have been applied in the treatment of sexual dysfunction.

Biofeedback has in common with psychoanalytic therapy the central process of making the unconscious processes available to the conscious. It has in common with behavior therapy the matching of precisely defined and quantifiable stimuli and responses, which are influenced by positive or negative reinforcement.

An example of a biofeedback method is that of the very sensitive measurement of skin temperature in the hand, demonstrated to the patient by the deflection of a needle on a scale. Patients may then learn "mentally" to increase the temperature of their hands. After initially learning to make this temperature change, a patient can then perform it even without the measuring device. Such techniques may be used in treatment of Reynaud's disease and migraine. The Greens (1977) of the Menninger Foundation describe programs in which 80 percent of migraine patients have obtained relief ranging from slight to excellent; some of them have achieved a migraine-free life. (The exact nature of this process is, of course, both complex and hypothetical, but the Greens' book is a good place to read more about it.)

Flooding

The directed exposure of a patient to anxious situations at high levels of intensity for prolonged periods is a technique for eventual reduction of anxiety. Flooding is usually done with the actual frightening situations, rather than as an exercise in imagination. It has been successful in agoraphobia and other conditions.

Aversive Control or Punishment

Aversive control or punishment involves the use of unpleasant stimuli (for an example, an emetic for an alcoholic, or electric shock for a homosexual) to reduce the frequency of undesirable behavior.

Assertiveness Training

Assertiveness training involves education, planning, and practice (for example, role-playing) in being neither submissive nor aggressive in various real-life situations, while constructively expressing one's own feelings and wishes in ways that produce useful practical results.

Negative Practice

In negative practice, a deliberate attempt is made to generate the problematic symptom with the goal of inhibiting it. A patient with a tic might be instructed to perform the tic movement many times during a number of sessions. This has been moderately successful in some cases in reducing the frequency of the tic.

Paradoxical Intention

Paradoxical intention involves a deliberate effort to inhibit a symptom by attempting to create it. This approach is an interesting, but somewhat manipulative technique that can have powerful impact in some situations. The process may be demonstrated by the example of a patient with panic attacks; the patient was told to keep notes about the situations in which the panic attacks occurred, and the intensity of his associated anxiety. He was also told that it was important that he have as many panic attacks as possible, in order to provide adequate data during the course of therapy. This resulted in complete cessation of panic attacks. The patient perceived the attacks as imposed on him and thought of himself as helpless to influence them; this apparently was an important factor in his distress.

Habit Reversal
The planned substitution of a new behavior for an older one, habit reversal can be applied to such problems as nail biting. The patient is taught to recognize the situations and feelings *preliminary to* the habitual behavior, and then to take some physical action incompatible with the unwanted behavior; in the case of nail biting, the person might grasp some object. This may be associated with use of a brief self-administered relaxation technique.

Cognitive Therapy
Cognition, or "thoughts," may be considered to be covert units of behavior, subject to the same rules of learning and relationships to stimuli as other forms of behavior. If this is so, then the stimuli leading to the gloomy cognitions may be reduced. Patients may be rewarded, or trained to reward themselves, for behavior incompatible with depression, such as goal-directed activity. Patients may set more realistic goals for themselves, and they may learn to reward themselves more with pleasant thoughts or events and punish themselves less.

Cognitions may also be seen as processes that modify the relationship between stimulus and response, determining *mood*. As such, they may be disturbed, irrational, wrong, untrue, but learned and maintained by some reinforcing factors. According to Burns (1980), the cognitions of depressed patients "nearly always contain gross distortions," and the patient can become aware of these.

Some of the idiosyncratic cognitive patterns or characteristic ways of thinking of an individual may be controlled by stressful stimuli that may dominate his or her thinking. However, the person may learn to recognize such patterns, correct the distortions, deprive them of their force, and bring them under more voluntary control. The overlap between cognitive behavior therapy and some aspects of psychoanalytic therapy is evident here.

Substitute Symptoms
The issue of the possible occurrence of substitute symptoms after successful behavior therapy is an important one. Initially, behavior therapists sometimes claimed that symptom substitution did not take place when one symptom was removed. As we have become more sophisticated, we have begun to deal with more realistic questions regarding the circumstances in which, and the symptomatic patients in whom, substitute symptoms are likely to appear.

Applications of Behavior Therapy
Behavior therapy is reported to be highly effective in the treatment of certain disorders, including phobias (especially agoraphobia), habit disorders, anxiety reactions, enuresis, stuttering, and tics. According to the 1974 APA Task Force Report, some improvement with behavior therapy has been reported in persons suffering from obsessive-compulsive disorders, hysteria, encopresis, psychological impotence, homosexuality, fetishes, frigidity, transvestism, exhibitionism, gambling, obesity, anorexia, insomnia, and nightmares; success was also reported in children with temper tantrums, head bobbing, thumb sucking, refusal to eat, and excessive scratching.

More practitioners probably consider behavioral techniques when symptom patterns are better defined and narrower in scope, or when specific behavorial techniques have been demonstrated to be dramatically effective. Psychodynamic therapeutic techniques are probably used more often when the clarification of the treatment issues, goals, and purposes may be expected to take a fair amount of time and where the character of the patient must be considered.

Among the problems in synthesizing behavioral and psychodynamic approaches is the fact that the therapist's role is quite different, requiring different personality traits and different technical expertise. Therapists who perform behavior therapy are extremely active and responsible for the success of the treatment. They must make decisions and intervene quickly in ways that feel strange to one whose experience has been in cautious observation over extended periods of time. There are, also, unsettling new philosophical viewpoints for psychodynamic therapists. Behavior theory states that symptoms may be the result of coincidences that have no significance in terms of the character or personality of the patient. An intensely anxiety-producing event may have occurred coincidentally with some aspect of the patient's life, resulting in symptoms that are characterologically meaningless, at least in psychodynamic terms. On the other hand, there is freedom in behavior therapy to intervene, to devise and innovate techniques, to ignore the analytic posture and assumptions about the patient's unconscious ambivalence, and to find flexible and practical applications.

Relationship of Dynamic Psychotherapy and Behavior Therapy

There are several possible relationships between behavior therapy and dynamic psychotherapy.

1. One is truth, the other heresy.
2. They are really the same; the therapist is doing the same thing in either case, but calling it by different names. That is to say, the effective part of psychotherapy is the unconscious, subtle reinforcements and punishments provided by the therapist in his or her reactions or verbalizations; alternatively, the important thing in behavior therapy is the relationship with the therapist, and the formal mechanical arrangements are incidental.
3. Each is effective in some kinds of cases, and both must be included in the therapeutic armamentarium.
4. Theoretical considerations (if not technical ones) of both are useful in every case, may help in different ways toward different goals, and may potentiate or facilitate each other.
5. In cases where either will be effective or neither will be very effective, one may be more comfortable for the patient or the therapist. Sometimes the utilization of a behavior therapy approach makes it clear to the patient and therapist that any progress is up to the patient. This leaves the therapist feeling less mystified and frustrated than does an obscure arrangement in which he or she may feel responsible for treatment failure. A patient, for example, who complains of anxiety but will not even attempt progressive muscle relaxation is making an important clarifying statement.

Behavior therapy is not appropriate for patients who refuse the techniques, choose psychotherapy, are unable to cooperate with behavior therapy, or are so unstable that the therapist cannot formulate behavior sufficiently specific enough to be relevant and inclusive. This last criterion may apply to patients with broad, diverse areas of psychopathology rooted in their entire character. Sometimes, therapy will largely be interpersonal and supportive. During a transition or crisis, changing behavior may not be as important as personal reassurance. Also, there are special issues to be considered regarding behavior therapy when control and obedience (or submission) are central issues for the individual.

Aside from their clinical usefulness, behavior therapy concepts may prove helpful in clarifying issues, dramatizing resistance, and facilitating thinking about the usefulness to a patient of pathologic adjustments. Sequences of behavior therapy and dynamic psychotherapy may be considered.

Indications for Psychological Therapies

The selection of patients for psychological therapies is fortunately simple. Every patient receives psychological therapy (whether good or bad). This may be in a relationship with an attending physician who works intuitively, or it may be a more purposeful approach of a general physician or specialist who is a student of the art of human relationships.

A decision may be necessary to refer the patient for specialized psychiatric care. This should be done (1) if the patient's distress or disability is not promptly alleviated; (2) if more time will be required for effective management than can be provided by the nonpsychiatric physician; (3) if the case requires specialized equipment or programs such as are usually developed only by specialists (for example, biofeedback, group psychotherapy, or hospital treatment); (4) if the patient needs long-term specialized psychiatric treatment approaches (for example, psychoanalysis); (5) if the case is complex, mysterious, or severe, and requires the attention of an experienced specialist; or (6) if the patient has human potential for growth and contribution to society and his or her own welfare that cannot be realized because of obstructive emotional handicaps.

Many physicians are overly hesitant to prescribe psychiatric treatment. Steinberg et al. (1980) found that in hospitalized patients with psychiatric problems, "physician resistance to consultation was involved in more than 50 percent of cases not referred, usually because the physicians believed there was no psychiatric problem or that psychiatry could not help, and less often because a physician thought the patient might become upset or the patient-doctor relationship would be destroyed." The physicians' resistance was generally found not to be justified, and most of the patients benefited from later psychiatric involvement.

Frequently, the physician may think that a patient would be horrified at the idea of psychiatric consultation, but the patient usually turns out to be relieved. All patients should know that sources of help are available so that they do not unnecessarily lose hope.

A patient referred for psychiatric treatment may at times be managed primarily in a pharmacologic or organic way. The psychological aspects of treatment may again be either intuitive and incidental or planned as a conscious part of the treatment program.

Psychiatrists may tend sometimes to administer whatever treatment they are expert in to any patient who comes under their care. It is certainly good for a final decision about treatment to be made by the therapist who will be providing it; it is also good for that therapist to use techniques with which he or she is most skilled. It does not, however, make sense for a treatment method to be selected by the accident of which psychiatrist a patient is referred to. Comprehensive evaluation and referral among psychiatrists with specialized skills and differing approaches would be most desirable. This is more frequently the case now than it was in the past.

Recent advances in biologic psychiatry have led in the last five to 10 years to a swing in the pendulum; psychological therapies are probably currently underprescribed.

In view of recent findings in neurochemistry, psychopharmacology, genetics, and neuroendocrinology, it would be unwise to consider any cases purely psychological, at least from a theoretical point of view. It is equally unwise to apply any biologic treatment without proper consideration of the meaning of the treatment to the patient, the challenge of adaptation that the patient has been given, and his or her unique characteristics and disabilities with or without medication—not to mention the issue of compliance. Biologic and psychological therapies (as well as sociological ones) must be considered in all cases, and justification for deemphasizing or eliminating one or more must be based on deliberate consideration of clinical factors as well as patient preference and practical considerations.

One factor determining the role of the psychological therapies is the degree to which other therapies are effective. Many patients benefit enough from biologic treatment that it is doubtful whether formal psychotherapy is needed. On the other hand, patients with great personal potential may be so overwhelmed and discouraged by intense anxiety or depression that they do not have the ability to undertake psychological therapy. Proper use of medication may make this technique possible, with great advantage for the individual. The old idea that medication interferes with psychotherapy is useful only in an extremely limited type of case and situation. The assumption that effective biologic treatment makes psychological factors insignificant can be maintained only by cruelly truncating the scope of our patients' humanity.

References and Further Reading

Alexander, F.G., Selesnick, S.T. *The History of Psychiatry*. New York: Harper & Row, 1966.

American Psychiatric Association, Council on Research and Development. *A Report of the APA Task Force on Behavior Therapy*. 2nd printing. Washington, D.C.: APA, 1974.

American Psychiatric Association. *Psychiatric Glossary*. 4th rev. ed. New York: Basic Books, 1975.

Bion, W.R. *Experience in Groups and Other Papers*. New York: Basic Books, 1959.

Brenner, C. *An Elementary Textbook of Psychoanalysis*, rev. ed. New York: International Universities Press, 1973.

Brill, A.A. (ed.). *The Basic Writings of Sigmund Freud*. New York: Random House, 1938.

Burns, D.D. *Feeling Good: The New Mood Therapy*. New York: William Morrow, 1980.

Clark, D.H. *Administrative Therapy: The Role of the Doctor in the Therapeutic Community*. London: J.B. Lippincott, Tavistock Publications, 1964.

Cumming, J., Cumming, E. *Ego and Milieu: Theory and Practice of Environmental Therapy*. New York: Atheneum, 1962.

Green, E., and Green, A. *Beyond Biofeedback*. New York: Dell, 1977.

Gunderson, J.G. Defining the therapeutic processes in psychiatric milieus. *Psychiatry* 41:327–335, 1978.

Jones, M. *The Therapeutic Community*. New York: Basic Books, 1953.

Steinberg, H., Torem, M., Saravay, S.M. An analysis of physician resistance to psychiatric consultations. *Arch. Gen. Psychiatry* 37:1007, 1980.

Wolpe, J. *The Practice of Behavior Therapy*, 2nd ed. Pergamon General Psychology Series. New York: Pergamon Press, 1973.

Yalom, I. D. *The Theory and Practice of Group Psychotherapy*, 2nd ed. New York: Basic Books, 1965.

Psychopharmacologic Treatment

KENNETH A. KESSLER, M.D.
STEVEN D. TARGUM, M.D.

During the 1950s several developments combined to form the basis of modern psychopharmacology. A precursor of chlorpromazine that was investigated for use as an antihistamine turned out to be an effective antipsychotic. The tricyclic iminodibenzyl was found to be a potent antidepressant after being tested as an antipsychotic. Iproniazid, a precursor of the monoamine oxidase (MAO) inhibitors used in the treatment of tuberculosis, was observed to be effective in the treatment of anxious depressives. Lithium carbonate, initially used as a salt substitute for hypertensives, proved to be a remarkably specific treatment for major bipolar affective disorders. These serendipitous findings were made by astute clinicians testing these drugs for other uses. The next 15 years saw the validity of their findings confirmed through a series of well-controlled studies with large patient populations. Consequently, there is no longer any serious question about the efficacy of these drugs or about the value of psychopharmacology in psychiatric practice.

Current research is oriented to finding a new generation of psychotropics that can selectively target a diagnostic subpopulation, be equally effective with fewer side effects, and have a more rapid onset of therapeutic action. Effective antipsychotics that do not cause tardive dyskinesia, antidepressants without the customary lag time of 7 to 21 days, and MAO inhibitors free of the potential for causing hypertensive crisis are but a few of the agents being actively investigated. Psychopharmacology will be able to offer more specific treatments for patient subpopulations while causing fewer side effects. These developments will make skillful handling of psychotropic agents essential for the practicing psychiatrist.

An empathic understanding of the patient's perception is an often-overlooked prerequisite for successful psychopharmacologic treatment. Patients resist taking medication and frequently do not comply with their physicians' instructions. This resistance may reflect their fear of losing autonomy (for example, "I don't want to be controlled by a drug"), unwillingness to recognize the seriousness of their problem ("I'll just snap out of it soon"), or previously unsatisfactory experience with psychotropics ("I don't want to feel like a zombie"). Resistance can be managed by supportive education, a thorough explanation of the necessity for medication, and a description of the anticipated course of treatment. This explanation should include a discussion of side effects, the lag time before the onset of therapeutic effects, and the expected duration of treatment. The possibility of a failure to respond to one drug and the necessity for switching to another should also be introduced. A thorough history should be obtained, including the dosage and duration of previous drug therapy, and related side effects experienced. A patient's history of unresponsiveness to medication can often be traced to a failure to prescribe an adequate dose for a sufficient time.

Patients and their families should be made aware of potential risks. We do not recommend a detailed list of *all* potential side effects because it may unnecessarily alarm patients and focus their attention on the risk, rather than the potential gain from treatment. When starting outpatients on medication, encourage them to call if they have any questions or experience an untoward reaction. Many patients may initially call once or twice. Patients should also be instructed to check with you if they are starting another medication. The risk of drug interactions is often overlooked, especially in patients who are reluctant to acknowledge to their other doctors that they are seeing a psychiatrist.

Drug treatment of the geriatric patient presents special problems. There are more than 30 million Americans who are over the age of 60, and their numbers are increasing by 300,000 to 400,000 each year. The use of psychotropic agents increases significantly with age. In one survey, 75 percent of nursing home patients were receiving one or more psychotropics. Geriatric patients are more vulnerable to side affects and adverse reactions. Age-related decreases in physiologic functioning and the higher incidence of other medical conditions demand special precautions.

Since the elderly are not a homogeneous group, treatment must be individualized. Changes in organ receptor sensitivity and drug metabolism, which are related to biologic aging, vary widely among individuals. While some drugs may have their metabolism reduced by as much as 50 percent among geriatric patients (requiring significant reductions in dose), other drugs are not affected at all. A safe way of initiating treatment of older patients is to start with smaller doses to assess the patient's sensitivity. Small doses will suffice for many geriatric patients, although full treatment doses may be required for others. Depression among the elderly is widespread and frequently undiagnosed. Contrary to popular thought (which views depression as a corollary to aging), geriatric depression is often responsive to drugs. Diagnosis may be obscured by the presentation, which can take the form of apathy and disturbed cognition (pseudodementia). With these precautions in mind, psychopharmacology can do a great deal to alleviate the problems of the often-neglected geriatric population.

The pediatric patient is also the subject of special attention in modern psychopharmacology. Although paradoxical reactions are occasionally noted, pediatric psychopharmacology utilizes the same psychotropic drugs as used in adults, but the monitoring is more thorough.

Drug Management of Psychotic Disorders

In the years since chlorpromazine was introduced, drug therapy has come to be recognized as a fundamental part of any comprehensive treatment program for schizophrenia. The annual census of chronic care institutions steadily declined after chlorpromazine came into widespread clinical use in 1956. By 1967, despite an increase in the general population, the inpatient psychiatric census was 25 percent less than in 1955. While the shift to community-based services has abetted this trend, it would not have been possible without effective antipsychotic agents.

Although antipsychotic medications do not cure schizophrenia, they make it possible, in many cases, to manage the disease successfully. A good analogy would be the role of insulin in diabetes or phenytoin in epilepsy. Chronically institutionalized patients can be discharged, and the length of stay for acute first-break admissions has been dramatically reduced. Antipsychotics have also been shown to exert a prophylactic effect, substantially reducing the frequency of psychotic episodes. Many of the more subtle and pervasive disturbances in thinking that are present in the interval between acute psychotic exacerbations can likewise be helped by antipsychotic drugs. The downward drift that has historically characterized chronic schizophrenia can, in many instances, be arrested.

Antipsychotic agents were initially called tranquilizers and were later redesignated major tranquilizers to distinguish them from diazepam, chlordiazepoxide, and meprobamate. This term was something of a misnomer since they are only weak tranquilizing agents—the major pharmacologic property of these drugs is their antipsychotic activity. They decrease the manifestations of psychotic thinking, such as hallucinations, delusions, and loose associations, and they lessen the diversely disturbed behavior that often accompanies disordered thinking. Antipsychotic agents can both calm an agitated patient and activate a blunted, withdrawn schizophrenic. These seemingly opposite effects suggest that such drugs are not so much tranquilizers as specific antipsychotic agents. Since the antipsychotic drugs in clinical use often cause extrapyramidal side effects, they are also called neuroleptics.

MECHANISM OF ACTION

Research on the mechanisms by which the antipsychotics work has tended to support Carlson's hypothesis of dopaminergic blockade. The dopamine hypothesis of schizophrenia was generated from the observation that neuroleptics block dopamine receptors in animals and reverse schizophrenic symptoms in humans. The various clinical effects of the neuroleptics appear to correlate with their dopamine-blocking activity in different regions of the brain. The antipsychotic action of these drugs may be due to dopamine receptor blockade in the mesolimbic and mesocortical areas of the brain, while extrapyramidal effects results from blockade of nigrostriatal neurons. There are significant differences among neuroleptics in the potency of their effects on both dopaminergic and nondopaminergic systems, such as alpha-adrenergic, cholinergic, and histaminergic neurons. These varying actions may determine both the antipsychotic and the extrapyramidal profiles of a given drug.

Snyder (1976) correlated the affinity of various phenothiazines for dopamine receptor sites with the antipsychotic potency of these drugs. The more potent phenothiazines closely resemble the physical configuration of dopamine, allowing them to bind readily to (or "fit") the receptor site. Other researchers have found a correlation between a drug's antipsychotic potency and the degree of dopamine receptor blockade it caused.

Despite the impressive body of evidence supporting the dopamine hypothesis, no one has yet been able to demonstrate a specific abnormality of dopamine in schizophrenic patients. Current formulations of the hypothesis include: (1) an excess of dopamine at the receptor; (2) a hypersensitive receptor; (3) an underactive antagonist to dopamine, such as acetylcholine; and (4) an impaired conversion of dopamine to norepinephrine.

CLASSIFICATIONS OF ANTIPSYCHOTICS

Since chlorpromazine was introduced in 1952, a large number of antipsychotic agents have been marketed. Unfortunately, they have not become more specific in their effects or been proved to be more effective than the first antipsychotic.

Antipsychotic agents are classified in several ways, most commonly by chemical structure. There are seven chemical classes of antipsychotics, but only three of these groups, the phenothiazines (for example, chlorpromazine), the thioxanthenes (such as chlorprothixene), and the butyrophenones (for example, haloperidol) are widely used. The other four are the rauwolfia alkaloids (reserpine), the benzoquinolines (butaclamol), the phenylpiperazines (oxypertine), and the indolic derivatives (molindone).

Another classification system that has recently come into use groups drugs by their milligram potency. More potent drugs are not more effective, but it is possible to achieve comparable clinical results with fewer milligrams per dose. High-potency agents such as haloperidol are given in small dosages and generally cause more extrapyramidal side effects. Low-potency drugs, such as chlorpromazine, are given in large dosages and tend to cause more sedation and have more antiadrenergic and anticholinergic side effects.

All of the antipsychotic drugs, when given in adjusted doses based on their potency, have essentially equivalent antipsychotic activity.

TREATMENT OF AN ACUTE EPISODE

Drug Selection

Although some newly admitted patients show a response within two or three days, therapeutic effects often are not evident for up to two weeks. Chronic schizophrenics may require as long as 12 to 24 weeks to show a response. Ninety-five percent of acute schizophrenics treated with a drug given in adequate doses will show some improvement within six to eight weeks. More than 50 percent of these patients will be moderately to markedly improved. There is some preliminary evidence that a dysphoric response to a test dose of chlorpromazine may help identify those patients less likely to have a positive drug response. No drug has been convincingly demonstrated to be either safer or superior for any schizophrenic subgroup or target symptom. There has been a belief that agitated patients respond best to a sedating drug like chlorpromazine while those who are withdrawn do better with an alerting drug like prochlorperazine, but this theory has not been supported by controlled studies.

Drug selection can be based on the compatability of a drug's side effects with a patient's needs. For instance, an outpatient who must remain alert in his or her work, will more easily tolerate drugs such as fluphenazine or haloperidol, which have a low incidence of sedative side effects. Conversely, the patient who has had repeated problems with extrapyramidal effects may do better on chlorpromazine or thioridazine. There is some evidence that molindone, alone among antipsychotics, causes weight loss rather than gain; this may be a crucial factor for ensuring compliance by certain patients concerned with physical appearance.

Initiating Treatment

A thorough history—including dose, side effects, and clinical response to previous medications—is essential since patients who have previously responded well to a drug usually improve when treated again. The only consistent difference between drugs is in the side effects they cause. It is useful to set specific treatment goals that can be monitored to assess drug response. Target symptoms that respond to drug treatment include agitation, hallucinations, combativeness, sleep disturbance, tension, and paranoid behavior. Impaired judgment, lack of insight, depression, withdrawal, and poor motivation are symptoms that are less likely to respond to drugs. It is good practice to avoid giving more than one drug for the same purpose. While there is no evidence that antipsychotic drug combinations are superior to either drug used alone, adverse drug reactions probably increase with the number of drugs used.

In general, an acutely ill patient who has not shown a response after four to six weeks on an adequate dose should be switched to another drug. Certain conditions, such as severe agitation, may require an earlier change. A patient who fails to respond to one drug may well respond to another. As a patient improves, the reemergence of side effects, especially sedation, may be a clue that the dosage needs to be evaluated. The goal is to find the lowest dose that will sustain impovement.

Dosage

General clinical practice, supported by double-blind studies, has shown the effective dosage range of chlorpromazine for hospitalized schizophrenics to be 400 to 1,200 mg daily. Smaller doses tend to be ineffective, while larger doses usually do not bring additional benefits. For drugs other than chlorpromazine, an equivalent dose should be used. Because there are large differences between individuals in drug absorption and metabolism, the dose must be individualized, taking into account clinical condition, age, drug response, and side effects. Larger doses are often required for patients who are agitated, more psychotic, younger, heavier, and male.

There are a number of advantages to giving antipsychotic drugs either in a single dose at bedtime or on a twice-a-day regimen, including greater patient compliance, fewer side effects during waking hours, and less need for hypnotics. The dose can be increased every three to four days until improvement occurs or serious side effects intervene. Extremely agitated patients may require more frequent increases. If speed of onset is crucial, intramuscular injections can be helpful. The oral dose should be halved when giving medication by this route. If a patient is not showing a response, the problem may be that he or she is not swallowing the pills. In such cases, liquid concentrate, given with a nurse's supervision, should be tried. The most common cause of treatment failure in the management of an acute psychotic episode is the prescription of an inadequate dosage or the failure of the patient to comply with the prescribed regimen.

Psychotolysis

Psychotolysis is a treatment that offers the possibility of a prompt resolution of psychotic episodes. The treatment regimen involves giving substantial intramuscular doses of a potent antipsychotic every hour until clinical control has been achieved. In one study, 78 percent of 124 agitated patients were stabilized within 72 hours. Donlon and co-workers (1979) reviewed seven open and seven double-blind studies done over the past 15 years; the studies included more than 650 patients. All studies had favorable outcomes, with moderate to marked improvements in the first 24 hours ranging from 50 to 83 percent. Improvement was measured in assaultiveness and agitation, as well as in the areas of core psychotic symptoms such as disorganized thinking, hallucinations, and delusions. In assessing these outcomes, one should note that half of these were open studies done with few controls; more rigorous studies are clearly needed.

Psychotolysis should be reserved for acutely disturbed psychotic patients treated under close supervision in a hospital setting. The only dangerous adverse reaction is severe hypotension associated with the use of chlorpromazine. Therefore, it is safer to use a potent antipsychotic that is individually titrated by clinical conditions, response, and side effects. Sedation is most often the limiting factor. Contraindications include a history of seizures and cardiovascular disorders. A suggested regimen would be haloperidol, 5 to 10 mg every hour, with a maximum daily dose of 40 to 60 mg. If severe side effects ensue, the dose can be decreased. If this dosage does not relieve the problem, it may be necessary to stop treatment. Otherwise, treatment should be continued until unmanageable symptoms are significantly improved. Oral medication can be started four to six hours after the last intramuscular dose. The daily oral dose should be about twice the total intramuscular dose given in the previous 24 hours.

MAINTENANCE TREATMENT

Drug Discontinuance Studies

There have been more than 100 well-controlled studies of schizophrenic relapse and drug maintenance completed over the past 15 years. The preponderance of evidence supports the conclusion that schizophrenia is a chronically relapsing disease, with two out of three patients decompensating within one year of drug discontinuance. Drug maintenance reduces this relapse rate by more than 50 percent. Three of these studies are briefly summarized below.

Hogarty and Goldberg randomly assigned 374 recently discharged schizophrenic patients to one of four treatment plans. At 12 months, 31 percent of patients who received drugs and 67 percent of patients given placebos had relapsed. After two years, the relapse figures were 48 percent of drug patients and 80 percent for those taking placebo. Drug maintenance approximately halved the chance of relapse. These figures probably understate drug effect, since over 50 percent of the patients reported as drug failures had not taken their medication, according to reports from their families. Excluding these noncomplying patients, the true relapse rate for drug patients taking medication was 20 percent at one year. Assessments of the overall level of social adjustment showed little improvement, suggesting that the only effect of drugs was to forestall relapse. Two other groups can be identified from these data. There is a substantial minority of schizophrenic patients who are not helped by drugs, and a somewhat small minority who do not need drugs. The former will relapse despite drug maintenance, while the latter will do well in the community without drugs. As yet, we cannot identify these patients except in retrospect.

Davis (1976b) reviewed 24 double-blind, random assignment studies involving more than 1,000 subjects. Among relapsed patients, 56 percent had been taking placebo, while only 15 percent had been taking drugs. A broader survey of the literature was completed by Docherty, who reviewed 100 English-language reports involving more than 8,000 patients. In 35 double-blind, well-controlled studies, the relapse rates were 22 percent for patients who received drugs and 54 percent for those given placebos. In fact, only one study failed to show a positive drug effect. Overall, drug maintenance reduced schizophrenic relapse by over 50 percent.

Patients Not Requiring Maintenance
The reports reviewed have all studied recently recovered patients who were randomly assigned without regard to their potential for relapse. Hogarty attempted to identify and study the group of schizophrenic patients who can survive in the community without medication; the study included 43 patients who were selected as having a low risk of relapse. One year after their medication had been discontinued, 66 percent of these low-risk patients had relapsed. This finding suggests that drug discontinuance, whether at two months or two years, eventuates in relapse for two out of three schizophrenic patients in the first year. Doctors' global impression, psychological testing, and a history of successful drug maintenance for two years were not helpful in identifying schizophrenic patients who could do well after drug discontinuance.

A systematic review of the field points to one conclusion: there is little evidence to define a group of schizophrenics who can survive in the community without medication. No variable, whether age, level of pathology, premorbid history, acute treatment dose, or any other factor, has emerged so far to define such a group. Does this mean that all schizophrenics should be maintained indefinitely? The answer at this time is no. In addition to the danger of tardive dyskinesia, which will be discussed later, we know too little about psychological and other medical implications of long-term drug use. In view of these possible complications, it is advisable to give some patients a period of time without medication, especially if they can be closely monitored. There is some evidence that patients over 60, in whom the disease process may burn out, and patients with very poor prognoses may do as well without medication. Maintenance regimens must be individualized, but a useful model might by the following: after the first episode, medication should be continued for six months; when a second episode occurs, this period is lengthened to between one and two years, depending on the individual; and, finally, patients who have experienced three or more episodes should probably be maintained on medication indefinitely.

MEDICATION MAINTENANCE PROGRAM
The implementation of a drug maintenance program should begin before discharge. Patients and their families can be prepared by educating them to the importance of continuing medication as prescribed. After a patient has stabilized, the acute treatment dose can be decreased 25 percent every three months. The goal is to find the smallest possible dose that will prevent relapse. The dose must be individualized, but for many patients, a suitable target might be one-third to one-fifth of the acute treatment dose. If a patient shows signs of decompensating, the dose should promptly be increased. A number of reports suggest that, in general, maintenance doses are too large.

Noncompliance
The most common cause of relapse is drug discontinuance. About 20 percent of schizophrenic inpatients taking oral medication do not actually swallow their pills. For outpatients, the range of drug defaulting is between

40 and 70 percent. Ayd (1975) found that medication noncompliance increased with the number of doses and the number of drugs. If there is a question, compliance can be monitored by checking prolactin levels. The neuroleptics have been shown to increase serum prolactin threefold to fourfold within 72 hours. Proper preparation of the patient and his or her family can improve the compliance rate, as can a single dose at bedtime. Even so, there are a substantial number of schizophrenic outpatients who do not take their medication and run a high risk of relapse. One way of reaching this population is through the use of injectable long-acting phenothiazines (LAP).

Long-Acting Phenothiazines
Fluphenazine enanthate and fluphenazine decanoate have been in clinical use for more than a decade. Despite early concerns, long-lasting undesirable side effects have not been a problem. The profile of an LAP side effect is quite similar to that of other phenothiazines of the piperazine subgroup, although there may be a higher incidence of akinesia. The two drugs differ only in the fatty acid side chain that determines how slowly they are released into the bloodstream. Enanthate has a duration of action of between 10 days and two weeks, while decanoate lasts three to four weeks. Both drugs are comparable in clinical efficacy, although decanoate has been reported to have a lower incidence of extrapyramidal effects. Since the clinical effects do not occur before one to four days after the initial injection, an oral supplement is often needed in the first several days. Some patients with chronic schizophrenia may require up to six months for maximal improvement.

The standard dose range of depot fluphenazine is 12.5 to 100 mg, while the usual starting dose is 12.5 to 25 mg. Agitated, younger, and heavier patients, or those already receiving large doses of another agent, can be given higher initial doses. Injections should be given every 10 days to two weeks for enanthate, or every three to four weeks for decanoate. Clinical observation will reveal whether the dose and duration, which must be individualized, are adequate. If a dose is not preventing symptoms it should be supplemented with oral medication; the next injection should be increased. Once an optimal response is achieved, the physician can begin increasing the duration between injections and lowering the dose. The goal is to maintain the patient at the lowest dose, given at the longest interval, that prevents relapse.

Several new long-acting drugs are currently being used in Europe. Penfluridol is especially interesting because it is an oral agent, similar to haloperidol, that lasts up to seven days on a single dose. Unfortunately, it has recently been reported to be associated with tumors in rats; therefore, its future is uncertain. Pipothiazine palmitate has the longest duration of action, lasting four to six weeks. Within the next several years, we are likely to see a number of new drugs approved for use in the United States.

Very-High-Dose Therapy
Another development for the chronic schizophrenic population is very-high-dose therapy. Howard reported treating 95 patients with chronic schizophrenia that was refractory to treatment; the mean duration of illness was over 17 years, spent mainly in custodial care. The average medication dose had been haloperidol, 10 mg daily, or its equivalent. Howard increased the dose by 50 percent each week until either improvement occurred or serious side effects intervened, up to a maximum of 75 mg a day. Five months after beginning the program, 81 of 95 patients had responded sufficiently to be discharged. The average daily dose of haloperidol at discharge was 35 to 40 mg. The annual return rate during the next two and one-half years of follow-up was five percent, compared with 80 percent before the study.

Several other open studies have reported impressive results working with chronically hospitalized schizophrenics. The dosage range for haloperidol was 35 to 150 mg, and that for fluphenazine hydrochloride was 600 to 1,200 mg. We should note that these studies were open, and that results were less impressive in recent double-blind studies. There does appear to be a subgroup of chronic schizophrenics who are refractory to standard regimens but who will respond to very high doses. Further study of this promising theory is needed.

Explanation of Results
The explanation for these results is unclear. Cole speculated that prolonged exposure to phenothiazines in certain patients may induce hyperactive microsomal enzymes that rapidly metabolize neuroleptics. Treating these patients with intramuscular fluphenazine, or with very large oral doses, may be accomplishing the same objective—elevating the tissue concentration of active drug in a population of schizophrenic patients who are unresponsive because their absorption or metabolism renders standard oral doses inadequate.

The neuroleptics have a wide range between clinically effective doses and toxic levels. The studies previously cited used doses 25 to 100 times greater than those recommended in the *Physicians' Desk Reference* (1983) (PDR), with no untoward reactions or increased side effects. High-dose treatment should be reserved for treatment refractory chronic schizophrenic patients who can be closely observed, and it is contraindicated in patients with a history of seizures, cardiovascular disorders, or organic brain damage. Before administering very high doses of a medication, the physician should try three to four times the standard dose. Fluphenazine is probably the drug of choice because there has been more evidence of its safety in megadoses. Once a patient has improved, which may take up to six months, the dose should be decreased as tolerated.

PLASMA LEVELS
Techniques to measure neuroleptic serum levels have been developed during the past 10 years. Because of interindividual differences in the absorption and metabolism of drugs, patients on the same dose may have very different plasma concentrations. It is not clear whether antipsychotic drug levels correlate with clinical efficacy, as they appear to do with tricyclic antidepressants. One impediment is the complex metabolism of most antipsychotic agents, which yield numerous pharmacologically active metabolites. Patients with very low drug plasma levels generally have poor clinical responses. However, further studies are needed to determine the relationship between clinical response and drug plasma level once a minimum level has been exceeded.

Measuring dopamine receptor binding in plasma appears to be a more promising lead. This technique may offer a relatively inexpensive method for measuring total plasma concentration of pharmacologically active compound, including both parent and active metabolites. Further studies correlating serum dopamine-receptor binding with clinical outcome would be of great interest.

TARDIVE DYSKINESIA
Tardive dyskinesia is a potentially irreversible syndrome of hyperkinetic involuntary movements produced by the use of antipsychotic medication. The clinical syndrome consists of repetitive and purposeless movements typically involving the mouth, lips, tongue, and jaw, but sometimes including the limbs and trunk. Severity can range from barely detectable movements of the tongue to severely incapacitating movements of the axial musculature. The dyskinetic movements, which have an insidious onset, are typically made worse by stress and intentional motor activity. Although initially thought to be confined to older chronic patients with underlying organic brain disease, the syndrome has now been found among younger patients and those whose condition is more acute. While it has been reported to appear as early as three months after the patient begins the medication, the syndrome most commonly occurs after at least two years of treatment. Although the movements usual-

ly appear while the patient is receiving the medication, the symptoms may not become clinically evident until the drug is either decreased or discontinued.

Tardive dyskinesia has been diagnosed after treatment with all currently approved antipsychotic medications. The incidence among older chronic patients who have been maintained on medication for many years is conservatively estimated to be 20 percent. For younger acute patients receiving medication for less than two years, the incidence is much lower; if medication is stopped, the syndrome is less likely to become chronic in these patients. In one study, 88 percent of long-term maintenance patients with tardive dyskinesia were found to have an irreversible condition. Another study showed a 92 percent reversal rate among younger patients in whom tardive dyskinesia was detected early.

The mechanism by which currently used antipsychotic agents cause tardive dyskinesia is not known. The most widely accepted explanation is that antipsychotic-induced blockade causes dopamine receptors to become hypersensitive. Research has focused on the reciprocal relationship between acetylcholine and dopamine, which may be unbalanced. Strategies for treatment generally involve attempts to rectify this balance, either by decreasing dopamine activity or by increasing cholinergic balance. Agents that have been reported to be helpful in reducing the severity of the movements include lecithin, deanol, choline, reserpine, L-dopa, alphamethyl paratyrosine, tetrabenazine, pyridoxine, clonazepam, and gamma-aminobutyric acid. Raising the antipsychotic dose can have a temporary ameliorating effect but may eventually lead to a worsening of the condition. Anticholinergic drugs used for the treatment of parkinsonian side effects tend to exacerbate the dyskinesia. Although this area is under active investigation, as yet there is no satisfactory treatment for tardive dyskinesia.

Tardive dyskinesia raises difficult clinical, ethical, and medicolegal questions. As discussed earlier, it is recommended that every schizophrenic patient have a trial period without the medication after his or her first and second acute episode. If medication is to be continued, the lowest maintenance dose that will sustain improvement should be used. Maintenance patients ought to be evaluated at least every three months for the development of tardive dyskinesia. As part of the examination, the patient is asked to keep his or her tongue extended since movements of the tongue are commonly the first sign. If early signs of tardive dyskinesia are detected, the risk of psychotic deterioration if the drug is withdrawn must be weighed against the danger of permanent neurologic damage if the drug is continued. This is a difficult decision that should be shared with the family and documented in the record. Given these risks, there is little justification for using antipsychotic agents for patients who are not actually psychotic.

REVERSIBLE EXTRAPYRAMIDAL SYNDROMES
Reversible extrapyramidal side effects (EPS) caused by antipsychotic drugs include acute dystonic reactions, akathisia, parkinsonian side effects, and catatonia. The incidence of the EPS varies with the type and amount of drug, duration of treatment, route of administration, sex, age, and individual sensitivity. The likelihood of EPS appears to depend on the balance between anticholinergic and antidopaminergic effects of a given drug. Drugs that have primarily antidopaminergic effects, such as haloperidol, commonly cause EPS. Conversely, drugs with high anticholinergic activity, such as thioridazine, infrequently cause EPS.

As EPS emerge clinically, they should be treated promptly. There is evidence that untreated EPS contribute to the high rate of noncompliance in schizophrenic outpatients. Akinesia, because of its undramatic nature, is common, disturbing to patients, and often neither diagnosed nor treated. Whether antiparkinsonian drugs should be used prophylactically remains an unresolved question. The arguments against prophylactic antiparkinsonian medication include cost, inconvenience, reduced compliance, drug interactions, and increased anticholinergic side effects. Antiparkinsonian drugs also have abuse potential. One school of thought recommends prophylactic use during the first four days in which a high-potency antipsychotic drug is prescribed for outpatients. Studies have shown that 60 to 90 percent of patients who initially needed antiparkinsonian drugs can be successfully withdrawn after three months.

Drugs used to treat EPS include agents that are primarily anticholinergic (for example, benztropine), agents with both antihistaminic and anticholinergic activity (such as diphenhydramine), and amantadine, an agent with primarily dopaminergic activity. Amantadine has the advantage of being only weakly anticholinergic, and thus does not compound the anticholinergic effects of the neuroleptics.

High-potency antipsychotics may cause catatonic reactions, characterized by posturing, waxy flexibility, withdrawal, and regression. The syndrome develops gradually and is usually accompanied by parkinsonian side effects. Making the correct diagnosis is critical because emerging catatonic features may be misdiagnosed as a worsening of the schizophrenic process; that diagnosis can lead the clinician to increase the drug dose, which in turn worsens the catatonic reaction. Once the diagnosis is made, the antipsychotic should be stopped.

OTHER SIDE EFFECTS

The antipsychotic agents vary considerably in their effects on cholinergic, alpha-adrenergic, beta-adrenergic, and histaminergic systems. In general, low-potency agents cause more anticholinergic side effects, while high-potency drugs cause more extrapyramidal reactions. Cholinergic blockage causes the atropinelike effects of urinary hesitation, exacerbation of closed-angle glaucoma, constipation, blurred vision, and dry mouth. Anticholinergic side effects and their management are described more fully in the discussion of the side effects of tricyclic agents. Low-potency drugs, such as chlorpromazine and thioridazine, also produce more alpha-adrenergic blockage, which may lead to hypotension. Among antipsychotics, thioridazine has the highest affinity for the cholinergic receptor (120 times that of haloperidol) and is more likely to cause cardiac effects. Caution should be used in prescribing thioridazine for patients with cardiac disorders. In contrast to high-potency agents, which are fairly safe even in massive overdoses, thioridazine has a small margin for safety, making it a poor choice for the suicidal patient. Thioridazine is also reported to cause retinitis pigmentosa when given in doses exceeding 800 mg daily. The extrapyramidal side effects associated with high-potency agents have already been discussed.

Antipsychotic agents cross the placenta and have been shown to produce transitory neurologic side effects in newborns of mothers taking phenothiazines. However, there is no evidence to date that antipsychotics are teratogenic. A large prospective study found that the incidence of congenital malformations among newborns whose mothers took antipsychotic medications did not differ from that in unexposed newborns. Furthermore, there was no difference between the two groups in perinatal mortality, mean birth weight, and IQ at age 4. A recent review concluded that the amount of phenothiazines passed in the milk is essentially safe for breast-feeding neonates.

Patients may be using other medications that can complicate their management. Interactions between drugs can potentiate or diminish antipsychotic effects. Studies of antipsychotic plasma levels have shown that antacids, antiparkinsonian agents, lithium, and barbiturates may lower serum levels of antipsychotics. Conversely, antipsychotic agents may antagonize the effects of L-dopa, guanethidine, and amphetamines. They also can potentiate the central nervous system depression produced by narcotic analgesics, minor tranquilizers, barbiturates, alcohol, and other psychoactive agents. Low-potency antipsychotic medications may potentiate the hypotensive effect of anesthetics, hypotensive diuretics, beta-adrenergic agonists (epinephrine), and alpha-adrenergic blocking agents (phentolamine).

NEW PHARMACOLOGIC TREATMENTS

One of the new areas of investigation has been the role of endogenous opioid compounds in schizophrenia. Opiate receptors have been found in several areas of the human brain that are unrelated to pain sensory pathways. Opiates have been shown to induce hallucinations in healthy human volunteers and to cause a prolonged muscular rigidity resembling catatonic schizophrenia when injected in rats. These effects are promptly reversed by the opiate antagonist, naloxone. Beta-endorphin, an endogenous peptide that binds to opiate receptors, has been isolated in the pituitary and other areas of the human brain, and it has been assayed in the cerebrospinal fluid and peripheral blood. These findings have led to the hypothesis that some mental disorders may be related to a disturbance in the endorphin levels at key receptor sites in the central nervous system. The reports to date have varied widely in their assessment of the effects of naloxone and beta-endorphin on schizophrenic symptoms. Further double-blind drug trials are needed to assess the relationship of the endorphins to schizophrenia.

Since lithium was introduced by Cade in 1949, its efficacy in the treatment of bipolar affective disorders has been firmly established (lithium is discussed more fully in the section dealing with the treatment of affective disorders). More recently, it has been tried in a variety of other psychiatric syndromes. There are convincing data that lithium can reduce the morbidity in schizoaffective illness. It appears that lithium may ameliorate the nonaffective or schizophrenic component of this disorder, in addition to stabilizing mood fluctuations. The role of lithium in the treament of schizophrenia, either alone or in combination with antipsychotic agents, remains to be clarified by further study.

Beta-adrenergic blocking agents, such as propranolol, have been reported to be useful in the treatment of angina pectoris, hypertension, thyrotoxicosis, and migraine. Several authors have reported that propranolol, given in doses of 500 to 3,500 mg, may have a beneficial effect on some schizophrenics unresponsive to antipsychotics. These are preliminary findings and await confirmation.

Another area of investigation is the search for a drug that possesses antipsychotic properties without causing extrapyramidal side effects. Such a drug theoretically would have less potential for causing tardive dyskinesia. As yet, there is no drug with such selective regional effects that it exclusively blocks the mesolimbic and mesocortical neurons related to antipsychotic activity, while sparing those in the nigrostriatal area associated with extrapyramidal effects. Two agents with some promise of selective antipsychotic activity are sulpiride and apomorphine. There is some evidence that they may function as presynaptic dopamine agonists, which decrease dopamine transmission by activating inhibitory presynaptic mechanisms.

These experimental treatments are being investigated in part to further uncover the mechanism by which drugs ameliorate schizophrenic psychosis. None of them are currently of clinical use, but in the coming years, the leads they produce may yield a therapeutic agent that does not cause tardive dyskinesia.

Drug Management of Affective Disorders

Depression is the most common disorder treated by psychiatrists. In the general population, the average prevalence of depression is close to ten percent, while five percent suffer from a serious disorder that requires treatment. The lifetime prevalence of depression in this country is estimated to be as much as 27 percent; about 15 percent of those depressed patients will go on to commit suicide. Many of these people do not respond to psychotherapy and will require pharmacologic treatment. There are three principal classes of antidepressant drugs in widespread clinical use: the tricyclic agents, lithium salts, and the monoamine oxidase (MAO) inhibitors. Several new classes of antidepressant drugs are currently being tested in Europe but are not yet available in the United States.

TRICYCLIC AGENTS
Iminodibenzyl, the parent compound of the tricyclic agents, was synthesized in 1899 and then was largely neglected for the next 50 years. Because of its structural resemblance to chlorpromazine, Kuhn began studying the drug in 1951 for use as an antipsychotic. Although schizophrenic psychoses showed little response, the depressive features of these patients improved markedly. Subsequent clinical trials confirmed the drug's antidepressant effects, and the Food and Drug Administration (FDA) approved imipramine in 1959.

Mode of Action
The catecholamine hypothesis was formulated in the 1960s as a unitary explanation of the affective disorders. It proposed that depression may be related to a functional deficiency of catechol neurotransmitters at central adrenergic receptor sites, while mania was associated with a functional excess. One of the earliest findings that suggested this hypothesis was that reserpine, which tended to cause depression, depleted intraneuronal stores of norepinephrine and serotonin. Further research led to the hypothesis that drugs causing depletion or inactivation of brain norepinephrine could produce depression, while drugs which raise or potentiate brain norepinephrine could have antidepressant effects.

The mechanism of action common to all tricyclic agents is thought to be the inhibition of reuptake of norepinephrine and serotonin. These two biogenic amines are released by the presynaptic neuron and traverse the synaptic cleft to stimulate the receptor. They then reenter the presynaptic cell, where they are either stored or metabolized. By blocking reuptake, tricyclic agents increase the amount, and thereby restore the putative deficiency of norepinephrine and serotonin available at the receptor site. For a more detailed description, the reader is referred to Schildkraut's (1970) review of the subject.

Most clinicians have observed that some patients respond better to one drug than another. Some endogenously depressed patients respond to both amitriptyline and imipramine, other patients to one drug but not the other, while some patients respond to neither. This heterogeneity of clinical response suggests that tricyclics vary in their effects on different neurotransmitter systems. There is evidence that imipramine works more on the norepinephrine system, while amitriptyline acts primarily on serotonin. Among tricyclic agents currently being investigated, maprotiline is the most specific blocker of norepinephrine and trazodone is the most specific for serotonin.

Maas (1975) and others attempted to correlate these heterogeneous pharmacologic actions with biologic measures and clinical outcome. The most reliable measures of central norepinephrine metabolism may be 3-methoxy,4-hydroxyphenylglycol (MHPG). Maas proposed that there are at least two groups of depressives. Group A is characterized by: (1) low pretreatment 24-hour urinary MHPG; (2) a favorable clinical response to imipramine; (3) response to a test dose of dextroamphetamine with a brightened mood; and (4) a poor response to amitriptyline. Group B is characterized by: (1) high or normal 24-hour urinary MHPG; (2) no response to imipramine; (3) no response to a test dose of dextroamphetamine; and (4) a positive response to amitriptyline. Maas theorized that the pathophysiology of group A primarily involves a disorder of norepinephrine metabolism, while group B has a disorder of serotonin metabolism. It should be noted that these studies involved retrospective analysis and had relatively small numbers of patients. In addition, some have questioned the usefulness of urinary

MHPG as a measure of central norepinephrine activity. Another promising attempt to correlate drug response with a biochemical lesion involves measuring the concentration of 5-hydroxyindoleacetic acid (5-HIAA), a serotonin metabolite, in the cerebrospinal fluid. There is some evidence that patients with low 5-HIAA levels are less likely to respond to nortriptyline, while those with higher levels have more improvement. These results suggest that the former group was deficient in serotonin, and, therefore, was less likely to respond to nortriptyline, a drug that primarily blocks norepinephrine reuptake.

While these findings are interesting, they are primarily of research interest. Their clinical usefulness remains to be confirmed in larger scale, prospective clinical trials. Much work remains to be done to identify and define subgroups in the depressed population in order to match the patient to a specific drug.

Some recent developments raise questions about the validity of the biogenic amine hypothesis and its corrolary, the reuptake blockage theory of tricyclic action. Both iprindole and mianserin have been shown to be as effective as amitriptyline, but they are only very weak blockers or either serotonin or norepinephrine. The mechanism by which these two agents exert antidepressant effects remains to be explained. Additional research is required to identify the neurophysiologic lesion in depression, and the mechanism of action of tricyclic antidepressants.

Treatment of Acute Depression
The clinical efficacy of the tricyclic antidepressants has been well established in numerous studies. Morris and Beck reviewed 146 double-blind, random assignment studies that used control groups. The result showed the tricylic agents to be significantly more effective than placebos in 61 of 93 comparisons (60 percent). Klein and Davis (1969) reviewed only double-blind studies of imipramine and combined the data. They found that of 734 patients treated with imipramine, 70 percent improved, compared with only 39 percent improvement in 606 patients receiving placebos.

Choice of Drug. There are currently over a dozen tricyclic agents that have been approved by the Food and Drug Administration (FDA); a number of new antidepressants that are being tested in Europe may offer significant clinical advantages. While not yet of proved efficacy and safety, several (maprotiline, trazodone, alprazolam, and amoxapine) were approved by the FDA in the early 1980s. Maprotiline and mianserin appear to have much milder side effect profiles than found with reference tricyclics. Both zimelidine and trazodone reportedly are effective broad-spectrum antidepressants with negligible anticholinergic side effects and very low cardiac toxicity. Amoxapine, alprazolam, and trazodone appear to have quicker onset of action than does imipramine or amitriptyline. It is worth noting that there is no conclusive evidence that any of the newer drugs are more effective than either imipramine or amitriptyline, the most thoroughly studied and widely used of the group.

Plasma levels of tricyclic agents should always be determined in patients who fail to respond to standard treatment, to avoid cardiotoxicity in geriatric patients: this determination also helps in the management of an overdose.

While blood levels are a more accurate measure of tissue concentration than is the dose, reliable measurements have not been widely available. The presence of autonomic side effects is a clinical alternative method for gauging drug response. A patient who fails to develop autonomic effects on standard dosage may be a rapid metabolizer who will require higher-than-average dosage. Conversely, the patient who evidences an abundance of autonomic side effects on lower dosages may have reached a therapeutic plasma level and not require an increase.

Predictors of Clinical Response. The problem of predicting drug response has also been approached by examining clinical features. Bielski and Friedel reviewed the literature for predictors of response to amitriptyline and imipramine. They included only prospective, double-blind studies done with a control group. In five of five studies, neurotic, hypochondriacal, or hysterical personality traits were associated with a negative response. This is consistent with the widely held belief that "neurotic" (characterologic) depressives do not respond well to tricyclic antidepressants (see the section on MAO inhibitors). In fact, two of three studies found that this diagnosis was itself associated with a negative response. Conversely, the diagnosis of major depression (with melancholia), as well as many of the individual features of this disorder, was associated with a positive drug response. These features include insidious onset, anorexia, weight loss, middle-of-the-night or late-night insomnia, diurnal variation, and psychomotor disturbance. A history of multiple prior episodes was associated with a negative response in three of three studies, perhaps suggesting a subpopulation of patients who are candidates for lithium maintenance. The clinical impression that the presence of delusions augurs a poor response to tricyclics was supported by four of four studies. The use of electroconvulsive therapy or phenothiazines is often effective with these patients.

Maintenance Treatment

As many as 15 percent of patients who experience an episode of acute depression go on to a chronic, unremitting course. Almost one-half of patients who have a single episode will suffer a recurrence sometime in their lives. After two episodes, the probability of future recurrence increases, and the time interval between episodes decreases. These findings suggest that a majority of patients presenting with acute, severe depression have a recurrent illness requiring long-term management. Failure to recognize the recurrent nature of many depressions has been a clinical shortcoming.

The evidence for the recurring nature of depression is quite convincing. In a series of nine double-blind, random-assignment studies, the mean relapse rate for patients experiencing an acute depression approached two-thirds. This finding raises the question about when the cessation of active drug treatment is indicated. A series of controlled studies examining the effect of drug maintenance on relapse rate showed a 50 percent reduction. The mean relapse rate in all the studies was reduced from 64 to 28 percent. Davis combined the data from these studies and calculated that the probability of the occurrence of this prophylactic effect by chance was 1.6×10^{-8}. Two conclusions seem warranted: The tricyclic agents appear to be effective in the prophylaxis of unipolar affective illness, and lithium is clearly effective in the prophylactic treatment of patients with bipolar disorders. Further studies are needed to compare the efficacy of lithium with that of the tricyclic agents for patients with unipolar disorders.

The literature has been ambiguous about the distinction between continuation and maintenance treatment. Prevailing clinical practice is that continuation treatment to prevent a relapse of the index episode should last six months. For patients with a history of three or more severe relapses, maintenance treatment should probably be indefinite. Further systematic study of this subject is needed. Two pressing questions are: Is six months the optimal duration of continuation treatment, and how can clinicians identify and define the subgroup that should be offered indefinite maintenance treatment? Psychoneuroendocrine challenge studies may prove to be useful predictions of the potential for relapse (see Chapter 3). This point is illustrated by a British study of 116 hospitalized depressive patients who had responded to drug treatment. Patients continued to receive either amitriptyline or imipramine for the first six months after discharge, and they did well. After another 12 months (18 months after hospitalization), follow-up studies were done. The mean recurrence rate was almost 60 percent, while rehospitalization was necessary for about one-fourth of these patients.

If a patient is to continue to receive medication, the dose should be reduced to a range of 75 to 150 mg daily. Some argue against this practice, pointing out that tricyclic agents do not accumulate over time. A reduction in dose will result in decreased plasma levels, which have been shown to be ineffective in the treatment of an acute episode. Whether lower plasma levels are also associated with reduced effectiveness in preventing relapse remains to be demonstrated by systematic study. If the dose is lowered, the patient's ability to tolerate this decrease should be closely monitored. Any serious worsening is an indication that the dose should be raised to the levels used for acute treatment.

Side Effects
The tricyclic agents cause a host of side effects. Attention to the patient's complaints and successful management of the side effects will often determine whether or not he or she stays in treatment. Side effects are simply unwanted pharmacologic actions—neither therapeutic nor toxic, but intrinsic to the drug. Most of them are related to the dual adrenergic and anticholingeric actions of tricyclic agents. Although often uncomfortable, the majority of side effects are mild and transient, with tolerance frequently developing within one to three weeks. Individual susceptibility to side effects varies markedly; the aged are more vulnerable to these problems, especially adynamic ileus, atonic bladder, and cardiac disorders.

Many of the side effects of the tricyclic agents are also symptoms of depression (that is, sleep disturbance, fatigue, or constipation) or anxiety (that is, sweating, dry mouth, or palpitations). It is often difficult to separate side effects from concurrent symptoms of the disease process.

Cardiac Side Effects. The tricyclic antidepressants have a number of cardiac effects; the most threatening of these actions are on cardiac condition. The effects of these drugs result from the interaction of age, the presence of heart disease, drug concentration, duration of treatment, and the specific characteristics of a given drug. Nortriptyline, for example, causes no detectable cardiac changes when given in a therapeutic range to young, healthy adults. However, when this range is exceeded, intraventricular conduction delays become prominent. Among older patients with preexisting cardiac disease, imipramine, even in small doses, routinely causes conduction delays. Most patients, even those with cardiac disease, can tolerate tricyclic antidepressants well. The group of patients in greatest jeopardy are those with preexisting bundle branch block, who can progress to complete heart block and develop tachyarrhythmias. These patients may account for the occasional reports of sudden death among patients taking tricyclic agents. Older patients and those with a history of cardiac problems should routinely have electrocardiograms performed. Doxepin has been the drug of choice for such patients since it causes little manic reaction. Temporarily discontinuing the drug during the course of electroconvulsive therapy is recommended.

Interactions Between Drugs. A number of interactions of tricyclic agents with other drugs have been reported. Because the list is long, only several of the more common interactions will be reviewed. The tricyclic antidepressants block the transport system that concentrates guanethidine within the sympathic neuron terminal, thereby diminishing the latter's effect. This problem may be compensated for by increasing the dose of guanethidine, but this increase may abruptly become excessive if the tricyclic agent is discontinued. The same phenomenon occurs with the hypotensive action of reserpine. Barbiturates decrease tricyclic plasma levels, while methylphenidate raises them. The tricyclic agents potentiate the sedative effects of alcohol, and patients should be cautioned against combining the two. The phenothiazines have atropinelike side effects that are additive to those of the tricyclics. Patients receiving more than 1 g of ethchlorvynol, a commonly prescribed hypnotic, may experience transient delirium. Nitroglycerine in combination with tricyclic drugs has been reported to cause a sudden fall in blood pressure.

A great deal has been said about the dangers of combining MAO inhibitors with tricyclic antidepressants. The FDA has advised against this combination. Several reviews have concluded that there is no evidence that combination treatment is unsafe when taken orally in therapeutic doses. Shopsin and Kline (1974) reported treating over 500 patients with combination therapy; they found no fatalities, and the side effects were about what one would expect for either drug used alone. Several British investigators have reported treating more than 2,000 patients with a combination of MAO inhibitors and tricyclic antidepressants without change in intraventricular conduction time. Imipramine has a quinidinelike suppressant effect, making it the drug of choice for cardiac patients with premature atrial and ventricular contractions.

The tricyclic antidepressants, especially imipramine, have a direct effect on the myocardium. By decreasing cardiac contractility, they decrease cardiac reserve and can lead to cardiac insufficiency. Older patients who have barely achieved cardiac compensation may be thrown into frank congestive heart failure by the addition of a tricyclic agent. In such patients, digitalization is often necessary.

Autonomic Side Effects Unrelated to the Heart. The side effects patients complain about are frequently related to the potent antimuscarinic action of the tricyclic agents. Perhaps the most common is dryness of the mucosa, which patients experience as "cotton mouth." This discomfort is often relieved by taking eight full glasses of fluids daily and by using agents that stimulate saliva, such as hard candies and chewing gum. Urinary retention is related to dosage, duration of treatment, and the individual patient's susceptibility (the elderly are the most vulnerable). Symptoms may include incomplete voiding, frequency, and complete inhibition of micturition. To avoid catheterization, one must treat this side effect promptly and vigorously. The treatment of choice is bethanechol (Urecholine), 10 to 25 mg three times a day. Another autonomic side effect is elevated intraocular pressure, which may worsen glaucoma. Constipation, a common symptom of depression, is made worse by the tricyclic agents. Early treatment is recommended as the condition may progress to paralytic ileus, especially in older patients or when the antidepressant is given in combination with other anticholinergic agents. Increased sweating may occur at night, or there may be acute attacks during the day. At times, the sweating is limited to the upper body.

Blurred vision is a frequent problem. Patients may complain of trouble reading, while distant vision is usually unaffected. The blurring is caused by an atropinelike effect that impairs the response of the sphincter and ciliary muscle of the eye. The patient should be warned of this side effect and reassured that it will clear once the drug has been stopped. Another common autonomic effect is hypotension. At smaller doses, tricyclic antidepressants may elevate blood pressure by reinforcing adrenergic mechanisms. In larger doses, an adrenergic blockade decreases blood pressure. Postural hypotension is a common clinical problem. Patients should be warned to get up slowly from a reclining position. In one study, 39 percent of patients had such severe problems with ataxia and falling that the drug had to be discontinued. No tolerance was noted after four weeks. In patients with preexisting cardiovascular disease, hypotension may precipitate congestive heart failure or myocardial infarction. Individual tricyclics vary widely in their anticholinergic activity—amitriptyline and doxepin cause more intense side effects.

Miscellaneous Side Effects. The tricyclic antidepressants also cause a variety of side effects unrelated to their action on the autonomic nervous system. Women may complain of amenorrhea and other menstrual irregularities; a reduction in dose often resolves the problem, but pregnancy should be ruled out. Although the data are inconclusive, tricyclic agents should probably not be given in the first trimester of pregnancy. Blood sugar may be decreased, especially in diabetics; this change may reflect an effect of the drug on carbohydrate metabolism, since patients are also subject to weight gain and carbohydrate craving. A variety of neurologic effects have been reported. In addition to lowering the seizure threshold, tricyclic agents may cause a fine or coarse tremor. Neurotoxic reactions, which are rare, usually occur only with very large doses; these reactions can include nystagmus, dysarthria, slurred speech, hyperpyrexia, and decreased levels of consciousness.

The tricyclic agents may cause a variety of hematopoietic changes. Transient eosiniphilia, which is very frequent in the first several weeks, is of no clinical significance. Leukopenia is another benign and transient side effect of the tricyclic antidepressants. Agranulocytosis is a rare and possibly fatal complication that is thought to result from an allergic hypersensitivity reaction; it usually occurs in the second month of treatment and more frequently affects women and the elderly. Routine ordering of blood tests is not recommended, but a complete blood count should be ordered promptly if a patient develops an infection or temperature. Another rare complication is an obstructive jaundice syndrome that resembles phenothiazine toxicity. It is idiosyncratic, occurs in the first three months of treatment, and clears once the drug has been stopped. An allergic skin reaction over the upper body that may occur in the first two months is harmless and rarely necessitates discontinuing treatment.

In the category of chemical side effects, the tricyclic agents cause a number of false results on laboratory tests, including spuriously elevated values of several measures of liver function, such as alkaline phosphatase, bilirubin, serum glutamic oxaloacetic transaminase (SGOT), serum glutamic pyruvic transaminase (SGPT), and sulfobromophthalein (BSP) retention. Cholesterol levels may be falsely low, while fasting blood sugar can be either high or low.

Effect of Medical Condition

The pharmacologic action of the tricyclic antidepressants has an adverse effect on certain medical conditions. There is only one absolute contraindication (after a myocardial infarction), but several other conditions are relative contraindications that require a clinical judgment of possible risk and potential gain. The potent anticholinergic action of many tricyclic agents may exacerbate preexisting problems with urinary retention. Older men with prostatic hypertrophy are particularly vulnerable. As mentioned before, such patients may be helped by betharechol, which should be instituted early to avoid catheterization. Autonomic side effects may increase intraocular pressure. Patients with glaucoma, especially the closed-angle type, will require close supervision by an ophthalmologist. Tricyclic antidepressants, like the phenothiazines, tend to lower the seizure threshold; patients with epilepsy may require increased anticonvulsant medication. Tricyclic agents have potentially toxic cardiovascular effects that make them absolutely contraindicated in the early recovery period following a myocardial infarction. These effects also make them hazardous for patients with congestive heart failure, preexisting hypotension, or advanced cardiovascular disease. Older patients with bundle branch block are the most susceptible to developing atrioventricular block, which may be dose related.

Tricyclic antidepressants may have toxic behavioral effects that exacerbate several psychiatric conditions. Schizophrenic patients may become agitated and more psychotic. A patient who appears depressed but is latently schizophrenic can become agitated and develop overt delusions and hallucinations. This is thought to be related to a general activating effect of these drugs rather than a specifically psychotogenic action. This complication may respond to a reduction in dose, but initiating or increasing antipsychotic drug therapy is a more reliable treatment. Patients with bipolar affective disorders may switch into mania when treated with a tricyclic agent. Occasionally, this switch will occur in cases with no previous history of mania. Patients experiencing a manic episode while being treated with one tricyclic drug will not necessarily have the same reaction to another. The combination of electroconvulsive therapy and tricyclic antidepressants may also result in a therapy without fatality or untoward side effects. Combination therapy should be reserved for refractory cases, and certain guidelines adhered to. The drugs should be given orally and in moderate doses; the tricyclic agent should be given first; and other drugs that act on the central nervous system should be avoided.

Acute Anticholinergic Syndrome

More widespread use of psychoactive drugs has led to an awareness of the acute anticholinergic syndrome, which often results from an excessive increase in the dose of a drug with strong antimuscarinic effects, or a combination of several such drugs. These include tricyclic antidepressants, phenothiazines, and antiparkinsonian agents, three categories of medication that are often combined in the treatment of an agitated depression. The clinical picture is that of an acute toxic confusional psychosis. Signs of central anticholinergic toxicity include delirium, hyperactivity, anxiety, hallucinations, and disorientation. Peripheral anticholinergic toxicity is manifested by tachycardia, mydriasis, facial flushing, hyperpyrexia, urinary retention, and decreased bowel motility. When tricyclic antidepressants are involved, there is the additional risk of cardiac conduction abnormalities. This syndrome is promptly reversed by 2 mg of physostigmine, given intramuscularly or by slow intravenous push. Physostigmine salicylate is a reversible anticholinesterase that crosses the blood-brain barrier. If there is no response initially, a repeat dose should be given in 15 to 30 minutes. The earliest signs of a positive response are decreased pulse, increased bowel motility, and clearing of the mental status. Since physostigmine has a very short half-life, repeat doses should be given every 30 minutes to two hours until the patient has improved and is stable.

Treatment of Overdose

Because tricyclic agents are prescribed for depressed patients, the risk of intentional overdose is high. Approximately 15 percent of these patients make a serious suicide attempt. As little as 10 times the daily dose can be fatal. One of the most common errors in treating an overdose is in underestimating the seriousness of the problem. Since tricyclic antidepressants are rapidly absorbed and quickly accumulate in tissue, plasma levels are often unreliable in acute overdoses. Tissue levels may be ten times greater than plasma levels. Spikes proposed that the only reliable measure of the severity of a tricyclic overdose is the duration of the QRS interval; serious overdoses generally are associated with a QRS interval longer than 0.1 second. Another indication of impending danger is when the ratio of parent compound to metabolite exceeds 2.1 despite a low plasma level. Treatment is symptomatic and generally conservative. Because the onset of symptoms is rapid, one should induce vomiting in a conscious patient only if it does not delay transporting him or her to the hospital. Life-threatening cerebral excitation, respiratory depression, and myocardial toxicity are problems for the first 24 hours. If the patient survives this period, recovery is likely. Early signs are usually those of anticholinergic poisoning such as hyperpyrexia, confusion, agitation, and hyperreflexia. Electrocardiographic changes from sinus tachycardia to various atrial arrhythmias are anticholinergic in origin, and respond well to physostigmine, 2 mg intravenously. Ventricular arrhythmias, which have a different etiology, are best treated with lidocaine or procainamide. A profound hypotension follows the initial presentation. Norepinephrine should be avoided, as its effects are directly potentiated by tricyclic agents. Correcting cardiac arrhythmias will generally restore the blood pressure. Excessive cerebral stimulation may produce convulsions. Intravenous diazepam is the preferred treatment because it minimizes respiratory depression. Controversy surrounds the use of either (1) forced diuresis, which may cause cardiac failure, and (2) hemodialysis, which is largely ineffective. The patient should be monitored on the medical service for at least 72 hours because symptoms can rebound later. Cardiac arrhythmias may persist for up to one week. This is probably related to the finding among patients with serious overdoses (plasma concentrations 100 ng/ml) that the mean plasma level at 96 hours was 630 ng/ml, which is well into the toxic range.

LITHIUM

Lithium salts have essentially revolutionized the treatment of patients with affective disorders, much as the introduction of chlorpromazine dramatically changed the treatment of schizophrenia 20 years ago. Lithium has been found to be an effective prophylactic agent against the recurrence of affective episodes and has altered the course of the illness for many patients. Further, the apparent specificity of lithium for affective disorders, in contrast to schizophrenic disorders, has caused psychiatrists to seek greater precision in the diagnosis of psychiatric syndromes.

Lithium salts were not accepted in American psychiatry until 1970, although the drug had been introduced for the treatment of affective disorders 20 years before. J.F. Cade, in Australia, noted that lithium salts produced a quieting effect on animals in his research on purine metabolism; he recognized a similar calming effect in acutely manic subjects as well. As a result of this rather serendipitous finding, several European investigators studied the efficacy of lithium in manic-depressive illness (later redesignated as bipolar and unipolar illness) through the 1950s and 1960s. American physicians were reluctant to accept lithium because they were skeptical about its safety. Several cases of severe intoxication and deaths had been reported in the United States among patients using lithium chloride as a salt substitute during treatment for cardiac or renal failure. The fear of lithium toxicity delayed the ultimate acceptance of research investigations that confirmed the efficacy of lithium in the treatment of affective illness. Ultimately, it became clear that lithium has a very narrow margin of safety and requires careful blood monitoring, and that sodium restriction and enforced diuresis exacerbates its potential toxicity. However, the carefully monitored use of lithium has yielded dramatic improvements in patients who were previously untreatable and for whom the burden of affective illness was great. Today, it is recognized that lithium may be effective in the treatment of patients experiencing acute manic syndromes, in the maintenance treatment of patients with affective disorder, and in the management of some patients with acute depressions as well. Lithium has been shown to reduce the intensity and duration of affective episodes, to prolong the symptom-free interval between episodes in many patients, and, in some patients, to entirely extinguish the course of illness. While lithium is primarily indicated for patients with affective illness, it has also been used successfully with some schizoaffective patients, reactive depressive patients, those with premenstrual tension syndromes, and some emotionally unstable adolescents as well.

Pharmacology and Mechanism of Action

Lithium is readily absorbed by the gastrointestinal tract, making oral administration acceptable. Lithium is not bound by protein molecules; unlike sodium and potassium ions, it is generally distributed rather evenly throughout the total body water space between blood and tissues. There is a difference between intracellular and extracellular lithium measures within tissues. In fact, the assay of lithium in the red blood cell (erythrocyte) in comparison with that in the plasma (red blood cell–to-plasma ratio) has been suggested as an indicator of brain cell lithium levels. While there is some delay in the penetration of lithium into the cerebrospinal fluid, there is no actual blood-brain barrier that lithium has to cross and generally equilibration is reached within 24 hours.

Lithium is excreted primarily by the kidney, and most of it is reabsorbed in the proximal renal tubules, where it competes with sodium ions. Consequently, a sodium diuresis, or a sodium deficiency, will tend to increase the retention of lithium and to increase the predisposition to lithium toxicity. Similarly, dehydration will increase the risk of lithium toxicity because of the increased proximal reabsorption of lithium. Under normal circumstances, the half-life of lithium is about 18 to 20 hours in young adults; it increases to as long as 36 hours in elderly individuals. Thus, patients being treated with lithium must have adequate renal function because of the low therapeutic index and the importance of maintaining adequate renal excretion of the ion. Fortunately, the measurement of serum lithium levels is relatively inexpensive and commercially available, making management of patients using lithium quite feasible.

Psychobiologists are still unclear about the mechanism of action of lithium ions. Certainly, lithium is related to sodium and potassium, which have similar contributions to nervous transmission. Therefore, a great deal of attention has been given to electrolyte balance across the cell membranes. Lithium may effect the polarization of action potentials in the nerve membrane. In the brain, at clinical concentrations, lithium has been shown to interfere with the synaptic transmission of catecholamines (norepinephrine and dopamine), to antagonize the stimulation of adenylate cyclase, and to alter the cellular uptake and oxidation of glucose. It remains to be established, however, how lithium is able to reduce the intensity and frequency of manic or severe depressive episodes.

Dosage Forms

Lithium ions are available in the United States as capsules, in tablet form, and as syrup. The tablets and capsules are offered as 300 mg of the diabasic carbonate salt, lithium carbonate, containing 8.12 mEq of lithium. The syrup is prepared in solution from lithium hydroxide and citric acid as 8 mEq for every milliliter. The anionic partner (carbonate, chloride, sulfate, and so on) is only the inert vehicle for transportation of the lithium ion; thus, the choice depends on convenience and side effects. Although lithium chloride or lithium sulfate could be used, these substances appear to be more irritating to the gastrointestinal tract than is lithium carbonate. The citrate form is useful in those patients who are unable or unwilling to swallow tablets or capsules.

Treatment with Lithium

Lithium does not cure affective illness. A single dose has no therapeutic effect—lithium ions must be maintained at the right concentration in the right tissues over time, and the reduction of these levels may result in a reemergence of manic or depressive symptoms. Thus, the value of lithium depends on its continued presence at therapeutic levels in the body. Fortunately, lithium in the blood, or even in the saliva, can be reliably determined. When measuring lithium levels, it is important that blood samples be drawn when the patients are in the postabsorptive state, six to eight hours after their last dose. Generally, it is most practical to draw blood specimens in the morning before the day's initial dose is taken.

Prior to the initiation of lithium treatment, it is essential to complete a medical evaluation of the patient. Physical examination and history should concentrate on cardiovascular, endocrine, and renal function, and laboratory evaluation should include tests of renal, electrolyte, and thyroid function in particular. In practice, serum blood urea nitrogen (BUN) and creatinine are useful measures of renal function, although creatinine clearance measures may be necessary in patients who have some degree of renal or cardiovascular disease. In addition, a complete blood count, fasting blood sugar, and an electrocardiogram should be obtained at the time of initiation of lithium treatment.

The first demonstration of the value of lithium in the treatment of affective illness was for acute manic syndromes. Today a large number of controlled studies have demonstrated the efficacy of lithium in hypomania and acute mania; improvement occurs in 70 to 80 percent of patients within two weeks. Antipsychotic medications generally are used in the first two weeks to bring a faster symptomatic improvement, but they are subsequently discontinued when adequate lithium levels and control of initial acute symptoms have been achieved.

In the initial phase (stabilization period) in the treatment of acute mania, lithium levels in the range of 1.2 to 1.6 mEq/L may be expected. The specific dose will be determined by frequent measurement of serum lithium levels. Lithium levels above 2.0 mEq/L should be avoided. After the first week of treatment, the lithium level may be adjusted downward to the maintenance therapeutic range of 0.6 to 1.2 mEq/L (therapeutic ranges vary between laboratories). This approach has been recommended for patients who are acutely manic and require rapid stabilization. On the other hand, hypomanic patients and those who do not require rapid treatment should initially be given smaller doses of lithium in order to avoid undesirable early side effects. In these patients, the dosage may be increased by 150 mg a day until blood levels are in the desired range for lithium prophylaxis (about 0.6 to 1.2 mEq/L).

It should be noted that levels of lithium in the blood vary widely among patients receiving the same dose of lithium; therefore the ultimate dose requirements are idiosyncratic and cannot be judged empirically. In clinically stable patients, a prediction of the daily dose requirement can be made from the serum lithium level measured 24 hours after a 600-mg oral test dose of lithium via a logarithmic relationship (Cooper et al., 1976).

Lithium has been shown to have greatest value in the prophylactic management of patients with affective disorders. A reduction of the intensity and frequency of affective episodes has been established in numerous controlled studies of the prophylactic effects of lithium. In general, patients are maintained at lithium blood levels about 1.0 mEq/L with periodic lithium monitoring (usually once per month) as well as periodic measurement of thyroid, electrolyte, and renal function (at least twice per year). Patients who have been demonstrated to be lithium responders have also been shown to have a reappearance of affective symptoms with the same frequency and intensity as before if lithium is discontinued. On the other hand, it is not clear whether patients who are lithium responders will need to receive the medication for the rest of their lives. Recently, increasing concerns about long-term side effects of lithium on the kidney have led some clinicians to reconsider indefinite lithium prophylaxis. In trying to determine the necessity for continued lithium prophylaxis, it is important to consider the frequency of affective episodes, the burden that these episodes have for the individual patient, the presence or absence of side effects, and the patient's attitude towards continued use of medication, weighing the advantages and potential hazards.

Lithium has also been reported to be beneficial in acutely depressed patients. The use of lithium for acute depression usually follows tricyclic or MAO inhibitor antidepressant medications, but it can also be considered an alternative approach. In patients with unipolar depression who have a family history of bipolar illness, lithium may be the drug of choice. In one study, 90 percent of biologic relatives of bipolar patients who developed unipolar or bipolar illness were themselves shown to respond to lithium treatment. Some investigators believe that lithium is effective in the prophylactic management of unipolar depressive patients as well as bipolar patients.

Lithium has also been reported to be effective in patients with epilepsy, chronic schizophrenia, schizoaffective illness, and premenstrual tension syndromes, as well as in children and adolescents with extreme emotional lability. Controlled studies of the use of lithium in these disorders have not been entirely convincing. Schizoaffective illness in particular may be a heterogeneous disorder in which some individuals have a spectrum disorder of affective illness and may be responsive to lithium. Therefore, it is desirable to consider each patient individually and evaluate his or her family history in determining the need and the potential benefit of lithium treatment.

Side Effects

As with most pharmaceutical products, lithium has numerous reported side effects and potential toxicity as well. Because lithium is readily absorbed from the gastrointestinal tract, there are transient lithium peaks occurring shortly after administration of the drug that create potentially upsetting side effects. This is the reason that lithium is given in divided doses rather than simply as a single dose prior to going to sleep. These early side effects necessitate the cautious introduction of the medication for most patients. The peak occurs between one and three hours after the medication is taken and may sometimes cause intestinal discomfort, including nausea, stomach pain, and indigestion.

Early Side Effects. Many patients treated with lithium experience initial side effects that subside after a few days. The most commonly encountered side effects are those affecting the gastrointestinal system; as already noted, the patient may experience nausea and stomach pain, as well as vomiting, diarrhea, and muscle weakness. In addition, many patients complain of thirstiness (polydipsia) and frequent urination (polyuria); some report feeling dazed or fatigued; and hand tremors are noted as well. The occurrence of these side effects is apparently related to the steepness of the rising concentration of lithium in the blood and to the transient peak effects of the lithium ions when it is absorbed. For most patients, these side effects diminish as soon as the peak effect begins to fall.

Late Effects. Of greater concern are the later side effects of lithium treatment. Sometimes the early side effects may extend into the prophylactic period—hand tremor, in particular, is one undesirable side effect that is seen in many patients. Some investigators have suggested that propranolol in doses of 40 to 80 mg a day may be effective in reducing the incidence of hand tremor. The side effects of polydipsia and polyuria have been reported in as many as 25 percent of patients receiving long-term lithium prophylaxis. The effect may be due to lithium's interference with the antidiuretic hormone (vasopressin) in its action on the proximal renal tubules.

Another nonspecific effect of lithium, similar to that of many other psychotropic medications, is weight gain. This problem is also noted in patients receiving long-term tricyclic antidepressant medications and antipsychotic medications. Sometimes diets are ineffective in helping patients maintain their desired weight. Lithium treatment precludes starvation dieting or excessive sodium restriction because of its interference in lithium excretion. Consequently, many patients may want to stop lithium treatment because they are concerned about their weight gain.

Lithium treatment on a long-term basis also has an effect on the thyroid. Lithium appears to interfere with thyroid functioning causing a decrease in the amount of thyroxine which is secreted by the gland. Periodic thyroid screening is therefore necessary while patients are maintained on lithium prophylaxis. Small doses of thyroxine or thyroid extract may be given along with lithium when the patient develops hypothyroidism that is apparently lithium induced. Patients with latent hypothyroidism may be the ones most vulnerable to this form of benign diffuse nontoxic goiter. There may be an increase in the circulating levels of the thyroid-stimulating hormone (TSH), but rarely will significant functional hypothyroidism or myxedema occur.

Dermatologic side effects of lithium have also been reported. Edema, skin eruptions (folliculitis), and even skin ulcerations have been noted. Sometimes the use of concomitant antihistamine medication may be helpful for the rashes or for the rare skin ulcers. Lithium has not been found to affect the bone marrow significantly, and only mild elevations of the peripheral leukocyte count have been noted in some patients. Thus, effects on the skin are largely reversible and innocuous, although irritating.

Renal Damage. The greatest current concern to clinicians is the effects of lithium on the kidney. Severe renal tubular damage due to lithium may be a consequence of long-term lithium use, and anatomic changes in the proximal tubules have been noted in recent pathologic studies of patients after lithium treatment was instituted. These effects are not necessarily reversible. Consequently, the potential hazard of renal pathology must be weighed against the patient's severity of illness. The appearance of renal dysfunction in a patient requires a reconsideration of the need for continued lithium treatment. Many patients have chosen to remain on lithium treatment despite the risk of renal damage because they perceive manic illness to be the greater burden.

Use in Pregnancy. A review of women who took lithium during pregnancy revealed an increased incidence of cardiovascular abnormalities in the newborn infant, particularly Ebstein's anomaly, which raised concern about the use of lithium in pregnancy. The first trimester appears to be the period of greatest risk. It would seem a logical course to withdraw lithium just before conception; however, the preconception period may be lengthy and create undesirably long intervals without prophylactic lithium treatment. The postpartum period is another high-risk time for lithium-taking women. In that period, a woman has such major alterations in fluid, hormone, and electrolyte balance that a sodium diuresis may result in an increased retention of lithium and consequently an increased risk of lithium toxicity. Further, the serum lithium level in the pregnant woman is not a good indicator of the fetal lithium level, which may become transiently high. Fetal distress has been reported in lithium-taking mothers, and instances of hypotonia, listlessness, cyanosis, neuromuscular weakness, and goiter have been reported in newborns. Finally, lithium crosses into the breast milk at concentrations approximately 50 percent of the mother's serum lithium level. Thus, newborn babies of breast-feeding lithium-taking mothers will receive a considerable dose of lithium.

While the preceding discussion about lithium and pregnancy does not preclude pregnancy in a lithium-taking woman, it does complicate the management of pregnancy and make these women high-risk obstetric patients. They require careful monitoring of the physiologic as well as mental status throughout pregnancy. It is our recommendation that lithium be withdrawn whenever possible just before conception and reinstituted shortly after delivery when clinical conditions permit. Postpartum mania has been reported in women who were withdrawn from lithium during pregnancy, and the disorder can occur quite suddenly. Therefore, increased vigilance of affectively ill women in the perinatal period is essential.

Treatment of Lithium Toxicity

The early signs of lithium intoxication include tremor, weakness, drowsiness (occasionally excitement), ataxia, slurred speech, blurring of vision, and occasionally tinnitus. The recognition of these early signs generally precedes the confirmation of increased lithium levels via blood measurement. The early signs are similar to the common side effects seen when lithium treatment is initiated, but they can occur at any time during the treatment. As the intoxication becomes more severe there is increased neuromuscular irritability revealed by hyperactive deep tendon reflexes, nystagmus, lethargy, and ultimately stupor, which may lead to coma and sometimes generalized seizures. There may be pulse irregularities with electrocardiographic changes that ultimately lead to peripheral circulatory failure and finally circulatory collapse in those patients who succumb.

Lithium toxicity may be noted at lithium levels between 2 and 4 mEq/L, and levels greater than 2 mEq/L may be fatal. However, the lithium level is not always a good indicator of lithium toxicity. Lithium levels less than 2 mEq/L may occasionally be associated with toxicity in individual patients. Therefore, clinical signs are more important than blood measurements in determining the necessity to initiate treatment.

Treatment of lithium toxicity is aimed at averting the complications of impaired consciousness, electrolyte imbalance, and potential cardiovascular collapse. Fatalities are often due to pulmonary complications. Treatment for lithium poisoning resembles that for barbiturate intoxications; thus, gastric lavage, support of vital functions, maintenance of electrolyte balance, careful nursing care, and attempts to increase the renal excretion of lithium should be utilized. Renal excretion of the lithium ion cannot be increased by the administration of thiazide diuretics, which may even increase the retention of lithium. Fluid loading, solute-induced diuresis (for example, with mannitol or urea), urine alkalinization with sodium bicarbonate, and the administration of theophylline may be helpful in increasing the renal excretion of lithium. Hemodialysis may be useful in some cases. It should be noted that the patient's lithium level may come down only to rise again at tissue redistribution of remaining lithium ions occurs. Therefore, constant vigilance for at least 48 to 72 hours is necessary to observe for rebound to high levels of lithium in the blood.

Although lithium toxicity can be avoided by careful management and serial monitoring of the serum lithium level, it should be remembered that changes in sodium concentration can alter lithium retention. Thus, excessive sweat, excessive use of diuretics, or unusual fad diets involving sodium restriction may increase the risk of lithium toxicity in otherwise cooperative patients.

Carbamazepine as a Potential Alternative to Lithium

Carbamazepine is an iminodibenzyl derivative that has been used for many years for treatment of patients with seizure disorders, trigeminal neuralgia, and dystonic disorders. Recently, some investigators have described the use of carbamazepine for the acute and prophylactic treatment of patients with major affective illness. Its mechanism of action differs from that of lithium in that it acts as a limbic system anticonvulsive, suppressing transmission across polysynaptic pathways; it thus suppresses afterdischarges and spontaneous or induced seizure discharges. As with lithium, serum levels of carbamazepine can be obtained, and maintenance between levels of 8.0 and 12.0 μg/ml have been recommended. Further clinical work with carbamazepine is necessary before it can be recommended as a general alternative to lithium treatment. While free of some of the disturbing side effects of lithium, carbamazepine treatment has been associated with bone marrow suppression and aplastic anemia. Thus, it is necessary to observe for signs of fever, sore throat, and petechiae or other signs of hemorrhage and to obtain complete blood counts. The blood counts should be determined weekly during the first few months of treatment and monthly thereafter; they are monitored for suppression of hematologic indexes, particularly the white cell count. Decreases of the white cell count below the normal range with associated rash or fever necessitates discontinuance of carbamazepine. Return of hematologic indexes to normal have been noted within two weeks after discontinuance. Thus it appears that reversal of the bone marrow suppression is possible if it is observed early enough.

MONOAMINE OXIDASE INHIBITORS

During the mid-1950s, tuberculosis patients being treated with iproniazid were observed to experience a brightening of their mood. Because of its hepatic toxicity, iproniazid was not investigated further, but other drugs of the MAO inhibitor class were subsequently developed and tested for antidepressant properties. By the late 1950s several British investigators reported successfully treating supposedly atypical depressives with MAO inhibitors. During the next two decades MAO inhibitors gained widespread acceptance as antidepressants in Britain and Europe, but their use in the United States remained very limited.

The principal reason why MAO inhibitors are not widely prescribed in this country is the early reports of fatal hypertensive episodes associated with use of these drugs. Most of these cases were subsequently found to be related to the ingestion of foods rich in tyramine. Even though hypertensive crises can be avoided by dietary restrictions, the MAO inhibitors continue to be underutilized in the United States.

Classification

The MAO inhibitors can be divided into two classes—the hydrazines and the nonhydrazines. Phenelzine is the most widely used hydrazine in the United States; the other drug in this class is isocarboxazid. The next most widely used MAO inhibitor is tranylcypromine, a nonhydrazine. Pargyline, another MAO inhibitor that is FDA approved, is not an effective antidepressant.

Current research is aimed at finding a drug that selectively inhibits MAO type B. The advantage of a selective drug is that it may not inhibit intestinal MAO, which is thought to be type A. Intestinal MAO metabolizes and thereby controls the amount of pressor amines that are absorbed through the intestinal wall. Hypertensive crises occur when intestinal MAO is inhibited, and sympathomimetics are allowed to enter the body unregulated. One drug currently being investigated is deprenyl, which is thought to be a selective MAO-B inhibitor. If deprenyl proves to be a clinically effective antidepressant without the threat of hypertensive crises, MAO inhibitors would undoubtedly enjoy a resurgence of interest in this country.

Indications for Use

It is difficult to evaluate the effectiveness of antidepressants because of the influence of intercurrent events and the natural history of the disease course. Many depressions wax and wane, and spontaneous remissions occur in more than 50 percent of cases at the end of a year. The subpopulation of depressives who are likely to have a more favorable response to an MAO inhibitor than to a tricyclic agent are generally outpatients diagnosed as *neurotic* or *atypical* depressives. Sargant was the first to describe a so-called atypical depression, which is characterized by increased appetite, fatigue, reversed diurnal variation, increased emotionality, somatic complaints, and hypersomnolence. These patients typically have mixed anxiety and phobic symptoms and probably overlap with another group known to be responsive to MAO inhibitors, agoraphobics. Neurotic depressives are usually middle aged and moderately depressed, lack endogenous features, have difficulty falling asleep, exhibit neurotic personality features, and have reversed or no diurnal variation. Because these two entities are not adequately defined, we will use the term *atypical neurotic depression* to indicate a group of nonendogenous depressives who are unlikely to have a positive response to tricyclic agents. This group closely resembles Paykel and associates' (1975) description of anxious depressives.

A series of studies by Robinson and others have demonstrated the value of the MAO inhibitors for this group of patients. In 11 studies that looked at the effect of treatment with phenelzine on neurotic or atypical depressives, 10 of the studies found phenelzine more effective than placebo.

Further systematic study aimed at establishing operational criteria may help define a more homogeneous group for whom MAO inhibitors are unequivocally the drug of choice. Since patients with endogenous features constitute only 10 percent of depressives, this clarification would clearly be a significant contribution. Quitkin and co-workers (1976) suggested that MAO inhibitors be used in depressed patients with the following symptom cluster: lethargy, hypersomnolence, increased appetite, rejection sensitivity, and reactivity of mood. Whether or not MAO inhibitors are the drug of first choice, there is enough evidence to support the efficacy in atypical depressives that they should be tried either first or after a tricyclic agent has been unsuccessful.

Clinical Use

Currently there are only three MAO inhibitors that the FDA approved for use in depression. Isocarboxazid is given in the range of 20 to 80 mg a day; phenelzine is given in doses of 45 to 90 mg; and tranylcypromine is prescribed at 40 to 80 mg daily. These dosage ranges exceed PDR recommendations. Higher doses may be required for certain patients to have a favorable response, as discussed later.

Is there a reason to prefer one drug over another? In a controlled study comparing four MAO inhibitors, Sargant was unable to find any significant difference in treatment outcome. Some investigators report that patients who are unresponsive to phenelzine may respond to isocarboxazid, while others have found tranylcypromine superior. Isocarboxazid may be the most potent of the three, but it is also thought to be the most toxic. Because most of the reports to date found phenelzine to be safe and effective, it would seem to be the MAO inhibitor of choice at this time. Additional double-blind comparisons of these three MAO inhibitors would be helpful in settling the issue of which, if any, offers important clinical advantages.

Monoamine oxidase inhibitors should be prescribed in either divided doses given either twice or three times a day. A single daily dose, as recommended for the tricyclic agents, is discouraged. Since MAO inhibitors often produce stimulation rather than sedation, they should be taken early in the day so as not to disturb sleep. There is usually a lag time of 7 to 21 days before improvement begins to occur.

Inhibition of Platelet Levels

One explanation for the wide variation in outcome that we see clinically may be related to the differences in the way individuals absorb and metabolize MAO inhibitors. It has been demonstrated that there is a tenfold variation in the rate at which individuals receiving standard doses concentrate tricyclic agents in their blood. Large variations have also been reported for the MAO inhibitors. Direct measures of MAO-inhibitor plasma levels do not correlate with the drug concentration at key receptor sites in the brain. However, inhibition of platelet MAO may be a useful alternative for estimating the level of brain MAO inhibition.

A number of studies have demonstrated that clinical response to MAO inhibitors is significantly improved when platelet inhibition levels exceed 80 percent. Seventy-nine percent of patients improved when platelet inhibition exceeds 90 percent. There was a two-week lag time before this degree of inhibition was achieved, which correlates clinically with the latency before antidepressant effects are apparent. While there is additional support for a correlation between response to phenelzine and the percentage of MAO platelet inhibition, at this time there is not enough evidence to support widespread clinical use. Because platelet MAO inhibition levels are not routinely available, treatment can proceed by increasing the dose until either side effects intervene or clinical improvement occurs.

Tyrer found that patients roughly divided into fast and slow acetylators. Slow acetylators, who metabolized MAO inhibitors more slowly and thus achieved higher plasma concentrations, had significantly greater improvement rates. Since many patients who fail to respond by four weeks are switched to another drug, one implication of this finding is that some nonresponders should either continue to receive treatment for six to eight additional weeks or be treated with higher doses. Either approach could allow fast acetylators to accumulate adequate tissue levels. This probably explains why one study found that the improvement rate doubled between the fourth and eighth week of treatment. Clinical factors may determine the nature of a patient's drug response, while genetic and biochemical factors appear to determine the rate of this response.

Hypertensive Crisis

As discussed earlier, the combination of food rich in tyramine and MAO inhibitors may lead to a severe elevation of blood pressure, or what has come to be known as the *cheese reaction*. This disorder is characterized by the onset (within minutes to hours after eating) of severe headaches, chest pains, palpitations, and a markedly elevated blood pressure. Substances that contain a high content of tyramine include cheese, wines (especially Chianti), chicken livers, sour cream, and cold remedies (containing vasoactive compounds). If a hypertensive reaction does occur, it can be successfully managed by giving 5 to 10 mg of the alpha-blocker phentolamine intravenously. Chlorpromazine, 50 mg intramuscularly, may be a useful adjunct in severe cases. A recent British study found that a significant minority of patients receiving MAO inhibitors were not observing dietary restrictions; even so, hypertensive reactions were relatively rare. In another series of 22,000 patients treated with MAO inhibitors, about 2 percent developed headaches, 0.3 to 0.5 percent had hypertensive crises, and less than 0.001 percent died.

With appropriate precautions, the MAO inhibitors have been safely used to treat thousands of cases without untoward reaction. Compared with the risk of suicide in untreated depressed patients, the threat of a hypertensive crisis is not adequate reason for withholding a treatment that has proved effective.

Other Side Effects

Jaundice has been reported in patients treated with hydrazine MAO inhibitors, although the frequency and causal relationship has not been established. The severe hepatic necrosis associated with iproniazid has not been reported with other MAO inhibitors. The MAO inhibitors cause a variety of anticholinergic side effects that resemble those of tricyclic antidepressants. The side effects include dry mouth, orthostatic hypotension, constipation, lightheadedness, and delayed micturition. (See the section on side effects of tricyclic agents for a fuller discussion.)

SECOND-GENERATION ANTIDEPRESSANTS

A variety of new antidepressant drugs have recently been or are likely to become FDA approved. All of these drugs have been evaluated in controlled studies in Europe, Japan, and the United States, and some have been in clinical use in Europe for several years. The chemical structures of these drugs differ from those of traditional tricyclic agents and MAO inhibitors. They range from a unicyclic (fluvoxamine) through bicyclics (zimelidine and viloxazine) and tricyclics (trimipramine and clomipramine) to tetracyclics (maprotiline, mianserin, and oxaprotiline). There is also a triazolpyridine (trazodone), a tetrahydroisoquinoline (nomifensine), and a dibenzoxazepine (amoxapine). Not surprisingly, these drugs seem to have different mechanisms of action from those of the older antidepressants, thus challenging our theories regarding the pathophysiology of depression. For instance, mianserin has negligible effects on serotoninergic and noradrenergic uptake, and it does not appear to have any effect on cholinergic neurons. Its mechanism of action may depend on presynaptic alpha-receptor blockade. Amoxapine is structurally very similar to loxapine, an effective antipsychotic, and appears to have significant dopamine-blocking activity. Alprazolam is benzodiazepine that may be an effective treatment for nonendogenous depression associated with anxiety features.

It appears that the second generation antidepressants are not more effective than reference tricyclic agents such as amitriptyline and imipramine. While there have been claims that some of these drugs act more rapidly than do earlier tricyclic agents, such reports should be viewed skeptically until they can be confirmed in controlled studies. There is widespread clinical support and some evidence that many of the new drugs cause fewer side effects. If so, this would be a significant clinical advantage in reducing patient noncompliance and dropout, especially among outpatients. It also appears that several of the new drugs may have a lower incidence of cardiotoxicity and may be less lethal when taken in overdose. While these drugs are not yet first choice agents in the treatment of depression, they should be considered in selected patients such as those with cardiac problems, geriatric patients, and refractory depressives.

The significance of the second-generation antidepressants is not that they are more effective or that they shorten the latency before clinical effects begin, but that many of them cause fewer side effects. There is also some advantage in having additional antidepressant drugs available to add to our clinical armamentarium, since some patients continue to respond well to only one antidepressant and not to any others. The new drugs may also speed up the process of uncovering the pathogenesis of depression by virtue of their more selective and variable mechanisms of action. At this time they seem promising, but only time will tell whether they offer enough significant advantages to become widely accepted.

Drug Management of Anxiety

Anxiety states, described in detail elsewhere in this book, are often accompanied by somatic and autonomic reactions including cardiovascular symptoms (tachycardia, palpitations, feelings of faintness) dryness of mouth, lack of appetite, indigestion, nausea, and not infrequently a free-floating feeling of dread or discomfort. Anxiety is a universal phenomenon that is often precipitated by identifiable environmental events, even though some individuals cannot identify a source or basis for their feelings. Occasionally anxiety is merely a symptom of a separate psychiatric disorder such as depression or schizophrenia, which should be considered whenever anxiety states persist without significant symptom relief.

In most cases, the treatment of anxiety can be achieved with support and occasionally the addition of an anxiolytic (antianxiety) agent. The benzodiazepines (and related antianxiety agents) have been identified by the FDA as one of the most frequently written prescriptions—most commonly by family practitioners and osteopaths, and less frequently by psychiatrists. These drugs have become the subject of widespread discussion in both the medical and lay communities because the apparent abuse has been recognized. In 1978, for instance, 68 million prescriptions for benzodiazepines were written in the United States for a total of about 10 million people. One of the reasons for the great popularity of the benzodiazepines is the rapid onset and general efficacy of a single dose, which distinguishes these drugs from lithium or antidepressant medications. The possibility of quick relief from anxiety is great temptation for people under stress. The benzodiazepines replaced a long list of medications that have been used for the treatment of anxiety. Bromides, alcohol, paraldehyde, and the barbiturates have all been used for the relief of anxiety. In 1951, a propanediol called meprobamate was introduced and shown to be effective in the rapid relief of anxiety. Meprobamate, however, is very addictive, has a low margin of safety, and can cause respiratory depression. Thus, a safer group of antianxiety agents was necessary, leading to the development and marketing of numerous benzodiazepines. Chlordiazepoxide was introduced in 1960 and numerous structural variants, including diazepam, have followed in the last 20 years. Today, research continues to seek agents that can separate antianxiety effects from sedative effects and that have less of an addictive potential than the current benzodiazepines. Experimental treatments of anxiety, including the use of beta-adrenergic blocking agents such as propranolol, have been introduced.

BENZODIAZEPINES

Benzodiazepines have antianxiety effects, sedative-hypnotic properties, anticonvulsant effects when given in appropriate dosages, and muscle-relaxing properties. The numerous benzodiazepine preparations on the market differ somewhat in their gastrointestinal absorption, distribution, metabolism, and elimination. Each of these drugs has the same clinical indications.

One group of benzodiazepines are metabolized by oxidative pathways including N-d-alkylation or N-d-methylation; aliphatic hydroxylation occurs in the liver. The drugs metabolized by oxidative pathways include chlordiazepoxide, diazepam, clorazepate, prazepam, flurazepam, and clobazam. A second group of benzodiazepines is metabolized by conjugative pathways; these drugs differ from the preceding group in that their metabolic products are pharmacologically inactive. The drugs metabolized by conjugative pathways include oxazepam, lorazepam, and temazepam. In the first group, the slowness of the oxidative transformation process affects the rate and extent of accumulation of drug and the time required to reach steady state (which may be as much as two weeks). Further, because the rate of elimination is slower in the first group, these agents may remain measurable for a month or more after discontinuance. The second group has a faster rate of accumulation, reaching steady-state levels in two to three days; rapid elimination occurs within two days. The advantage of the first group is that there will not be a rapid blood level decline to zero following discontinuance, and steady state blood levels are maintained for a longer period of time. The advantage of the second group is that steady-state blood levels can be reached quickly, and blood levels will decline rapidly when discontinuance and elimination are desirable. The first group of drugs may be desirable for anxious patients with bad compliance habits or poor memories who are likely to forget daily drug administration, whereas the second group may be preferential for the large group of patients for whom accumulation of drug is undesirable and rapid elimination a potential benefit.

Patients develop a physiologic tolerance (adaptation) to the effects of the benzodiazepines. Tolerance implies that the central depressant effects of the drug tend to decline as the duration of exposure increases and that chronic exposure and drug accumulation results in diminished sedative effects. Psychological and physical dependence can occur with prolonged use and can result in an abstinence syndrome if the drug is abruptly discontinued. Many of those who develop a physical dependence on a benzodiazepine are emotionally unstable people who often have misused alcohol or other sedative-hypnotic substances as well as benzodiazepines. If a patient has been taking a benzodiazepine at the usual therapeutic dosage for less than 20 weeks, there appears to be little or no risk of a withdrawal reaction even with abrupt discontinuance. When they do occur, withdrawal symptoms are generally mild and last for less than 48 hours. The data indicate that the larger the dosage and the longer the time during which the drug has been administered, the greater will be the risk for moderate or severe withdrawal reactions. Symptoms of withdrawal include depression, aggravation of psychoses, agitation, insomnia, loss of appetite, nausea, and vomiting; seizures may also occur seven or eight days after discontinuance of the benzodiazepine. The risk of a severe withdrawal reaction is greater if the patient has taken a substance with which the benzodiazepine is cross-tolerant in the weeks or months prior to the use of a benzodiazepine. Cross-tolerant drugs include alcohol, barbiturates, and meprobamate. Thus, short-term benzodiazepine use not accompanied by adjunctive sedative-hypnotic medications is unlikely to create a physical dependence on the drug.

Long-term users appear to be of two types: the single-drug user and the abuser of multiple drugs. In the former group many patients would meet criteria for borderline personality or dysthymic disorders; others suffer from chronic insomnia or chronic pain syndromes. In the latter group, abusers of multiple drugs are patients who add benzodiazepines to other medications and are usually willing to take whatever psychotropic drugs they can obtain. Patients in that group will often take benzodiazepines in excess of the usual therapeutic doses and may become dependent on other drugs as well. On the other hand, agoraphobic individuals who have taken benzodiazepines for a long time and who are then successfully treated with imipramine or MAO inhibitors (as described later) are often eager to discontinue chronic use of benzodiazepines.

Mechanism of Action

The benzodiazepines have widespread, diffuse inhibitory effects on the central nervous system. These drugs block stimulation of the brain stem reticular formation and depress the duration of electrical afterdischarges in the limbic system, including the septal region, the amygdala, and the hippocampus. The neuroanatomic selectivity of action promotes a greater antianxiety effect with less sedative effect than is found with other hypnotic-sedative agents. The diffuse effect of benzodiazepine is reflected in electroencephalographic changes, which include a slowing of the main frequency of the alpha rhythm and low voltage, fast (beta) activity.

Clinical Use of Benzodiazepines

The main indication for the use of anxiolytic agents is the short-term alleviation of anxiety and related symptoms of fear and tension. These drugs are also used as preoperative sedatives, in the management of pain syndromes and seizure disorders, and in caring for patients experiencing withdrawal from addictive substances such as barbiturates and alcohol, with which the benzodiazepines share cross-tolerance. The development of tolerance to the antianxiety as well as sedative effects of the benzodiazepines limits the clinical effectiveness of these agents over time. Further, the likelihood of reduced efficacy at an established dose increases the risk of self-induced dosage increases, resulting in a potential for abuse and addiction. Thus, the prolonged use of anxiolytic agents in the management of characterologic disorders is unacceptable because of the likelihood of physical dependence and abuse.

Favorable responses to anxiolytic medications have been associated with lower-socioeconomic-class patients who lack psychological sophistication and may have magical expectations of and dependencies on the physician. Patients who are very anxious and vulnerable to somatization disorders and who are less subject to obsessionalism or interpersonal or depressive complaints often respond best to anxiolytic medications. In fact, depressive symptomatology appears to be negatively correlated with outcome; patients suffering from anxiety with significant concomitant depression usually improve less than do those without depressive features.

Response to treatment within one week is another possible predictor of ultimate outcome to anxiolytic medications. There is a high correlation between early positive response and final outcome. In one study, 90 percent of the patients who responded with marked or moderate improvement during the first week showed sustained improvement after six weeks, whereas only 20 percent of patients who felt no improvement after one week had attained moderate or marked improvement after six weeks. Thus, the failure to show a good response after one week may indicate that one should consider an alternative treatment for the patient. Further, it appears that the improvement reached by the sixth week of treatment may be as much as can be expected even if treatment is continued for six months. Thus, if the level of improvement after six weeks of benzodiazepine treatment is unsatisfactory, an alternative form of treatment should be considered.

Recently, reliable assays of the steady-state plasma levels of diazepam and desmethyldiazepam have been developed. Higher plasma levels have been noted in patients reporting significant improvement. Thus, the evidence suggests that there is a significant correlation between adequate plasma levels and clinical improvement. The increased commerical availability of tests that can determine benzodiazepine plasma levels will enhance the clinical usefulness of these agents in the short-term treatment of anxiety disorders.

Overall, benzodiazepines have been shown to be the most efficacious agents for the control of anxiety currently available. An improvement of 70 to 75 percent has been demonstrated in many studies, as compared with 50 to 55 percent improvement in those using barbiturate medications and 35 percent with placebos. Currently, the most popular benzodiazepine is diazepam, which is used in dosages of 2 mg to 10 mg, three or four times per day. Diazepam has a rapid onset of action and has been reported to induce euphoria, which increases its abuse potential. Diazepam has a high lipophilic property, resulting in greater accumulation of the drug and increasing its dangerousness compared with other benzodiazepines. Chlordiazepoxide, the second most popular benzodiazepine, is used in dosages of 5 to 25 mg, three or four times a day, and has a similar onset of action and rate of accumulation as has diazepam. As described earlier, benzodiazepines in the conjugative group (for example, oxazepam) are more rapidly metabolized and cleared than are those in the oxidative group and may be preferable for the short-term treatment of anxiety. Oxazepam is prescribed in dosages of 15 to 30 mg, three or four times a day.

The lethal dose of the benzodiazepines is not well established but exceeds a week's supply of the ordinary dose. Fatalities have been reported after the ingestion of 700 to 1000 mg of diazepam or chlordiazepoxide. In general, these agents are less dangerous than are the barbiturates and the nonbarbiturate hypnotic-sedative alternatives.

In children and elderly patients, benzodiazepines may have value in reduced dosages. In these groups, excessive sedation, intoxication, or paradoxical excitement may occur, necessitating careful monitoring during pharmacotherapy. Alternative agents, such as diphenhydramine or other antihistamines, may be equally effective and are preferable in these patients.

Side Effects and Toxicity

The most commonly seen side effects in the use of benzodiazepines are sedation and drowsiness, decreased ability to concentrate, and occasional ataxia. Patients who are receiving benzodiazepines for the first time should be warned against driving or working with dangerous instruments until their specific idiosyncratic response can be assessed. These agents can interact with other medications, particularly barbiturates or alcohol, increasing the sedative effects and thereby increasing the risk of accidents.

As described earlier, a serious problem associated with the use of benzodiazepine is the tendency to develop a physiologic as well as psychological dependence on the agents. Patients may innocently increase their dosage via self-medication to the point of toxicity. Those with a previous history of substance abuse or alcoholism should be given very limited doses of benzodiazepines, if the medication is given at all. Characterologic problems that may require long-term therapy are generally not amenable to benzodiazepine therapy. The likelihood that a patient will become physically dependent on a benzodiazepine increases with increasing dose and with the length of time over which the medication is given. It is unlikely that patients who receive the medication in appropriate dosages will become physically dependent on the medication. However, it is still prudent to withdraw the medication gradually whenever the patient has taken a significant dose for more than a month. It is important to determine whether symptoms of agitation occurring following discontinuance of medication represent a withdrawal reaction or simply recurrence of anxiety symptoms. In general, mild withdrawal symptoms will subside within five days whereas a return of the underlying anxiety symptoms will emerge after the first week and continue beyond that time.

The safety of the benzodiazepines during pregnancy is not well established. There have been some studies demonstrating increased instances of cleft lip and cleft palate in the offspring of women who took diazepam during their pregnancy. It would be best to avoid the use of benzodiazepines during pregnancy; when necessary, one can prescribe low doses of barbiturates like secobarbital (Seconal). Barbiturates alter fetal hepatic metabolism and should be used sparingly.

Benzodiazepine toxicity and overdose can be potentially fatal, although this is rare. Patients have died from overdoses equivalent to about two weeks supply (or less if taken with cross-tolerated medications or alcohol). Treatment of overdoses should be similar to that of barbiturate overdose, including gastric lavage, maintenance of electrolyte balance, intensive monitoring and observation in an intensive care unit, and possibly hemodialysis when indicated.

Physical dependence on benzodiazepines can result in a withdrawal syndrome, as described earlier. While the withdrawal is generally mild, it is important to remember that delayed withdrawal response occurring as long as two weeks after withdrawal may include seizures and delirium. Therefore, patients who have been using large doses of benzodiazepines for a considerable time are best managed by gradual detoxification rather than abrupt management.

OTHER AGENTS FOR THE TREATMENT OF ANXIETY

As described in the preceding section, the benzodiazepine anxiolytic drugs are the current choice in the short-term treatment of anxiety symptoms. Historically, bromides, alcohol, barbiturate medications, and nonbarbiturate sedative drugs (glutethimide, methyprylon) have been used. Generally we do not recommend these medications for the treatment of anxiety. They possess addictive potential as well as related sedative properties that make them unsatisfactory for the treatment of anxiety. Meprobamate, in particular, has a more potent addictive potential and a more serious tendency to cause withdrawal problems and seizures than do the benzodiazepine derivatives. The addicting dose of meprobamate overlaps its therapeutic range, and physical signs of withdrawal can follow the discontinuance of doses as small as 1,200 mg per day. The antihistamine compounds diphenhydramine, hydroxyzine, and promethazine are potential anxiolytic medications. Generally, these compounds are less useful than the benzodiazepines, although they may serve a purpose in elderly or very young patients. Hydroxyzine has the potential of being more sedating than anxiolytic and may create ataxia and dizziness without producing substantial benefit. Diphenhydramine in doses above 50 mg may also have more sedating than anxiety reducing effects, although it may have value for some patients. These drugs are relatively safe, are nonaddicting and do not produce a physiologic or psychological dependence. Overall, these medications may be better sedatives than they are anxiolytics.

Propranolol

Propranolol, a beta-adrenergic blocking agent, has been proposed as a potential antianxiety medication. In blocking beta-receptors, propranolol has a substantial effect on the peripheral autonomic expression of anxiety. Propranolol may have value individually or in combination with a benzodiazepine medication. Propranolol has been shown to improve the somatic manifestation of anxiety, including palpitations, tremor, tingling, chest constriction, twitching, and cold sweat. These physiologic symptoms may be caused by a hyperawareness of normal adrenergic (epinephrine) functioning on a peripheral level. In fact, dextropropranolol, which lacks beta-blocking properties, has been shown to be ineffective in the treatment of patients with anxiety. Further, the specific peripheral beta-blocker practolol, which lacks central beta-blocking properties, does have antianxiety effects. The dose of propranolol that would be effective in the treatment of anxiety states will vary and may be determined on the basis of a 20 percent reduction of the patient's pulse rate. Starting doses of 40 to 80 mg per day with gradual increments would be recommended.

Propranolol is almost completely absorbed from the gastrointestinal tract, enters the blood, and is partially bound by the liver. Its peak effect occurs within one to one and one-half hours after the dose, and its biologic half-life is approximately two to three hours. Because propranolol is rapidly absorbed and metabolized, divided doses are essential to maintain a sustained antianxiety effect. Propranolol has been shown to decrease cardiac output, inhibit renin release, and diminish the tonic sympathetic nerve outflow from the central nervous system. These mechanisms result in an antihypertensive effect, which is the principal approved indication for propranolol use at the present time.

Beta-receptor blockade interferes with sympathetic stimulation, which may be vital in some conditions. Ventricular heart function, for example, is maintained by virtue of sympathetic drive; in the presence of atrioventricular block, beta-blockade may be dangerous. Further, beta-blockade results in bronchial constriction by interfering with bronchodilator activity and should therefore be avoided in patients who are subject to bronchospasms (as in asthma).

Therefore, propranolol is contraindicated in patients with bronchial asthma, allergic rhinitis during the pollen season, sinus bradycardia, greater-than-first-degree heart block, cardiogenic shock, right ventricular failure secondary to pulmonary hypertension, or congestive heart failure, and in patients receiving adrenergic-augmenting psychotropic drugs (including MAO inhibitors) and in those who have used those drugs within the previous two weeks. Propranolol should be withdrawn from patients 48 hours before surgical procedures because of its potential to impair the ability of the heart to respond to reflex stimuli. The withdrawal of propranolol should be done gradually over several weeks in patients who have been using dosages greater than 200 mg per day.

In clinical use, propranolol may cause some light-headedness, weakness or fatigue, and mild depressive symptoms, and it has been associated with disorientation, loss of short-term memory, emotional lability, and hallucinations. Patients may occasionally complain of nausea or vomiting, but this is rare. The use of propranolol, like the use of any other psychotropic medication, should be discouraged during pregnancy.

Propranolol toxicity may be accomplished by profound bradycardia, hypotension, and bronchospasm. Emergency measures involve the administration of atropine (0.25 to 1.0 mg) intravenously to reverse the bradycardia, digitalis and diuretics to manage cardiac failure, vasopressors (levarterenol or epinephrine) to reverse the hypotension, and aminophylline and isoproterenol to reverse the bronchospasms.

In closing, it should be recalled that the treatment of persistent anxiety should include psychotherapy; patients who experience pharmacotherapeutic failure may be suffering from depressive or schizophrenic disorders in which anxiety is just part of the syndrome.

PHOBIC ANXIETY STATES

The phobic anxiety states are discussed in detail in Chapter 9. A number of treatments have been tried in the management of phobic anxiety. Psychoanalytic therapy has generally not been successful in alleviating symptomatic attacks. Treatment with phenothiazines has also failed to yield favorable results; in several cases the phobia worsened. The modes of treatment currently recommended are behavioral and drug therapies. There are many reports of favorable outcomes using a variety of behavioral techniques, including desensitization, modeling, and flooding. In general, these have proved most successful with monosymptomatic phobias, such as to dogs or heights. The complex phobias, such as agoraphobia and social phobias, are frequently more resistant to behavior therapy, possibly because they are more diffuse and often associated with other personality handicaps. Attenuated panic attacks often persist after successful behavior therapy, even though phobic avoidance has resolved. During the past decade, a number of studies have concluded that agoraphobia, especially in adults, can be effectively treated with drugs.

The earliest report of successful drug therapy for what may have been agoraphobia appeared in 1958. Dally reported that iproniazid, an MAO inhibitor, was useful in treating mild depressive states with anxiety features, which were labeled *atypical depression*. Sargant and Dally subsequently reported that atypical depressions often overlapped with, and were sometimes indistinguishable from, anxiety neuroses. In 1962 the same authors reported an open study of 246 phobic patients. At the end of the month, 74 percent of those treated with MAO inhibitors were moderately to markedly improved. Other investigators were soon replicating these results.

In the United States Klein was simultaneously reporting favorable results using tricyclics. In 1962, he attempted to derive a descriptive-behavioral typology based on drug response. Imipramine was randomly given to psychiatric inpatients in doses ranging from 75 to 300 mg. Patients who had a positive response were then studied, leading to the identification of a group with similar behavioral changes after drug treatment and a common set of behavioral characteristics before treatment. These patients often had a history of episodic anxiety attacks that improved dramatically with imipramine. Typically, they had previously failed to respond to phenothiazines and sedatives.

A subsequent prospective study compared imipramine with tranylcypromine, phenelzine, chlorpromazine, and placebo. Panic attacks responded well to imipramine, sometimes ceasing in three to four days. Patients appeared to benefit from smaller doses and in less time than would be characteristic of antidepressant action. Half the patients relapsed after one month when imipramine was discontinued, but most recovered when the medication was resumed.

The results of these seminal studies were subsequently confirmed by other investigators. Both MAO inhibitors and tricyclic agents are now generally regarded as effective treatments for the phobic anxiety syndrome. Beta-blockers such as propranolol may also have some limited role to play in the management of phobias. They are especially helpful in alleviating the physical symptoms that accompany anxiety attacks, but they have little impact on the subjective sense of dread.

Monoamine Oxidase Inhibitors

More than two dozen studies have examined the use of MAO inhibitors in treating phobic anxiety. Virtually all found drug treatment superior to results with placebos, although in a number of studies the difference was only marginal. Double-blind comparisons of phenelzine with aversion therapy, systematic desensitization, and flooding found that phenelzine produced the fastest and most comprehensive improvement. Between 80 and 90 percent of phenelzine-treated patients were significantly improved after two months.

Comparisons of four MAO inhibitors (phenelzine, isocarboxazid, phenoxypropazine, and iproniazid) were unable to detect significant differences in treatment outcome. All drugs were superior to placebos. Each drug was shown in double-blind, random-assignment studies to relieve panic attacks, which recurred when the drug was discontinued and remitted when the drug was reinstituted. Some reports found that patients who were unresponsive to phenelzine subsequently responded to isocarboxazid. While isocarboxazid may be more potent, it is also considered more toxic. Because most studies in the field were done with phenelzine, which was shown to be safe and effective, it is the MAO inhibitor of choice at this time. The dosage range employed in most studies was 40 to 75 mg.

A review of the well-controlled studies reveals favorable outcome varied between 50 and 90 percent. Overall 40 to 50 percent of patients had a complete remission, while another 30 to 40 percent sustained a moderate to marked improvement. Some studies have been unclear in their criteria for a good drug response. A majority of patients in whom improvement was seen lost the autonomic component of their panic attacks, such as palpitations and faintness, but they still felt a subjective sense of impending doom. This residual symptom has been shown to be responsive to behavior therapy.

A disturbing finding that emerged in those studies with longer follow-up periods is the tendency of some patients who demonstrated positive responses to relapse when drugs were discontinued, even after one to two years. Current recommendations for continuation of treatment range between six months and one year. The vast majority of patients treated with this regimen will not relapse when medication is stopped.

Studies vary as to whether premorbid personality—especially hysterical features—is significantly related to treatment outcome. Slightly more than half of those reviewed found no correlation, but this may reflect a narrower measure of improvement. Studies that evaluate social adjustment and maintenance of improvement after drug discontinuance tend to support the presence of a negative relationship between treatment outcome and premorbid personality.

The clinical use of MAO inhibitors is discussed in the section covering the drug treatment of depression.

Tricyclic Agents
Following Klein's initial report on imipramine, more than two dozen studies have been published on the use of tricyclic antidepressants in the treatment of phobic anxiety. These studies have conclusively demonstrated that tricyclic agents are significantly superior to placebos in the treatment of phobic anxiety. Many of these reports concern clomipramine. A number of investigators, mostly in Britain, have found clomipramine to be effective in the treatment of both refractory phobic and obsessional illnesses. Some have theorized that phobic anxiety states and obsessional illness are on a continuum. Marshall (1971) studied several groups of patients with mixed phobic and obsessional symptoms; these patients had previously been refractory to behavior modifications, minor tranquilizers, phenothiazines, phenelzine, and leukotomy. Three weeks of daily intravenous treatment with clomipramine produced a complete remission in over half the cases, and a moderate or good response in another 25 percent. No relapses were found on follow-up after six months of oral clomipramine maintenance.

More than a dozen subsequent studies found an overall improvement rate that averaged 80 to 85 percent, with a relapse rate of 15 percent at 18 months. Many of these were uncontrolled studies, but several used random-assignment, double-blind methods and achieved comparable results.

A review of the studies done to date suggests that clomipramine produces a sixfold reduction in symptom severity among phobic patients, and a twofold to fourfold reduction for obsessives. Between 50 and 70 percent of these patients have either a complete cessation of or a marked reduction in symptoms. To consolidate these gains, patients should be given supportive-directive "encouragement" or behavior modification therapy.

The only study comparing several tricyclic agents found clomipramine to be superior. Imipramine-treated patients experienced more relapses and partial remissions on follow-up. MAO inhibitors, in comparison, produced an equivalent therapeutic response. Further well-controlled studies should be done comparing other tricyclic agents with clomipramine and tricyclic agents with MAO inhibitors.

Clinical Management
With evidence supporting the efficacy of both the tricyclic agents and MAO inhibitors, is there a reason to prefer one drug class over another? Only two controlled studies have compared the clinical outcome of two groups of patients, one treated with MAO inhibitors and the other with tricyclic agents. In both studies, no significant difference was found in treatment outcome between the two drug groups, although patients had less resistance to taking tricyclic agents because the MAO inhibitors involved dietary restrictions and the threat of hypertensive crisis. If this finding is sustained in further well-controlled studies, tricyclic agents would emerge as the preferred drug in treating phobic anxiety.

Both MAO inhibitors and tricyclic agents are effective in blocking panic attacks, but they offer little benefit for the two other components of agoraphobia—anticipatory anxiety and phobic avoidance. As previously mentioned, benzodiazepines and behavior therapy may be helpful in these areas. While benzodiazepines are of little benefit in the prevention of panic attacks, they have proved to be useful in treating the free-floating, anticipatory anxiety that is typically part of the phobic anxiety syndrome. This is the most likely explanation of the fact that the two studies making such a comparison found that MAO inhibitors combined with benzodiazepine were superior to MAO inhibitors alone.

Behavioral therapy may have its greatest impact on fearful avoidance, with relatively little effect on panic attacks. Conversely, successful drug treatment abolishes panic, but often does little to alleviate phobic avoidance. Klein (1964) noted this finding in his initial study. Many investigators have found that when supportive-directive psychotherapy is added to drug therapy—even for as little as two weeks—improvement is more generalized. Patients show a marked decrease in avoidant behavior, as well as substantial improvement on social scales.

Optimal management of phobic anxiety should incorporate all three of these treatments. Benzodiazepines are beneficial when used intermittently for free-floating anxiety; MAO inhibitors or a tricyclic agent can abolish panic attacks; and behavior therapy may help a patient overcome his phobic avoidance. With this multifaceted approach, improvement rates approach 70 to 90 percent.

Mechanism of Drug Action
The mechanism by which MAO inhibitors and tricyclic agents block panic attacks is unknown. Since these drugs are known primarily for their antidepressant action, it is conceivable that phobic anxiety syndrome is part of the spectrum of affective disorders. However, virtually all studies have found no correlation between a positve drug response and the presence of depressive symptoms. In addition, many phobic patients respond at dose levels significantly less than those associated with antidepressant activity. Thus, the evidence suggests that the ability of these drugs to block panic attacks is unrelated to their antidepressant effects.

The three drugs that are clinically effective in blocking panic anxiety—propranolol, tricyclic agents, and MAO inhibitors—have two known mechanisms of action in common: they block beta-adrenergic receptors and inhibit MAO systems. The effectiveness of these drugs in the treatment of panic attacks correlates with the degree to which MAO is inhibited. The MAO inhibitors are the most potent in this respect, and thus the most effective clinically, while propranolol is the least potent in both measures. One weakness in this interesting line of inquiry is that the MAO inhibitors and tricyclic agents appear to be roughly equivalent in clinical effectiveness, while their degree of MAO inhibition is not.

Some investigators have suggested that phobic patients may be biochemically different from normal people. Panic attacks have been experimentally precipitated in certain anxious patients by the use of intravenous sodium lactate, which causes a release of epinephrine. In one study, phenelzines reduce "lactate-induced" anxiety, suggesting that MAO inhibitors may block panic attacks by inhibiting central adrenergic activity via a blockade of MAO. To date, there is still uncertainty about the mechanism of action of the MAO inhibitors and tricyclic agents in mitigating the severity of panic attacks.

Since efficacy studies provide little support for a preference of one FDA-approved tricyclic over another, the choice may depend on a patient's tolerance for the drug's side effects. Doxepin and amitriptyline are thought to be the most sedative (with dose); patients who are particularly sensitive to side effects, have a cardiac history, or are older should be started on divided doses. The occurrence of frightening dreams or severe side effects is often relieved by switching to divided doses. If a drug has a stimulating effect on the patient, the larger portion may be given in the morning.

Another common cause of poor outcome is the failure to prescribe an adequate dose. A review of depressed patients referred to National Institute of Mental Health found that fewer than 40 percent of patients receiving tricyclic antidepressants received the minimum of 150 mg daily. Most studies have found that imipramine and amitriptyline are well tolerated up to and beyond 300 mg daily.

Suggested Dose Schedule

The majority of patients will respond to a daily dose range of 150 to 300 mg for amitriptyline, imipramine, and desipramine, and 75 to 150 mg for nortriptyline. A commonly used regimen is 75 mg daily during the first three days, 150 mg until day 14, 225 mg daily in the third week, and 300 mg a day beginning with the fourth week, as needed and as tolerated. If a patient improves or develops disabling side effects, the dose need not be increased. Older patients are often more sensitive to drugs and may metabolize them more slowly. They are vulnerable to the development of toxic side effects at low doses, including confusion and cardiac arrhythmias (this is especially true among the debilitated and organically impaired). It is prudent to begin the geriatric patient at a lower and divided dose, such as 20 mg after the evening meal and 30 mg at bedtime. The dose may be increased until either side effects occur or improvement intervenes. Some elderly patients may need larger doses. When a patient has been on high doses for more than two months, the drug is usually discontinued by progressive reductions of 25 percent every week. Abrupt termination may produce a withdrawal syndrome, characterized by muscle aches, gastrointestinal symptoms, anxiety, and akathisia.

Although side effects begin immediately, therapeutic response is often delayed for up to three weeks. There is no conclusive evidence that this lag time can be shortened by choice of drug, route of administration, or addition of an adjuvant agent. Some patients get discouraged and stop taking the medication prematurely. Educating the patient and his or her family to expect side effects and a delayed onset of improvement can help to avoid such an outcome. The addition of small doses of benzodiazepines during the first week or two of treatment will often relieve anxiety and restlessness before the tricyclic agent begins to work. When patients start to improve, they are usually slow to recognize it. Those around them may notice increased activity and attention to personal appearance. Subjective feelings of improvement usually follow within a week. Patients who have not shown any improvement after four weeks on an adequate dose should be given another drug.

Correlation of Plasma Levels with Clinical Outcome

Until recently it has been assumed that most patients handle drugs in much the same way. Scant attention was paid to differences among individuals in absorption and metabolism. Substantial variations in patients' ability to concentrate medications were first reported for the anticonvulsant medications and the cardiac drug digoxin. Research in the past several years has revealed a 10-fold to 20-fold variation in tricyclic plasma levels among patients taking the same dose. This variability may be explained in part by genetically determined differences in pharmacokinetics. Monozygotic twins have been shown to have similar plasma levels on a standard dose of nortriptyline, while dizygotic twins do not. Variability in plasma concentration may also be related to the intake of other drugs. Methylphenidate can raise tricyclic plasma levels by as much as 250 percent, while barbiturates may lower them by half. Both drugs act via their effect on hepatic microsomal enzymes involved in tricyclic metabolism. It appears that tricyclic plasma levels are determined by a variety of factors, including dose, genetically controlled pharmacokinetics, the concomitant intake of other drugs, and gastrointestinal absorption.

The variability in tricyclic plasma levels after a standard dose suggests that dosage alone is not a reliable indicator of how much active agent reaches the target site. Nortriptyline plasma concentration has been shown to correlate significantly with both actual side effects and amelioration of depression at four weeks. Dosage, however, did not correlate with either. Asberg reported an unexpected finding about plasma levels; she found that 18 of 21 patients with a nortriptyline plasma concentration below 175 ng/ml recovered, whereas only one of eight above this level responded. Similarly, levels below 50 ng/ml seemed to be ineffective. There is a curvilinear relationship between nortriptyline plasma concentration and therapeutic response. At plasma levels outside this "therapeutic window," this medication loses much of its specific antidepressant activity.

These findings about nortriptyline plasma levels have been confirmed by other investigators. Of 43 studies attempting to correlate tricyclic plasma levels with clinical response, about two-thirds showed a relationship between plasma level and clinical response. The most convincing data is for nortriptyline, which appears to have an inverted U-shaped response curve. There is some evidence that other secondary amine tricyclic agents such as desipramine have a similar biphasic curve. Tertiary amine tricyclic agents such as amitriptyline and imipramine appear to have a linear response curve, with positive outcomes increasing proportionately with plasma concentration. This has been shown most clearly for imipramine, which needs a minimum concentration to be effective but has no reported maximum. One report found that 93 percent of depressed inpatients recovered when their imipramine levels exceeded 225 ng/ml. There is less convincing evidence that amitriptyline also has a linear response curve. The evidence for the other tricyclic agents is contradictory, and no conclusions can be drawn about them at this time.

References and Further Reading

Appleton, W.S. Skin and eye complications of psychoactive drug therapy. In DiMascio, A., Shader, R.I. (eds.), *Clinical Handbook of Psychopharmacology*. New York: Jason Aronson, 1970.

Ayd, F.J. The depot fluphenazines: a reappraisal after 10 years' clinical experience. *Am. J. Psychiatry* 132:491–500, 1975.

Baldessarini, R.J. *Chemotherapy in Psychiatry.* Boston: Harvard University Press, 1977.

Baldessarini, R.J., Tarsy, D. Tardive dyskinesia. In Lipton, M.A., DiMascio, A., Killam, K.F. (eds.), *Psychopharmacology: A Generation of Progress.* New York: Raven Press, 1978.

Ballenger, J.D., Post, R.M. Carbamazepine in manic-depressive illness: a new treatment. *Am. J. Psychiatry* 137:782–790, 1980.

Benzodiazepines 1980: current update. *Psychosomatics* 21[Suppl.]:3–32, October, 1980.

Bigger, J.T., Kantor, S. Cardiovascular Effects of the Tricyclics. Paper presented at the American College of Neuropsychopharmacology Annual Meeting, New Orleans, Dec. 13–17, 1976.

Caroff, S. The neuroleptic malignant syndrome. *Am. J. Psychiatry* 141:79–83, 1980.

Coleman, J.H., Hayes, P.E. Drug induced extrapyramidal effects. *Dis. Nerv. Syst.* 36:591–593, 1975.

Cooper, T.B., Simpson, G.M. The 24-hour lithium level as a prognosticator of dosage requirements: a 2-year follow-up study. *Am. J. Psychiatry* 133:440–443, 1976.

Davis, J.M. Overview: maintenance therapy in psychiatry: I. Schizophrenia. *Am. J. Psychiatry* 132:1237–1245, 1975.

Davis, J.M. Recent developments in the treatment of schizophrenia. *Psychiatr. Ann.* 6:71–106, 1976a.

Davis, J.M. Overview: maintenance therapy in psychiatry: II. Affective disorders. *Am. J. Psychiatry* 133:1–13, 1976b.

DeSilva, F.R.P., Wijewickrama, H.S.S. Chlomipramine in phobic and obsessional states: preliminary report. *N.Z. Med. J.* 84:4–6, 1976.

DiMascio, A. Behavioral toxicity. In DiMascio, A., Shader, R.I. (eds.), *Clinical Handbook of Psychopharmacology.* New York: Jason Aronson, pp. 185–194.

Donlon, P.T., Stenson, R.L. Neuroleptic induced extrapyramidal symptoms. *Dis. Nerv. Syst.* 37:629–635, 1976.

Donlon, P.T., Hopkins, J., Tupin, J.P. Overview: efficacy and safety of the rapid neuroleptization method with injectable haloperidol. *Am. J. Psychiatry* 136:273–278, 1979.

Epstein, L.J. Anxiolytics, antidepressants, and neuroleptics in the treatment of geriatric patients. In Lipton, M.A., DiMascio, A., Killam, M.F. (eds.), *Psychopharmacology: A Generation of Progress.* New York: Raven Press, 1978.

Friend, D. Adverse cardiovascular and hematologic effects of psychotropic drugs. In DiMascio, A., Shader, R.I. (eds.), *Clinical Handbook of Psychopharmacology.* New York: Jason Aronson, 1970, pp. 195–204.

Gelenberg, A.J. Amantadine in the treatment of benztropine-refractory extrapyramidal disorders induced by antipsychotic drugs. *Curr. Ther. Res.* 23:375–380, 1978.

Glassman, A., Perel, J. Kinetics of Anti-Depressant Drugs and Clinical Response. Paper presented at the American College of Neuropsychopharmacology Annual Meeting, New Orleans, Dec. 13–17, 1976.

Greenblatt, D.J., Shader, R.I. Pharmacotherapy of anxiety with benzodiazepines and beta-adrenergic blockers. In Lipton, M.A., DiMascio, A., Killam, K.F. (eds.), *Psychopharmacology: A Generation of Progress.* New York: Raven Press, 1978, pp. 1375–1380.

Jarvik, M.E. (ed.). *Psychopharmacology in the Practice of Medicine.* New York: Appleton-Century-Crofts, 1977.

Jopsen, K., et al. Successful treatment of severe anxiety attacks with tricyclic antidepressants: a potential mechanism of action. *Am. J. Psychiatry* 135:863–864, 1978.

Kelly, D. Phenelzine in phobic states. *Proc. R. Soc. Med.* 66:949–950, 1973.

Klein, D.F. Delineation of two drug-responsive anxiety syndromes. *Psychopharmacologia* 5:397–408, 1964.

Klein, D.F., Davis, J.M. Review of antipsychotic drug literature. In Klein, D.P., Davis, J.M. (eds.), *Diagnosis and Drug Treatment of Psychiatric Disorders.* Baltimore: Williams & Wilkins, 1969, pp. 52–138.

Klerman, G.L. Drug therapy of schizophrenia: I. Nature of the disorder and the drugs used in treatment. *Drug Ther.* Jan: 9–106, 1973.

Klerman, G.L., DiMascio, A., Weissman, M., et al. Treatment of depression by drugs and psychotherapy. *Am. J. Psychiatry* 131:186–191, 1974.

Maas, J.W. Biogenic amines and depression. *Arch. Gen. Psychiatry* 32:1357–1361, 1975.

Marshall, W.K. Treatment of obsessional illnesses and phobic anxiety states with chlomipramine. *Br. J. Psychiatry* 119:467–468, 1971.

Marshall, W.K. Clinical experience in the treatment of phobic disorders. *J. Int. Med. Res.* 5[Suppl. 5]: 65–70, 1977.

May, P.R., Van Putter, T. Plasma levels of chlorpromazine in schizophrenia: critical review of the literature. *Arch. Gen. Psychiatry* 35:1081–1087, 1978.

Paykel, E.S., DiMascio, A., Haskell, D., Prirsoff, B.A. Effects of maintenance amitriptyline and psychotherapy on symptoms of depression. *Psychol. Med.* 5:67–77, 1975.

Prange, A.J. The pharmacology and biochemistry of depression. *Dis. Nerv. Syst.* 25:217–221, 1964.

Prien, R.F., Levine, J., Switzalski, M. Discontinuation of chemotherapy for chronic schizophrenics. *Hosp. Community Psychiatry* 22:4–7, 1971.

Prien, R.F., Carrey, E.M. Guidelines for Antipsychotic Drug Use. Research Report No. 95. Perry Point, Md.: Veterans Administration Central Neuropsychiatric Research Laboratory, 1974.

Quitkin, F., Rifkin, A., Kane, J., Klein, D. Amine biochemistry and treatment of depression. In Klein, D.F., Gittleman-Klein, R. (eds.), *Progress in Psychiatric Drug Treatment*, Vol. 2. New York: Brunner/Mazel, 1976, pp. 79–86.

Quitkin, F., Rifkin, A., Gochfeld, L., et al. Tardive dyskinesia—are first signs reversible? *Am. J. Psychiatry* 134:1–84, 1977.

Rivera-Calimlin, L., Nasrallah, H., Strauss, J. et al. Clinical response and plasma levels: effect of dose, dosage schedules and drug interactions on plasma chlorpromazine levels. *Am. J. Psychiatry* 133:646–652, 1976.

Schildkraut, J.J. Biochemical studies of drugs used in the treatment of the affective disorders. In DiMascio, A., Shader, R.I., (eds.), *Clinical Handbook of Psychopharmacology*. New York: Jason Aronson, 1970.

Schildkraut, J.J. Norepinephrine metabolites as biochemical criteria for classifying depressive disorders and predicting responses to treatment: preliminary findings. *Am. J. Psychiatry* 130:695–698, 1973.

Schuckit, M., Robins, E., Feighner, J. Tricyclic antidepressants and monoamine oxidase inhibitors: Combination therapy in the treatment of depression. *Arch. Gen. Psychiatry* 24:509–514, 1971.

Shader, R. L. Endocrine, metabolic and genitourinary effects of psychotropic drugs. In DiMascio, A., Shader, R.I. (eds.), *Clinical Handbook of Psychopharmacology*. New York: Jason Aronson, 1970.

Shopsin, B., Kline, N.S. *J. Pharmacol.* 5:103, 1974.

Simpson, G.M., Tee, J.H. A ten year review of antipsychotics. In Lipton, M.A., DiMascio, A., Killam, K.F. (eds.), *Psychopharmacology: A Generation of Progress*. New York: Raven Press, 1978. Pp. 1131–1137.

Slone, D., Siskin, V., Henoven, O.P. Antenatal exposure to the Phenothiazines in relation to congenital malformations—perinatal mortality rate, birth weight, and intelligence quotient scores. *Am. J. Obstet. Gynecol.* 125:486–488, 1977.

Snyder, S.A. The dopamine hypothesis of schizophrenia: focus on the dopamine receptor. *Am. J. Psychiatry* 133:197–202, 1976.

Tarsy, D. and Balderssarini, R.J. The tardive dyskinesia syndrome. In Klawans (ed.), *Clinical Neuropharmacology*, Vol. 1. New York: Faver Press, 1976.

Tune, C.E., Creese, Z., DePaulo, J.R., et al. Clinical state and serum neuroleptic levels measured by radio-receptor assay in schizophrenia. *Am. J. Psychiatry* 137:187–190, 1980.

Tyrer, P., Candy, J., Kelly, D. A study of the clinical effects of phenelzine and placebo in the treatment of phobic anxiety. *Psychopharmacologia* 32:237–254, 1973.

Tyrer, P., Steinberg, D. Symptomatic treatment of agoraphobia and social phobias: a follow-up study. *Br. J. Psychiatry* 127:163–168, 1975.

U.S. Public Health Service. Lithium in the treatment of mood disorders. USPHS Publication No. 2143 (74-73), Washington, D.C.: Government Printing Office, 1974.

Usdin, E., Bunney, W.E., Kline, N.S. *Endorphins in Mental Health Research*. London: Macmillan, 1979.

Van Praag, H.M., Korf, J. Importance of dopamine metabolism for clinical effects and side effects of neuroleptics. *Am. J. Psychiatry* 133:1171–1177, 1976.

Wheatley, D. Comparative effects of propranolol and chlordiazepoxide in anxiety states. *Br. J. Psychiatry.* 115:1411–1412, 1969.

Electroconvulsive Therapy

C. GIBSON DUNN, M.D.

Electroconvulsive therapy has been the object of much recent adverse comment, usually from poorly informed sources. Since its development in 1938 by Cerletti and Bine, electroconvulsive therapy (ECT) has been an established and accepted treatment in psychiatry. Today there is an increasing appreciation of the invaluable role ECT can have in alleviating severe mental disorders.

Indications

Electroconvulsive therapy remains the most effective treatment for severe depression and is clearly the treatment of choice for delusional depressions—that is, depression complicated by psychotic delusional ideation. It is also indicated for intensely suicidal patients, patients with medical conditions that make prolonged use of antidepressant medication hazardous, and patients inadequately responsive to psychotherapy and pharmacotherapy after adequate clinical trials. In many elderly depressed patients, ECT is a safer, more controlled treatment than any alternative. It is recognized as especially effective in patients with severely agitated depressions that occur in middle to late life, illnesses previously termed involutional melancholia. ECT also benefits certain patients with severe obsessive-compulsive disorders, especially when depression coexists as a complicating factor. There may also be a subgroup of schizophrenic patients with inadequate response to neuroleptic medication; they may benefit from a course of ECT, but usually a somewhat greater number of treatments is needed than would be required for depression.

Electroconvulsive therapy, like any medical procedure, should not be undertaken casually; however, it must be remembered that depression is a potentially lethal disorder. Inadequate or incomplete treatment can pose a very severe risk to the patient. It is my impression that patients and their families are generally very receptive to this treatment when it is presented by a well-informed clinician who is secure in its use.

Procedure

Today ECT is an essentially painless, extremely safe procedure with only transient side effects and few complications. After informed consent for the procedure and the requisite anesthesia has been obtained, a medical evaluation must be completed before ECT is administered; the evaluation includes physical examination, electrocardiogram, and serum electrolytes. Spinal x-ray studies are now optional, but they are indicated if there is some question of spinal pathology. The patient generally receives treatment two to four times per week; three times a week on alternating days is the most common schedule. The patient is not given oral intake on the night preceding the treatment, which is usually performed in the early morning to avoid risk of accidental ingestion of food or water.

To minimize secretions during anesthesia, the patient is given atropine 0.5 to 1.0 mg subcutaneously 30 to 60 minutes before treatment. The patient then empties his or her bowel and bladder to avoid incontinence during the seizure. The patient is dressed in a hospital gown, and any dentures are removed. The patient lies supine on a standard hospital bed or stretcher and an intravenous line of 5 percent dextrose in water is begun to allow access for anesthetic agents. Areas where stimulus electrodes are to be applied are cleaned with an alcohol swab to inprove electrical conduction.

Anesthesia today most often consists of intravenous administration of methohexital 0.75 mg/kg for sleep, followed by intravenous succinylcholine 0.5 mg/kg for neuromuscular blockade. The latter drug minimizes or eliminates significant muscle contractions during the brain seizure. This method avoids the risk of stress fractures, especially in osteoporotic, elderly individuals. The patient is well ventilated with oxygen until maximal neuromuscular blockade is achieved, and a rubber biteblock is then inserted. The stimulus electrodes are put in place, either bitemporally or unilaterally over the nondominant hemisphere (temporal and frontal). An electric current is delivered for 1.0 to 2.0 seconds. The presence of a bilateral seizure determined either by observation of residual muscle contractions or by the simultaneous recording of a two-lead electroencephalogram, now increasingly used on certain treatment apparatuses. A seizure duration of 60 to 120 seconds is sought, although variations occur in both directions. The patient is ventilated throughout the seizure and until spontaneous respirations resume. An electrocardiogram may or may not be recorded throughout. The patient is usually awake and responsive within 10 minutes from the beginning of the procedure. Postictal confusion and somnolence may persist for one to two hours. Bed rest is generally indicated for this time, but not a great deal longer. Rapid reinvolvement in the hospital routine is preferable to maximize the therapeutic benefit.

Multiple seizures may be induced during one anesthesia session, for the purpose of hastening recovery. The discussion of this alternative is beyond the scope of this text, but this approach does not seem to have any major contraindications or complications and may act more rapidly as intended.

Mechanism of Action
The mode of action of ECT remains uncertain. It is generally believed that there is a major effect on the brain monoamine systems, including serotonin, dopamine, and norepinephrine. It is also quite possible that ECT alters central nervous system endorphins and calcium metabolism. The precise sites of such effects remain unknown.

Response and Complications
Clinical response appears to result from the cumulative effects of the brain seizures. The stimulus itself does not appear to be therapeutic. The total seizure time necessary for maximum therapeutic response remains under investigation. Maletsky (1979), studying patients treated with multiple ECT, found that virtually no clinical improvement could be expected from a total seizure time of 300 seconds or less, while more than 75 percent of patients responded well to a total seizure time of 750 seconds. Generally, the patient's response is assessed solely on clinical observation, with the average number of treatments being 6 to 12; however, there is no arbitrary limit on the total number as long as continued improvement can be observed. Recent research suggests that the dexamethasone suppression test (see Chapter 3) may be of use in assessing response. If the dexamethasone suppression test is abnormal prior to ECT, a normalization in the test is sought before completion of the series. This appears to have a highly significant predictive value—a low rate of relapse occurs in patients with a normalized test.

Complications include nausea and muscle aches from the anesthesia, rare bone fractures from inadequate anesthesia, and extremely infrequent death (less than five per 100,000 treatments) from cardiac arrhythmias. There has been a serious question about memory impairment. It is definite that memory processes are impaired immediately following each procedure. This effect builds during the course of a series of treatment, especially in elderly patients. The great majority of this acute effect, however, will clear within three weeks after the end of the series. Follow-up studies have been unable to show any residual, permanent cognitive impairment. A minority of patients do complain of persistent memory difficulties, and these reports cannot be dismissed despite the lack of objective data. Memory effects have been reduced further by the increased use of a unilateral placement of the stimulus electrodes over the nondominant hemisphere to avoid electric shock to the dominant temporal lobe. This treatment, however, may not be quite as effective as bitemporal placement.

Outcome

Electroconvulsive therapy is quite effective in the treatment of primary depressions and severe depressive components of other disorders. An absolute rate of response is of debatable value given the variability of patient populations studied, previously questionable methodologic procedures, and lack of standardization in treatment parameters. The most frequently cited figure for treatment response by primarily depressed patients is 80 percent and greater. Patients with melancholia appear to have a response rate that may exceed 90 percent when ECT is properly administered. A significant issue has been the high rate of relapse during the year following treatment—figures as high as 50 percent have been cited. To decrease relapse, patients now are routinely given an antidepressant medication or lithium carbonate (which is a second choice in unipolar disorders). If these are ineffective, maintenance ECT on a regular basis (monthly to quarterly) may prove necessary. As noted earlier, the dexamethasone suppression test may prove of significant benefit in predicting relapse.

References and Further Reading

American Psychiatric Association: Electroconvulsive Therapy, Task Force Report 14. Washington, D.C.: APA, 1978.

Avery, D., Lubrano, A. Depression treated with imipramine and ECT: the De-Carole's study reconsidered. *Am. J. Psychiatry* 136:559–562, 1979.

Avery, D., Winokur, G. Mortality in depressed patients treated with electroconvulsive therapy and antidepressants. *Arch. Gen. Psychiatry* 33:1029, 1975.

Fink, M. Efficacy and safety of induced seizures (EST) in man. *Compr. Psychiatry* 19:1–18, 1978.

Greenblatt, M., Grosser, G.H., Wechsler, H. Differential response of hospitalized depressed patients to somatic therapy. *Am. J. Psychiatry* 116:935–943, 1964.

Maletzky, B.M. Seizure duration and clinical effect in electroconvulsive therapy. *Compr. Psychiatry* 19:541–550, 1979.

Squire, L.G., Chace, P.M. Memory functions six to nine months after electroconvulsive therapy. *Arch. Gen. Psychiatry* 32:1557–1564, 1975.

Index

Abstract reasoning, on mental status examination, 13
Acetaminophen, 65
Acetylcholine, 112, 128, 189
Acting out, 200, 202, 263
　in adolescence, 220, 225
　treatment of, 225
Addiction, 60. *See also* Drug abuse; Substance use disorders
Addison's disease, 125
Adenosine diphosphate, 94
Adenylate cyclase, 300
Adjustment problems
　depressed mood with, 124–125
　elderly and, 242
　psychiatric interview on, 8, 9
Adolescence psychiatric disorders, 217–232
　acting out in, 220
　adult psychiatric disorders different from, 217
　bipolar disorder in, 111
　case examples of, 228–229
　diagnostic evaluation of, 220–225
　DSM-III categories related to, 230–232
　family interview in, 224–225
　family participation in therapy for, 227–228
　hospitalization for, 226–227
　narcissistic and omnipotent defenses in, 218–220
　parent interview and, 221–222
　pharmacotherapy for, 225–226
　psychiatric disorders found in, 229–230
　psychiatric interview for, 9, 222–223
　psychological testing of, 223–224
　psychotherapy and, 220
　residential treatment for, 227
　schizophrenia in, 226, 228, 229
　social history in, 222
　special characteristics of, 217–220
　suicide risk in, 227, 248
　treatment of, 225–228
　violent behavior and, 261
Adolescent turmoil, 217
Adrenal gland disorders, 50, 125
Adrenocorticotropic hormone (ACTH), 28, 50, 247
Affect
　blunting or flattening of, 120
　mental status examination of, 12

Affective disorders. *See also* Bipolar disorder (manic-depressive illness); Depression and depressive disorders
　adolescent, 229
　depersonalization disorder with, 154
　drug management of, 291–308
　violent behavior and, 260
Affective syndrome, organic, 45, 48, 50
Age, and suicide risk, 253
Aged. *See* Elderly
Age phobia, and anorexia nervosa, 209
Aggresive behavior. *See also* Passive aggressive personality disorder
　object relations and, 262
　psychotherapy and, 263
　violent behavior and, 261
Aging process, 233–235
　biologic features of, 234
　psychologic features of, 234–235
Agitated depression, 241
Agoraphobia, 133, 135–136, 195
　case examples of, 148–150
　course of, 142–143
　depressive disorders with, 125
　DSM-III criteria for, 136
　onset of, 134
　panic anxiety disorder and, 136, 142
　treatment of, 277, 310, 314, 316
Agras, S., 134
Al-Anon, 82, 83
Alcohol abuse and alcoholism, 59, 61–64
　adolescent, 229
　aftercare in, 82
　alcoholism intoxication in, 62–63
　alcohol withdrawal syndrome in, 63
　amnestic syndrome with, 53, 64
　anorexia nervosa and, 209, 212
　anxiety disorders with, 140, 143, 146, 147, 308, 312
　bipolar disorder with, 109, 112
　case example of, 83–84
　clarification of problems by patient in, 81–82
　confrontation in, 78–79
　cross-dependence in, 60
　delirium with, 51
　denial of, 78–79

depressive disorders with, 125–126
diagnosis of, 77–83
differential diagnosis of, 50, 73–74
disulfiram (Antabuse) in, 76
DSM-III criteria for, 61–62, 63
engaging patient in treatment of, 79–80
etiology of, 75
families and, 75, 82–83
hospitalization for, 70–71, 80–81
illness model of, 73
Michigan Alcoholism Screening Test in, 77, 78, 84–86
Minnesota Multiphasic Personality Inventory (MMPI) in, 19
mixed abuse patterns with, 66, 295
onset of, 59
parental, 9
patient reaction to, 78
personality disorders and, 189, 192
physician in treatment of, 75–76
recovery period in, 82
referral or consultation in, 79
rehabilitative model of treatment in, 77–83
results of prolonged, 64
selection of treatment setting in, 80
suicide risk and, 255, 257–258
treatment of, 70–71, 75–76, 310, 311
violent behavior and, 259, 261
Alcoholics Anonymous, 73, 76, 80, 81, 82, 83, 84, 258
Alexander, Franz, 175, 176–177, 181, 208, 215
Alexithymia, 178, 181, 182
Alprazolam, 293, 307
Alzheimer's disease, 45, 51, 52, 236
Amantadine, 290
Amitriptyline, 32
　depressive disorders with, 128, 240, 294
　mode of action of, 292, 293, 317
Amnesia. *See* Psychogenic amnesia
Amnestic syndrome, 45, 47–48
　alcohol abuse with, 53, 64
　etiology of, 53
　DSM-III criteria in, 48
　management and treatment of, 54
Amotivational syndrome with marijuana, 68
Amoxapine, 293, 307

325

Amphetamine abuse, 59, 61, 66–67
  acute effects of, 66–67
  anxiety disorders and, 140
  bipolar disorder and, 110, 112
  depressive disorders with, 125, 241
  drug interactions with, 67, 290
  treatment of, 72
  withdrawal from, 50, 72
Anemia, 248
Anger, during psychiatric interview, 4, 5
Anhedonia, and depression, 119, 123
Animals, phobias concerning, 137
Anorexia nervosa, 179, 207–216, 231
  case example of, 215
  clinical features of, 208–209
  diagnostic criteria in, 207–213
  early work in, 207–208
  etiology of, 209
  family and, 208–209, 210–211
  follow-up to treatment for, 213
  hospitalization for, 211
  physical and laboratory findings in, 209–210
  treatment of, 210–213, 277
Anticholinergic syndrome, acute, 298
Antidepressant drugs. *See also* Tricyclic antidepressant drugs; *specific drugs*
  adolescent disorders with, 226
  bipolar disorder treatment with, 114–115
  bulimia and, 214
  depressive disorders with, 122
  electroconvulsive therapy (ECT) and, 323
  geriatric disorders and, 240–241
  manic episode precipitated by, 110–111, 112
  second-generation, 307–308
Antiinflammatory drugs, 125
Antiparkinsonian drugs, 290, 298
Antipsychotic drugs, 282–291. *See also specific drugs*
  bipolar disorder with, 114
  choosing, 283–284
  classification of, 283
  dissociative disorders and, 155
  dosage with, 284–285
  drug interactions with, 290–291
  geriatric psychotic conditions and, 241–242
  initiating treatment with, 284
  maintenance treatment with, 285–288
  mechanism of action of, 283
  plasma levels in, 288
  psychological factors affecting illness and, 182
  psycholysis with, 285
  reversible extrapyramidal syndromes with, 289–290

  schizophrenia and, 36, 260–261
  side effects with, 288–291
  tardive dyskinesia with, 288–289
Antisocial personality disorder, 189, 193
  clinical features of, 193
  differential diagnosis of, 193
  intelligence tests and, 17
  treatment of, 203–204
  violent behavior and, 260
Anxiety. *See also* Separation and anxiety
  amphetamine abuse and, 72
  bipolar disorder with, 109
  castration, 169
  depressive disorders and, 119, 125, 308
  drug management of, 307–318
  homosexuality and, 168
  hypochondriasis and, 152
  medical disorders causing, 246, 247, 248, 249
  organic brain syndromes with, 45
  psychosexual disorders and, 161, 162, 171, 173
  sexual dysfunction and, 167
  somatization disorder with, 151
  substance abuse and, 74
Anxiety disorders, 133–150. *See also specific anxiety disorders*
  adolescent, 229, 231
  atypical, 139
  case examples of, 147–150
  classification of, 135–139
  complications with, 142–143
  course of, 142–143
  cultural factors in, 135
  differential diagnosis of, 140–142
  drug management of, 308–318
  DSM-III criteria in, 135, 137, 138, 139, 140
  early work in, 133
  elderly and, 242
  epidemiology of, 134–135
  etiology of, 143–144
  generalized, 138
  hospitalization for, 147
  onset of, 134
  personality type and, 142
  physical and mental disorders and, 141–142
  physician-patient relationship in, 144–145
  precipitating events in, 144
  psychological therapy in, 146–147, 271
  signs and symptoms in, 133–134
  substance use disorders and, 74, 140
  treatment of, 144–147, 242, 275, 276, 277
Anxiety neurosis, 133, 138, 229
Apomorphine, 291

Arteriosclerosis, 52, 245
Assertiveness training, 147, 204, 272, 276
Asthmatic disorders, 246, 276
Atherosclerosis, 64, 122
Attention deficit disorders, 193, 198, 230, 261
Autonomic balance, 182–183
Autoregulatory techniques, in psychosomatic syndromes, 182–183
Average evoked response (AER) studies, 31
Aversive conditioning, 276
  ego-dystonic homosexuality with, 170, 173
  paraphilias with, 170
Aversion relief, 170, 173
Avoidant personality disorder, 190, 194, 209
  adolescent, 231
  clinical features of, 194
  differential diagnosis of, 194, 195
  treatment of, 204
Ayd, F.J., 287

Barbach, L., 173
Barbiturate abuse, 59, 61, 64–65
  anxiety disorders with, 140, 308, 312
  case example of, 84
  cross-dependence with, 60
  drug interactions with, 66, 290–291, 295, 309, 318
  geriatric disorders and, 242
  treatment for, 71–72, 310
  violent behavior and, 261
  withdrawal from, 65
Bateson, Gregory, 92
Beck, A., 127
Behavior modification
  personality disorders in, 202
  psychosexual disorders with, 171, 172–173
Behavior therapy, 269, 274–278. *See also specific therapies*
  applications of, 147, 205, 277–278, 314, 316
  definition of, 274
  psychological factors affecting illness and, 181
  psychotherapy and, 278
Bellack, L., 15
Bender Visual Motor Gestalt Test, 19, 22–23, 24
Benzodiazepines
  abuse of, 65, 261
  alcoholism treatment with, 70, 71
  anxiety disorders and, 140, 145–146, 308, 309–312, 316
  dependence on, 311–312
  geriatric disorders with, 242

mechanism of action of, 310
psychological factors affecting illness and, 182
side effects of, 311–312
somatoform and dissociative disorders with, 155, 156
tolerance to, 309, 310
withdrawal from, 65, 312
Benzoquinolines, 283
Benztropine, 290
Bereavement, uncomplicated, 124
Beta-blocker drugs, 249, 291
Bethanechol, 296, 297
Binet, Alfred, 16
Bion, Wilfred R., 272
Biofeedback, 183, 275–276
Biogenic amine hypothesis in depression, 127–128, 293
Biologic rhythms, and stress, 180
Bipolar disorder (manic-depressive illness), 105–117
  adolescent, 229
  anorexia nervosa and, 209
  antidepressant drugs precipitating, 110–111
  case examples of, 116–117
  classification of, 107–109
  complications in, 111–112
  course of, 111
  differential diagnosis in, 109–111, 125
  DSM-III on, 105, 108
  early work with, 105
  elderly and, 239, 241
  epidemiology of, 107
  etiology of, 112–113
  family and, 115–116
  genetic factors in, 33, 39, 107, 112–113
  hospitalization for, 113–114
  interviewing techniques in, 109
  length of manic episodes, 112
  lithium carbonate in, 37, 113, 114–115, 116, 117, 241, 299, 301–302
  medical disorders causing, 111
  mixed state, 107
  onset of, 111
  paranoid type, 105, 109
  physician-patient relationship in, 115–116
  prognosis for, 112
  psychological markers in, 36, 37
  schizophrenia variants and, 97, 108, 109–110
  signs and symptoms of manic episode, 105–107
  substance abuse and, 74
  suicide risk and, 112, 254–255
  treatment of, 113–116, 241
  unipolar affective disorder differentiated from, 110
  use of term, 105, 123
  violent behavior and, 260
  visual average evoked response (AER) studies in, 31
Bissell, LeClair, 78
Blacker, K.H., 98
Bleuler, Eugen, 87
Blindness, hysterical, 180
Blunting of affect, 120
Body image, and anorexia nervosa, 207
Boll, T.J., 23
Borderline personality disorder, 188, 189, 193–194, 198
  anxiety disorder and, 140
  clinical features of, 193–194, 196
  differential diagnosis of, 155, 191, 192
  Rorschach techniques in, 20
  treatment of, 204, 310
  violent behavior and, 260
Bowen, M., 210
Bowers, M., 98
Brain damage. *See also* Organic brain syndrome
  intelligence tests and, 17
  psychiatric manifestations of, 248
  schizophrenia and, 94
Brief reactive psychosis, 87, 97, 102
Briquet's syndrome, 151
Bromides, 308, 312
Bronchial asthma, 175, 180
Brown, G.W., 101
Bruch, H., 207, 208
Buchsbaum, M.S., 36
Bufotenin, 94
Bulimia, 207, 213–214, 231
  case examples of 215–216
  clinical features of, 213–214
  diagnostic criteria in, 213–214
  treatment of, 214
Burns, D.D., 277
Butaclamol, 283
Butyrophenones, 155, 283

Cade, J.F., 291, 299
Caffeinism, 140
Cancer
  personality profile in, 176
  psychiatric manifestations of, 248
  somatoform disorders and, 152–153
Cannabis. *See* Marijuana
Carbamazepine, 57, 114, 304
Carbon dioxide inhalation, 275
Cardiovascular system disorders, 245–246
Carlson, G.A., 106, 283
Carpenter, W.T., 90
Carroll, B.J., 33, 123
Case examples
  adolescent disorders, 228–229
  anxiety disorders, 147–150
bipolar disorder, 116–117
dementia, 58
depressive disorders, 129–130
dissociative disorders, 157–158
eating disorders, 215–216
geriatric disorders, 244
psychiatric interview, 7–8
psychobiologic evaluation, 39–41
psychological factors affecting physical condition, 183–185
psychotherapeutic approaches, 269
schizophrenia, 103–104
somatoform disorders, 157–158
suicide risk, 257–258
violent behavior, 264–265
Castration anxiety, 169
Catatonic features, in mania, 110
Catatonic schizophrenia, 96–97
Catecholamines, and affective disorders, 27, 292
CAT scan. *See* Computerized axial tomography (CAT)
Central nervous system dysfunction, 18, 246
Cerletti, 321
Charcot, Jean-Marie, 155
Child abuse, 259, 262
Childbirth, depressive disorders after, 122
Childhood
  antisocial personality disorder in, 193
  anxiety disorders of, 231
  gender identity issues in, 163–164
  intelligence tests in, 17, 18
  petit mal seizures in, 56
  pica in, 214
  psychiatric interview information on, 8–9
  rumination disorder of, 214–215
  separation anxiety in, 144, 231
  sexual dysfunction and, 167–168
  suicide risk in, 248
  violent behavior and, 261
Chloral hydrate, 70
Chlordiazepoxide (Librium), 65, 70
  anxiety disorders with, 308, 309, 311
  geriatric disorders with, 242
Chlorpromazine, 281, 282, 283, 284, 307
  anxiety disorders with, 314
  bipolar disorder with, 113
  schizophrenia and, 93, 98
  substance abuse treatment with, 72
Chodoff, P., 121
Cholesterol, and stress, 177, 178
Chronic factitious disorder with physical symptoms (CFDPS), 180–181
Chronic obstructive pulmonary disease, 246–247

Cirrhosis, 247
Class, and schizophrenia, 89, 92
Clobazam, 309
Clomipramine, 307
Clonidine, 72
Clorazepate, 242, 309
Cocaine abuse, 61, 66
  bipolar disorder and, 110, 112
  depressive disorders with, 125
  differential diagnosis and, 50
  patterns in, 66, 67
  treatment of withdrawal in, 72
Codeine, 65, 84
Cognitive functioning
  mental status examination of, 12–13
  organic disorders and, 22
  somatoform and dissociative disorders and, 156
Cognitive therapy, 129, 268, 277
Cola beverages, 140
Cold tablets, 140
Command hallucination, 11
Commitment. *See* Hospitalization
Complex partial seizures, 56
Compulsions, 138, 139. *See also* Obsessive compulsive disorder
Compulsive personality disorder, 190, 195
  clinical features of, 195
  differential diagnosis of, 195
  intelligence tests and, 17
  treatment for, 205
  violent behavior and, 260
Computerized axial tomography (CAT)
  dementia on, 52
  use in geriatric organic brain disorders, 236, 240
  preventive psychiatry with, 38
Conduct disorders, 230–231, 261
Connective order diseases, 249
Conversion disorder, 151–152, 275
  diagnosis of, 152
  psychological factors in illness and, 180
Core schizophrenia, 89, 90
Cornelison, Alice, 91
Coronary artery disease, 176
Corticosteroids, 50, 247
Cortisol, 28, 177
Countertransference, 256, 268
Crime, 259. *See also* Violent behavior
Crisis intervention, 256, 263–264, 274
Crisp, R.H., 209, 211, 213
Cross-dependence in substance abuse, 60
Crow, T.J., 94
Cultural factors
  anxiety disorders and, 135
  intelligence tests and, 18

Cushing's disease, 111, 125, 247
Cyclothymic disorder, 35, 157

Da Costa, J.M., 133
Dangerousness, concept of, 264
Davis, J.M., 128, 286, 293, 294
Day care centers, 243
Defense system
  adolescence and, 218–220
  illness and inadequacy of, 178–179
  personality disorders and, 199–201, 263
  physical reactions and, 177–178
  specific mechanisms in, 200–201
  stress and, 177–179
  violent behavior and, 263
Delirium, 45–46, 51
  alcohol withdrawal and, 63
  causes of, 51
  clinical picture in, 45–46
  course of, 51
  dementia resembling, 46
  differential diagnosis in, 49
  DSM-III criteria for, 45, 46
  management and treatment of, 54
  medical disorders and, 247, 248, 249
  suicide risk and, 255
Delirium tremens (DT), 63, 71
Delusions
  bipolar disorder with, 106, 109
  depressive disorders with, 120
  dissociative disorders with, 155
  electroconvulsive therapy (ECT) in, 321
  on mental status examination, 11
  organic delusional syndrome with, 48, 50
  organic disorders and, 22
  schizophrenia with, 87, 88–89, 260, 297
  tricyclic antidepressants and, 294, 297
Dementia, 45, 46–47, 51–53
  alcohol abuse and, 64
  atrophy of unknown cause in, 51
  case example of, 58
  categories of, 51, 52
  causes of, 51
  clinical picture in, 46–47
  course of, 46
  delirium resembling, 46
  differential diagnosis in, 49, 247
  DSM-III criteria in, 46, 47
  elderly and, 235–236, 241, 242
  intellectual deterioration in, 46–47
  multiinfarct, 52
  primary degenerative, 52
  treatment of, 54, 242

Dementia praecox, 33, 87, 91, 105
Denial
  as defense mechansim, 201, 263
  substance abuse and, 78–79
Dependence, in substance use disorders, 60
Dependent personality disorder, 188, 190, 194–195
  clinical features of, 195
  differential diagnosis of, 195
  treatment of, 204–205
Depersonalization disorder, 11, 151, 153, 154
Depot phenothiazines, 287
Depression and depressive disorders, 119–130. *See also* Major depressive disorders
  adjustment disorder with, 124–125
  adolescent, 227
  alcoholism and substance abuse and, 74, 75, 125–126
  anxiety disorders with, 142
  biogenic amine hypothesis in, 127–128, 293
  case examples of, 129–130
  classification of, 123–125
  complications of, 122
  course of, 121–122
  dexamethasone suppression test (DST), 27–28, 36
  differential diagnosis in, 50, 125–126, 237
  drug management of, 291–308
  DSM-III criteria in, 123, 124–125, 188–189
  early work with, 119
  elderly and, 237, 240–241, 282
  electroconvulsive therapy (ECT) in, 321
  environmental factors in, 126, 180
  epidemiology of, 121
  etiology of, 126–128
  familial, 36
  genetic factors in, 33
  hospitalization for, 129
  loss and grief and, 126
  medical disorders and, 247, 248, 249
  melancholia with, 124
  monoamine oxidase (MAO) inhibitors in, 305, 306
  neuroendocrine abnormalities and, 27
  organic brain syndromes with, 45
  personality patterns and, 121, 125, 127
  postpartum period and, 122
  post-psychotic, 99–100
  psychobiology in prediction of, 37–38
  psychological factors in, 126–127

psychological markers in, 35–36, 37
psychotherapy in, 128–129
signs and symptoms of, 119–120
social factors in, 126
somatoform disorders with, 151, 152, 153
suicide risk and, 120, 121, 122, 128, 129
treatment of, 128–129, 240–241, 275
tricyclic antidepressant drugs in, 37
violent behavior and, 260
Depressive spectrum disorder, 122, 127
Derealization, on mental status examination, 11
Desensitization. *See* Systematic desensitization
Desipramine, 40, 317
  depressive disorders and, 128, 237, 240
  plasma level measurements for, 32
Desmethylclomipramine, 32
Desmethyldiazepam, 311
Detre, T.P., 56
Developmental disorders, adolescent, 232
Developmental history
  Erikson's stages of, 198–199, 233
  personality disorders and, 198–199
  in psychiatric interview, 8–9
  sexual dysfunction and, 167–168
  violent behavior and, 262
Dexamethasone suppression test (DST), 27–28
  clinical uses of, 36, 40, 49, 123
  electroconvulsive therapy (ECT) in, 322, 323
  techniques in, 28, 33
Dextroamphetamine, 226, 249, 261, 292, 313
Diabetes mellitus, 247
Diagnosis
  adolescent disorders and, 220–225
  formulation of, 14
  intelligence tests and, 18
  psychiatric evaluation and, 13–14
  psychodynamic formulation in, 14
  recommendations for treatment and, 14
  Rorschach techniques in, 20
  summary of interview findings in, 14
Diagnostic and Statistical Manual of Mental Disorders, Third Edition, (DSM-III), 14
  adolescent disorders and, 230–232
  alcohol abuse and alcoholism, 61–62, 63
  anorexia nervosa, 207

anxiety disorders, 135, 137, 138, 139, 140
axis I disorders in, 188
axis II disorders in, 189
axis III disorders in, 245
bipolar disorder in, 105, 108
bulimia in, 213
depressive disorders in, 123, 124–125, 188–189
dissociative disorders in, 153
geriatric disorders and, 235
hypochondriasis, 238
melancholia in, 123, 124
organic brain syndromes in, 45, 46, 47, 48
paranoid disorders, 87–88, 102–103
personality disorders in, 187–188, 189, 190, 191, 192, 193, 194, 195, 196, 198
psychological factors affecting physical condition (PFAPC), 175, 177, 180
psychosexual disorders, 161, 163, 164
schizophrenia in, 87, 90, 95, 96, 97
somatoform disorders in, 151, 152
substance abuse disorders in, 59, 60, 69
Diazepam (Valium), 185, 275, 299
  abuse of, 65
  anxiety disorders with, 148, 309, 311
  geriatric disorders with, 242
  substance abuse treatment with, 70, 73
Dihydromorphone, 65
Dimethoxyphenylethylamine, 94
Dimethyltryptamine (DMT), 67, 94
Diphenhydramine, 290, 312
Disorganized schizophrenia, 96
Disorientation, on mental status examination, 12
Dissociation (defense mechanism), 200
Dissociative disorders, 151, 153–155
  atypical, 153, 154
  case examples of, 157–158
  cognitive style in, 156
  differential diagnosis in, 155
  DSM-III classification of, 153
  early work with, 151
  etiology of, 155–156
  specific syndromes in, 153–154
  treatment of, 156–157, 271
Disulfiram (Antabuse), 76
Diuretics, 210, 291
Dizygotic twin studies
  anxiety disorders in, 143

bipolar disorder in, 112
drug plasma levels in, 318
psychobiologic evaluation with, 34, 35, 38
schizophrenia in, 93
Donlon, J.T., 98
Donlon, P.T., 285
Dopamine, 288
  bipolar disorder and, 112
  depressive disorders with, 127–128
  electroconvulsive therapy (ECT) with, 322
  lithium and, 300
  schizophrenia and, 93–94, 283
  stress and, 179
  tardive dyskinesia and, 289
Doxepin, 32, 237, 240, 317
Dreams, 267
Drug abuse. *See also* Substance abuse
  anxiety disorders with, 142, 147
  bipolar disorder and, 110
  delirium with, 51
  Minnesota Multiphasic Personality Inventory (MMPI) in, 19
  narcissistic personality disorder with, 192
  organic mental disorders with, 45, 49
  parental, 9
  violent behavior and, 259, 261–262
Drug therapy. *See* Psychopharmacology; *specific drugs*
DSM-III. *See Diagnostic and Statistical Manual of Mental Disorders,* Third Edition (DSM-III)
DST. *See* Dexamethasone suppression test (DST)
Dual matings, 38–39
Dunbar, Flanders, 176
Dysmorphobia, 152
Dysphoria, and depression, 119
Dysthymic disorder, 195
  DSM-III description of, 125
  elderly and, 240, 242
  genetic factors in, 35
  treatment of, 310

Eating disorders, 207–216. *See also* Anorexia nervosa; Bulimia
  adolescent, 231
  case examples in, 215–216
  DSM-III criteria in, 207, 213
  pica and, 214
  rumination disorder of infancy and, 214–215
ECT. *See* Electroconvulsive therapy (ECT)
Eczema, 180
EEG. *See* Electroencephalography (EEG)

Ego defenses. *See* Defense system
Ego-dystonic homosexuality
  DSM-III criteria for, 168
  etiology of, 168–169
  treatment of, 170, 171, 173, 277
Elderly. *See also* Geriatric disorders
  aging process and, 233–235
  bipolar disorder in, 107
  dementia in, 49
  depressive disorders in, 121
  psychometric issues for, 24
  self-medication in, 240
Electroconvulsive therapy (ECT), 130, 294, 321–323
  geriatric disorders with, 237, 242
  indications for, 321
  mechanisms of action of, 322
  memory and, 323
  outcome with, 323
  procedures in, 321–322
  response and complications with, 322–323
  thyrotropin-releasing hormone (TRH) stimulation test with, 33
Electroencephalography (EEG)
  seizure disorders on, 55, 56, 57
  sleep analysis on, 30–31, 124
Electrolyte imbalances, 247
Empty nest syndrome, 234, 240
Encephalitis, 248
Encounter groups, 272
Endocrine disorders, 50, 247
Endorphins, 94, 291, 322
Engel, G.I., 178
Environmental factors
  anxiety disorders and, 144
  biologic rhythms and, 180
  depressive disorders and, 126, 180
  exogenous toxins, 249
  homosexuality and, 169
  personality disorders and, 198–199
  psychological factors affecting physical condition (PFAPC), 175
  schizophrenia and, 92
  twin studies in genetics and, 34, 35
Epilepsy, 55–57, 248. *See also* Seizure disorders
  causes of, 55–56, 248
  diagnosis of, 56–57
  management of, 57, 276, 302
  violent behavior and, 261
Epileptogenic focus, 56
Epinephrine, 291
Episodic dyscontrol syndrome, 261
Ergoloid (Hydergine), 242
Ergotamine tartrate, 185
Erikson, Erik, 198–199, 233
Ethchlorvynol, 65, 242, 295

Evaluation, 1–41. *See also* Psychiatric evaluation; Psychobiologic evaluation; Psychometric evaluation
Exhibitionism, 164, 170, 277

Factitious disorder with psychological symptoms, 49–50
Family
  adolescent disorders and, 221–222, 225–226, 227–228
  alcoholism and, 75
  anorexia nervosa and, 208–209, 210–211
  bipolar disorder and, 115–116
  bulimia and, 214
  defensive inadequacy in illness and, 179
  double bind in, 92
  elderly and, 242
  enmeshment in, 210
  homosexuality and, 169
  interview of, 221, 224–225
  schizophrenia and, 91–92, 101–102
  somatoform and dissociative disorders and, 156
  therapy and, 268
  violent behavior in, 259, 262
Family history
  anorexia nervosa and, 210–211
  psychiatric interview on, 8–9
  psychobiologic evaluation in, 33–39
  somatoform and dissociative disorders and, 156
  violent behavior and, 262
Family therapy, 272–273
  anorexia nervosa and, 209, 211, 212
  personality disorders and, 202
  schizophrenia and, 101–102
Fantasy (defense mechanism), 200–201
Feinbloom, D.H., 174
Fetishism, 164, 170, 277
Fielding, C., 15
Fiorinal-Plus, 65
Flattening of affect, 120
Fleck, Steven, 91, 210
Flight of ideas, in bipolar disorder, 106, 108
Flooding, 276, 314
Fluphenazine, 237, 284
Fluphenazine decanoate, 287
Fluphenazine enanthate, 287
Fluphenazine hydrochloride, 288
Flurazepam, 65, 242, 309
Fluvoxamine, 307
Focal lobe epilepsy, 55
Folie à deux, 238
Forer Structured Sentence Completion Tests, 21

Fraternal twin studies. *See* Dizygotic twin studies
Free association, 267
Freud, Sigmund, 91, 126–127, 133, 155, 198, 271
Fugues, 56. *See also* Psychogenic fugue

Gamma-aminobutyric acid (GABA), 94, 289
Gastrointestinal disorders, 247
Gender identity issues, 163–164. *See also* Transsexualism; Transvestism
Generalized anxiety disorders, 135, 138, 143
Genetic factors
  adoption studies, 35
  alcoholism and, 75
  anxiety disorders and, 143
  bipolar disorders with, 33, 39, 107, 112–113
  counseling and, 38–39
  degree of relatedness and risk in, 34
  dual matings and, 38–39
  homosexuality and, 168
  markers for vulnerability, 35–37
  personality disorders and, 198
  preventive psychiatry and, 37–39
  psychobiologic evaluation and, 33–39
  psychological factors in illness and, 180
  and psychiatric interview, 9
  schizophrenia and, 33, 34, 35, 38–39, 92–93, 198
  twin studies, 34, 35
  violent behavior and, 262
Geriatric disorders, 233–244
  aging process and, 233–235
  assessment in, 239–240
  case example of, 244
  drug therapy in, 281–282
  electroconvulsive therapy (ECT) in, 242
  and functional psychiatric disorders, 237–239
  living alone and, 239, 243
  organic mental disorders in, 235–237
  psychotherapy and, 242–243
  self-medication and, 239
  single women and, 234–235
  treatment of, 240–244
Gestalt therapy, 272
Giving up/given up syndrome, 178, 180, 181
Glasser, A.J., 17
Glithero, E., 152
Globus hystericus reaction, 157, 158
Glutethimide, 65, 242, 312

Goodwin, F.K., 106
Gottesman, I.I., 93
Grandiosity
    bipolar disorder with, 105, 106, 109
    on mental status examination, 11
Grand mal seizures, 55, 56
Green, A., 276
Green, E., 276
Green, R., 170
Grief, and depressive disorders, 126
Group therapy, 271–272
    antisocial personality disorder and, 204
    anxiety disorders and, 147
    avoidant personality disorder and, 204
    compulsive personality disorder and, 205
    concepts of, 271
    depressive disorders and, 129
    ego-dystonic homosexuality and, 173
    elderly and, 243
    evaluation of, 272
    personality disorders and, 202
    psychological factors affecting illness and, 182
    psychosexual disorders in, 170–171, 173
    schizoid personality disorder in, 203
    schizophrenia with, 100
    somatoform and dissociative disorders and, 156
    types of, 271–272
Guanethidine, 290, 295
Gull, William W., 207–208
Gunderson, J.G., 273

Habit reversal, 277
Hallucinations
    with alcohol abuse, 63–64
    bipolar disorder with, 106, 109
    delirium with, 46
    depressive disorders with, 120
    dissociative disorders with, 155
    on mental status examination, 11
    multiple personality with, 154
    organic disorders and, 22
    organic hallucinosis with, 22, 45, 48, 50, 53, 54–55
    psychomotor seizures with, 56
    schizophrenia with, 87, 89, 254, 297
Hallucinogen abuse, 50, 61, 67–68, 73
Hallucinosis
    alcohol, 64
    organic, 22, 45, 48, 50, 53, 54–55
Haloperidol, 284
    bipolar disorder with, 114
    delirium treatment with, 54

dementia treatment with, 54
psychotolysis with, 285
schizophrenia and, 98, 261
substance abuse treatment with, 71, 73
very-high-dose therapy with, 287–288
violent behavior and, 264
Halstead-Reitan neuropsychological test battery (HRB), 22, 23–24
Hamilton Depression Scale, 41
Harrison, R., 21
Headache, 175, 185, 276
Head trauma, 50
Hebephrenic schizophrenia, 96
Hepatitis, 247, 248
Heroin, 65
History taking
    in psychiatric interview, 8–9, 13–14
    sexual, 161–163
Histrionic personality disorder, 189, 191–192
    clinical features of, 191–192, 196, 201
    differential diagnosis of, 192, 195
    dissociative disorders and, 155
    Rorschach techniques in, 20
    treatment of, 203
Homicide, 12, 259
Homosexuality. See also Ego-dystonic homosexuality
    definition of, 168
Hospitalization
    adolescent disorders and, 224, 225, 226–227
    alcohol abuse and, 70–71, 80–81
    anorexia nervosa and, 211
    anxiety disorders with, 147
    bipolar disorder and, 113–114
    depressive disorders with, 129
    schizophrenia and, 99
    suicide risk and, 254, 255, 257
Human leukocyte antigen (HLA), 37
Huntington's chorea, 50, 51, 52–53, 255
Hydrocephalus, normal pressure, 51, 53
6-Hydroxydopamine, 93
5-Hydroxyindoleacetic acid (5-HIAA), 293
Hydroxyzine, 312
Hyperadrenalism, 111, 141, 247
Hyperbaric oxygen, 242
Hyperkinesis, 198
Hypertension, 175, 245, 307
Hyperparathyroidism, 153
Hyperthyroidism, 141, 247
Hypnosis, 156, 267
Hypnotic drug abuse, 59, 61, 64, 65
    anxiety disorders with, 140
    withdrawal from, 249

Hypochondriasis, 151, 152, 195
    as defense mechanism, 201
    DSM-III criteria for, 238
    elderly and, 238–239
    psychological factors in illness and, 180
Hypoglycemia, 141, 247, 262
Hypomania, 301
    bipolar disorder with, 105, 106
    Minnesota Multiphasic Personality Inventory (MMPI) in, 19
    violent behavior and, 259
Hypothalamic-pituitary-adrenal (HPA) axis, 28, 128
Hypothyroidism, 125, 302
Hysteria, 151, 277
Hysterical blindness, 180
Hysterical disorders, 151, 155. See also Dissociative disorder; Somatoform disorder
Hysterical neurosis, conversion style, 151
Hysterical personality disorder. See Histrionic personality disorder
Hysterical psychosis, 97. See also Brief reactive psychosis
Hysteroid dysphoria, 156–157, 203

Iatrogenic disorders, 249
Ideas of reference, on mental status examination, 11
Identical twin studies. See Monozygotic twin studies
Illusion, on mental status examination, 11
Imagery techniques, 183
Iminodibenzyl, 281, 292
Imipramine, 40, 292
    anxiety disorders with, 146, 148–149, 150, 310, 314, 316
    case examples with, 148–149, 150
    depressive disorders and, 128, 240, 293, 294
    dosage for, 317
    plasma level measurements for, 32
    side effects of, 295, 296
Immunologic system, and stress, 180
Incoherence, on mental status examination, 11
Infancy, rumination disorder of, 214–215
Infectious processes, 248
Insanity, legal issues with, 24
Insight, on mental status examination, 13
Intellectual functioning
    dementia and, 46–47
    tests covering, 21–22
Intellectualization, 199, 200
Intelligence, definition of, 17
Intelligence quotient (IQ), 17

Intelligence tests, 15, 16–19
  cultural deprivation and, 18
  definition of intelligence in, 17
  diagnostic applications of, 18
  interpretation of, 17–18
  trends in use of, 16
  Wechsler Adult Intelligence Scale (WAIS) in, 16–17
  Wechsler Intelligence Scale for Children (WISC) in, 17
Interviewing techniques, 3–5
  accuracy empathy in, 4
  closing, 5
  feelings of interviewer in, 5
  politeness and courtesy in, 4–5
  psychiatric evaluation with, 3–5
  psychosexual disorders with, 162–163
  universal statements used in, 4
Intoxication. *See also* Alcohol abuse and alcoholism; Drug abuse
  organic mental disorders with, 45, 48
Introjection, 201
Iprindole, 293
Iproniazid, 281, 305, 315
IQ, 17. *See also* Intelligence tests
Isocarboxazid, 305, 306, 315
Isolation, 200

Jacksonian seizures, 55
Jakob-Creutzfeldt disease, 53
Janet, Pierre, 155
JD virus, 53
Johnson, Vernon E., 80
Johnson, Virginia, 165, 171–172
Jones, Maxwell, 273

Kalucy, R.S., 209, 213
Kaplan, Helen Singer, 167, 172, 173
Kety, S.M., 93
Kierkegaard, C., 33
Kiloh, L.G., 56
Klein, D.F., 123, 137, 293, 314, 316
Kline, N.S., 296
Korsakoff's psychosis, 48, 64, 70. *See also* Amnestic syndrome
Kovacs, M., 129
Kraepelin, Emil, 33, 87, 91, 96, 105, 107
Kuru, 53

La belle indifférence, 180
Lasègue, Ernest C., 207, 208
Latent schizophrenia, 191
L-dopa, 290
Learning, and organic disorders, 21–22
Learning theory, of homosexuality, 169
Legal issues
  insanity definition in, 24
  mental status examination and, 12
  psychometric evaluation and, 24
  violent behavior and, 264
Librium. *See* Chlordiazepoxide (Librium)
Lidz, Theodore, 91
Life change, and stress, 177–183
Lipowski, Z.J., 51, 54
Lishman, W.A., 56
Lithium carbonate, 87, 281, 290, 291, 299–304
  bipolar disorder with, 37, 113, 114–115, 116, 117, 241, 301–302
  case example with, 116, 117
  depressive disorders with, 301–302
  dosage forms of, 300
  early work with, 299
  electroconvulsive therapy (ECT) in, 323
  genetic factors in response to, 37
  maintenance treatment with, 294
  mechanism of action of, 299–300
  pregnancy and, 303
  psychological factors affecting illness and, 182
  schizophrenia and, 97, 291
  side effects of, 302–303
  somatoform and dissociative disorders with, 157
  toxicity with, 303–304
Lorazepam, 309
Loss, and depressive disorders, 126
Lysergic acid diethylamide (LSD), 67, 94

Maas, J.W., 128, 292
Major depressive disorders, 195
  dexamethasone suppression test (DST) in, 28
  differential diagnosis of, 236–237
  DSM-III criteria for, 124
  electroencephalographic (EEG) sleep analysis in, 30
  genetic factors in, 33, 34
  monoamine oxidase (MAO) studies in, 36
  psychobiology in prediction of, 37–38
  psychological markers in, 35–36
  suicide risk and, 254
  thyrotropin-releasing hormone (TRH) stimulation test in, 28, 29, 30
Maletsky, 322
Malingering, 181, 189
Mania and manic disorders
  differential diagnosis in, 49, 50, 247
  early work in, 87
  elderly and, 241
  mental status examination and, 12
  positron emission tomography (PET) in, 38
  schizophrenia variants and, 97
  substance abuse and, 74
  thyrotropin-releasing hormone (TRH) stimulation test in, 29
Manic-depressive disorder. *See* Bipolar disorder (manic-depressive illness)
MAO inhibitors. *See* Monoamine oxidase (MAO) inhibitors
Maprotiline, 293, 307
Marijuana abuse, 59, 61, 68–69
  amotivational syndrome with, 68
  differential diagnosis and, 50, 110
  treatment of, 73
Marital therapy, 129
Marmor, Judd, 168
Marriage
  psychiatric interview information on, 9
  stress and, 177
  suicide risk and status of, 254
Marks, P.S., 18
Marshall, W.K., 315
Masochism, 164
Masters, William, 165, 171–172
Maternity blues, 122
Measles virus, 53
Medical disorders
  DSM-III axis III for, 245
  mental changes caused by, 245–249
  psychiatric manifestations of, 245–250
  signs and symptoms caused by, 246, 249
  suicide risk and, 255
  treatment of, 249–250
Meditation, 183
Megavitamin therapy, 102
Melancholia, 119
  depression with, 124
  electroconvulsive therapy (ECT) in, 323
  DSM-III on, 123, 124
  electroencephalographic (EEG) sleep analysis in, 30
  tricyclic antidepressant drugs in, 32
Memory
  amnestic syndrome and, 47–48
  dementia and, 47
  electroconvulsive therapy (ECT) in, 322–323
  on mental status examination, 12–13
  organic disorders and, 21–22
  psychogenic amnesia and, 153
Mental retardation
  adolescent disorders and, 230
  differential diagnosis with, 193
  psychometric issues in, 24

use of term, 24
violent behavior and, 262
Mental status examination, 9–13
  adolescent disorders with, 223
  assessment areas in, 10
  attitude noted in, 10
  cognitive functioning in, 12–13
  general appearance noted in, 10
  insight about self on, in, 13
  mood and affect in, 12
  motor behavior noted in, 10
  perception noted in, 11
  psychiatric interview with, 9–13
  purpose of, 10
  sensorium and orientation in, 12
  speech noted in, 10
  thoughts noted in, 10–11
Meperidine, 65
Meprobamate, 65, 242, 308, 309, 312
Mescaline, 68, 94
Messina, J.A., 152
Metabolic disorders, 247–248, 262
Methadone, 72
Methaqualone, 65, 242
3-Methoxy,4-hydroxyphenyglycol (MHPG), 292–293
Methyldopa, 50
Methylphenidate, 226, 241, 261, 318
Methyprylon, 312
Methysergide maleate, 185
Meyer, Adolph, 91
Meyerowitz, S., 152
Meyerson, A.T., 153
Mianserin, 293, 307
Michigan Alcoholism Screening Test, 77, 78, 84–86
Migraine, 175, 185, 209, 276
Milieu therapy, 202, 273–274
  definition of, 273
  processes in, 273–274
Minnesota Multiphasic Personality Inventory (MMPI), 18–19, 23
  interpretation of, 18–19
  psychotic tetrad on, 19
  validity scales for, 19
Minority groups
  intelligence tests and, 18
  violent behavior and, 260
Minuchin, S., 179, 211, 213
Mitral valve prolapse syndrome (MVPS), 141
Mixed state in bipolar disorders, 107
Modeling, 314
Molindone, 283
Monoamine oxidase (MAO)
  genetic marker studies of, 36–37
  schizophrenia and, 94
Monoamine oxidase (MAO) inhibitors, 281, 305–307
  anxiety disorders with, 314–315, 316–317
  classification of, 305

clinical uses of, 203, 241, 306, 310
  indications for, 305–306
  platelet levels with, 306–307
  psychological factors affecting illness and, 182
  side effects of, 307
  tricyclic antidepressants with, 296
Money, John, 163, 169
Monozygotic twin studies
  anxiety disorders in, 143
  bipolar disorder in, 112
  drug plasma levels in, 318
  homosexuality and, 168
  psychobiologic evaluation with, 34, 35, 38
  schizophrenia in, 93
Mood, on mental status examination, 12
Mood disorders, 108. See also Affective disorders
Morphine, 66
Morton, R., 207, 215
Motor behavior, on mental status examination, 10
Mourning, 126, 234
Movement disorders, 231–232
Multiinfarct dementia, 52
Multiple personality, 151, 153, 154
Multiple sclerosis, 51, 53, 153
Münchausen syndrome, 180–181
Murder, 259
Murphy, G.E., 115, 122
Muscle relaxation, 182, 275
Mutism, 231, 248

Naloxone, 94, 291
Narcissistic defenses, in adolescence, 218–220
Narcissistic personality disorder, 189, 192–193, 198
  clinical features of, 192
  differential diagnosis of, 192–193, 195
  treatment of, 203
Narcotics Anonymous, 80, 81, 82
Negative practice, 276–277
Nervous system, and stress, 179
Neurodermatitis, 175
Neuroendocrine system
  depression and, 27
  stress and, 179–180
Neuroleptic drugs. See also Antipsychotic drugs
  anxiety disorders with, 146
  bipolar disorder and, 114
  delirium treatment with, 54
  dementia treatment with, 54–55
  paranoid disorders with, 103, 203, 238
  plasma levels of, 288
  schizophrenia with, 98–99, 100, 288

schizophreniform disorder with, 102
schizotypal personality disorder with, 203
substance abuse treatment with, 71, 72, 73
Neurologic disorders, 9
Neuropsychology, 21
Neurosyphilis, 248
Neurotic disorders in adolescence, 229
Neurotransmitters
  affective disorders and, 27, 292
  bipolar disorder and, 112
  depressive disorders with, 127–128
  electroconvulsive therapy (ECT) in, 322
  schizophrenia and, 93–94
  stress and, 179
Nicotinic acid therapy, 102, 248
Nitroglycerine, 295–296
Nomifensine, 307
Norepinephrine, 298–299
  anxiety disorders with, 143
  depressive disorders with, 127, 128, 292
  electroconvulsive therapy (ECT) in, 322
  lithium and, 300
  schizophrenia and, 94
  stress and, 179
Nortriptyline
  depressive disorders with, 128, 240
  dosage for, 317
  plasma level measurements for, 32–33, 318
  side effects of, 295
Nursing care for elderly, 243

Obesity, 181, 277
Object relations
  aggressive behavior and, 262
  schizophrenia and, 91
Obsessive compulsive disorder, 138–139, 277
  compulsion in, 138
  course and prognosis of, 143
  depressive disorders with, 125
  DSM-III criteria for, 139
  family of, 143
  onset of, 134, 135
Obsessive thinking
  anorexia nervosa and, 209
  on mental status examination, 11
Obstructive pulmonary disease, chronic, 246–247
Occupational status, and suicide risk, 254
Omnipotent defenses, in adolescence, 218–220
Opioid abuse, 59, 61, 65–66, 72
Opioid compounds in schizophrenia, 291

Index

Oppositional disorder, 231
Organic affective syndrome, 45, 48, 50, 55, 68
Organic brain syndromes, 45–50. *See also* Delirium; Dementia
  atypical or mixed, 45, 49
  case example of, 58
  categories of, 45
  differential diagnosis in, 49–50, 140
  DSM-III definitions in, 45, 46, 47, 48, 49
  functional disorders presenting as, 49–50
  intelligence tests and, 18
  management and treatment of, 53–55
  organic affective syndrome in, 48
  organic hallucinosis in, 48
  organic personality syndrome in, 48–49
  presenting as functional disorders, 50
  seizure disorders and, 55–57
Organic delusional syndrome, 45, 48, 50, 53, 54–55, 68
Organic hallucinosis, 45, 48, 50, 53, 54–55
Organic mental disorders, 45–58. *See also specific disorders and syndromes*
  Bender Visual Motor Gestalt Test for, 22–23
  case example of, 58
  differential diagnosis of, 236–237
  elderly and, 235–237
  Halstead-Reitan neuropsychological test battery (HRB) in, 23–24
  management and treatment of, 53–55
  seizure disorders and, 55–57
  Standardized Luria-Nebraska Battery (SLNB) in, 23–24
  suicide risk and, 255
  tests for diagnosis of, 21–24
Organic personality syndrome, 45, 48–49, 50, 53
  clinical picture in, 49
  DSM-III criteria for, 48
  management and treatment of, 55
Orgasm dysfunction, 165
  DSM-III criteria for, 166, 167
  etiology of, 167–168
  treatment of, 171–173
Orientation, on mental status examination, 12
Oxaprotiline, 307
Oxazepam, 70, 242, 309, 311
Oxazolidines, 56
Oxycodone, 65
Oxypertine, 283

Pain, 181; *See also* Psychogenic pain disorder
Palazzoli, M.S., 210
Panencephalitis, 53
Panic disorder, 137, 138
  agoraphobia and, 136, 142
  DSM-III criteria for, 138
  onset of, 134
  somatoform disorders with, 153
  treatment of, 146, 277, 314
Paranoid disorders, 102–103
  amphetamine abuse and, 66–67, 72
  bipolar disorder with, 105, 109
  course and prognosis for, 103
  differential diagnosis in, 50, 103, 190, 237, 238
  DSM-III on, 87–88, 102–103
  elderly and, 237–238, 241
  medical disorders and, 247, 248
  on mental status examination, 11
  Minnesota Multiphasic Personality Inventory (MMPI) in, 19
  treatment of, 103, 238
  types of, 102–103
Paranoid personality disorder, 188, 189, 190
  clinical features of, 190, 198
  differential diagnosis of, 190, 195
  DSM-III on, 189, 190
  treatment of, 202–203
Paranoid schizophrenia, 96, 97, 100
  amphetamine abuse in, 67
  bipolar disorder differentiated from, 109–110
  differential diagnosis of, 190
Paraphilia, 163, 164
  DSM-III classification of, 164
  treatment of, 170–171
Paraphrenia, 238
Parathyroid gland disorders, 125, 247
Parents. *See* Family
Pargyline, 305
Passive aggression (defense mechanism), 201
Passive-aggressive personality disorder, 190, 196
  clinical features of, 196
  differential diagnosis of, 196
  treatment of, 205
Paykel, E.S., 305
Pedophilia, 164, 170, 171
Penfluridol, 287
Pentazocine, 65, 72
Pentobarbital (Nembutal), 71
Peptic ulcer, 175, 183, 247
Perception, on mental status examination, 11
Percodan, 65
Performance ability, on intelligence tests, 17

Personality disorders, 187–205
  atypical, 190, 196
  classification of, 188–189
  clusters in, 189–190
  concept of, 187–189
  decision tree for, 196, 197
  definition of, 187–188
  depersonalization disorder with, 154
  DSM-III categories of, 187–188, 189, 190, 191, 192, 193, 194, 195, 196, 198
  ego defenses and, 199–201
  environmental and developmental factors in, 198–199
  etiology of, 196–199
  features of, 188
  genetic factors in, 198
  medical disorders and, 247, 248
  psychopathology and, 189
  specific disorders in, 189–199
  treatment of, 201–205, 263, 271
  violent disorders and, 260, 263
Personality types
  anxiety disorders and, 142
  depressive disorders with, 121, 125, 127
  organic disorders and, 22
  psychosomatic illnesses and, 176
  seizure disorders and, 57
Personality theory, and psychological tests, 15
Petit mal epilepsy, 53, 56
Phencyclidine (PCP), 61, 67, 68
  differential diagnosis with, 50, 67
  treatment of withdrawal from, 73
  violent behavior and, 261
Phenelzine, 146, 241, 305, 306, 314, 315
Phenobarbital, 71
Phenothiazines, 283, 294, 295
  dissociative disorders and, 155
  dopamine and, 283
  long-acting, 287
  phobic anxiety states with, 314
  schizophrenia with, 99, 287
  side effects of, 290, 298
  substance abuse treatment with, 72
Phenoxypropazine, 315
Phentolamine, 291, 307
Phenytoin, 71, 72
Phobic disorders, 135–137
  adolescent, 229
  anorexia nervosa and, 209
  DSM-III classification of, 135, 136, 137
  epidemiology of, 134
  on mental status examination, 11
  onset of, 134
  simple, 136–137
  social, 136–137

substance abuse and, 74
  treatment of, 275, 277, 314–318
Physical examination, in psychiatric interview, 13–14
Physostigmine, 298
Pica, 214, 231
Pick's disease, 52, 236
Pipothiazine palmitate, 287
Pituitary gland disorders, 50, 125
Placebo therapy, 181
Porphyria, 153, 247–248
Positron emission tomography (PET), 38
Postpartum period, and depressive disorders, 122
Post-psychotic depression, 99–100
Posttraumatic stress disorder, 135, 139
  course and prognosis for, 143
  DSM-III criteria for, 139
Practolol, 313
Prazepam, 309
Pregnancy
  depressive disorders after, 122
  drug therapy and, 290, 297, 303
Premature ejaculation
  DSM-III criteria for, 166, 167
  treatment of, 171, 172, 275
Premenstrual tension, 262, 302
Preventive psychiatry, and psychobiology, 37–39
Procaine, 242
Prochlorperazine, 284
Projection, 201
Projective tests, 15, 19–21
  mental retardation on, 24
  Rorschach technique in, 19–21
  sentence completion tests, 21
  Thematic Apperception Test (TAT), 21
Promazine, 72
Promethazine, 312
Propranolol, 73, 125, 291, 312–313
  mechanism of action of, 313, 316–317
  side effects of, 313
Propoxyphene, 65
Prostaglandins, and schizophrenia, 94
Protriptyline, 32, 240
Pseudodementia
  differential diagnosis of, 49, 236–237
  treatment of, 240
Psilocybin, 67
Psychiatric evaluation, 3–14
  accurate empathy in, 4
  case example of, 7–8
  chief complaints in, 6
  collation of data about present illness in, 7–8
  course of present illness in, 7

data gathering in, 3
developmental and family history in, 8–9
diagnostic formulation in, 14
doctor-patient relationship in, 3–5
effect of present illness in, 7
geriatric disorders and, 239
identifying data in, 6
interviewing techniques in, 3–5
mental status examination in, 9–13
onset of present illness in, 6–7
organization of, 6
past psychiatric and medical history in, 8
politeness and courtesy in, 4–5
precipitants of present illness in, 7
present illness information in, 6–7
sources used in, 3
treatment recommendations in, 14
universal statements used in, 4
Psychoanalysis, 158, 270–271
  borderline personality disorder and, 204
  compulsive personality disorder and, 205
  psychological factors affecting illness and, 182
  sexual development in, 167–168
Psychoasthenia, 19
Psychobiologic evaluation, 27–41. See also specific tests
  case example of, 39–41
  clinical assessment and, 27–31
  family predisposition and, 33–39
  genetic counseling and, 38–39
  geriatric disorders and, 239
  preventive psychiatry and, 37–39
  psychiatric genetics and, 33–35, 38–39
  psychological markers of vulnerability in, 35–37
  treatment issues and, 31–33
Psychogenic amnesia, 153
Psychogenic fugue, 153, 154
Psychogenic pain disorder, 151, 152, 180
Psychological factors affecting physical condition (PFAPC), 175–185
  case examples of, 183–185
  diagnosis of, 175
  differential diagnosis in, 180–181
  DSM-III criteria for, 175, 177, 180
  giving up/given up syndrome in, 178, 180, 181
  seven classic illnesses in, 175, 181
  stress and life change and, 177–183
  theories about, 176–177
  treatment of, 180–183
Psychological factors in depressive disorders, 126–127

Psychological factors in suicide risk, 255–256
Psychological factors in violent behavior, 262–263
Psychological tests, 15–16
  adolescent disorders with, 223–224
  advantages and disadvantages of, 16
  background to derivation of, 15
  elderly and, 24
  intelligence, see Intelligence testing
  predictive value of, 15–16
  psychiatric interview with, 14
  purposes of, 15–16
  reliability of, 15
  validity of, 15–16
Psychological therapies, 267–280. See also specific therapies
  basic concepts in, 267–268
  indications for, 279–280
  referrals for, 279
Psychometric evaluation, 15–25. See also Intelligence tests; Psychological tests
  elderly and, 24
  legal issues in, 24–25
  mental retardation in, 23
  organic disorders with, 21–23
  projective techniques in, 19–21
Psychomotor changes, in depression, 120
Psychomotor seizures, 56–57
  diagnosis of, 56–57
  management of, 57
Psychopharmacology, 281–318. See also specific drugs
  affective disorders in, 291–308
  anxiety disorders in, 308–318
  drug interactions in, 290–291, 295–296
  patient's understanding of, 281
  psychotic disorders in, 282–291
Psychosexual disorders, 161–173
  classification and diagnosis of, 163–169
  DSM-III on, 161, 163, 164
  etiology of, 167–168
  gender identity disorders in, 163–164
  interview in, 162–163
  paraphilia in, 164
  psychosexual dysfunction in, 164–168
  sexual history in, 161–163
  treatment of, 169–173, 276
Psychosexual dysfunction, 163, 164–168
  DSM-III criteria for, 166, 167
  etiology of, 167–168
  phases of sexual response and, 165–166

Psychosis and psychotic disorders
  atypical, 88
  depersonalization disorder with, 154
  differential diagnosis in, 49, 155
  drug management of, 282–291
  DSM-III categories for, 87
  elderly and, 237, 241–242
  medical disorders and, 247, 248
  Minnesota Multiphasic Personality Inventory (MMPI) in, 19
  psychobiology in prediction of, 38
  substance abuse and, 66–67, 73, 110, 261
Psychosocial factors, in twin (genetics) studies, 34
Psychosomatic illnesses. *See also* Psychological factors affecting physical condition (PFAPC)
Psychotherapy, 269–270
  adolescent disorders in, 220, 225, 227
  antisocial personality disorder in, 203–204
  anxiety disorders with, 146–147
  approaches used in, 268–269
  basic concepts in, 267–268
  behavior therapy and, 278
  borderline personality disorder and, 204
  compulsive personality disorder and, 205
  dependent personality disorder and, 204–205
  depressive disorders and, 128–129
  ego-dystonic homosexuality and, 173
  genetic counseling in, 38
  geriatric disorders and, 242–243
  histrionic personality disorder and, 203
  medical background of therapist, 270
  narcissistic personality disorder and, 203
  paranoid personality disorder and, 202–203
  passive-aggressive personality disorder and, 205
  patient's role in, 270
  personality disorders and, 201–202
  psychological factors affecting illness and, 182
  psychosexual disorders with, 171, 172–173
  schizophrenia and, 100–101
  somatoform and dissociative disorders and, 156
  therapist's role in, 278
  violent behavior and, 263

Psychotolysis, 285
Pulmonary disorders, 246–247

Quitkin, F., 305

Rape, 259
Rapid-eye-movement (REM) sleep, 30–31, 180
Raskin, M., 153
Rauwolfia alkaloids, 283
Reaction formation, 200
Referrals 79, 279
Regression (defense mechanism), 201
Reichmann, Frieda Fromm, 91
Relationship-oriented therapy, 269
Relaxation techniques, 182, 275
Reliability of psychological tests, 15
Religious fixation, 11
Repetitive ideas, on mental status examination, 11
Repression, 267
  as defense mechanism, 200, 201
  somatoform disorders and, 151, 155, 156
Reserpine, 50, 115, 249, 283, 289
Residential treatment
  adolescent disorders in, 227
  geriatric disorders in, 243–244
Residual schizophrenia, 97
Resistance in therapy, 268
Retirement, 177, 234, 240
Rheumatoid arthritis, 175, 180, 249
Rohde Sentence Completion Method, 21
Rorschach, Hermann, 19–20
Rorschach techniques, 19–21
  criticisms of, 20–21
  development of, 19–20
  diagnostic value of, 20, 24
  scoring criteria in, 20
Roth, M., 137
Rotter Incomplete Sentence Blank, 21
Rubella panencephalitis, 53
Rumination disorder of infancy, 214–215

Sadism, 164
Scatter concept, in intelligence testing, 17
Schildkraut, J.J., 128, 292
Schizoaffective disorder, 97
  bipolar disorder differentiated from, 110
  genetic factors in, 33
  lithium in, 291, 299, 302
Schizoaffective psychosis, acute, 97
Schizoid personality disorder, 189, 190–191
  adolescent, 231
  clinical features of, 190, 198

  differential diagnosis of, 190–191, 194, 195
  fantasy used by, 200
  treatment of, 203
Schizophrenia, 87–104
  acute phase, 89, 90, 98–99
  adolescent, 226, 228, 229
  antipsychotic drugs in, 36
  biologic theories of, 92–94
  bipolar disorder and, 97, 108, 109–110
  brain abnormalities and, 94
  case examples of, 103–104
  catatonic, 96–97
  categories of, 87
  complications with, 90
  course of, 89–90
  depression associated with, 125
  dexamethasone suppression test (DST) in, 28
  differential diagnosis of, 49, 50, 191, 193
  disorganized, 96
  drug management of, 282, 297–298
  DSM-III criteria for, 87, 90, 95, 96, 97
  early work with, 87, 105
  elderly and, 237–238, 239, 241
  electroconvulsive therapy (ECT) in, 321
  electroencephalographic (EEG) sleep analysis in, 30
  epidemiology of, 89–90
  etiology of, 91–94
  family and, 101–102
  genetic factors in, 33, 34, 35, 38–39, 92–93, 198
  intelligence testing and, 18
  lithium in, 97, 291, 302
  maintenance treatment in, 285–288
  medical disorders and, 247, 248, 249
  Minnesota Multiphasic Personality Inventory (MMPI) in, 19
  monoamine oxidase (MAO) studies in, 36
  neurotransmitters and, 93–94, 283
  noncompliance with medication in, 286–287
  onset of, 89–90
  organic disorders and, 22
  positron emission tomography (PET) in, 38
  post-psychotic depression in, 99–100
  praecox feeling in, 89
  psychobiology in prediction of, 37–38
  psychological markers in, 35, 36
  psychosocial theories of, 91–92
  recovery phase in, 99–100

residual phase of, 100–101
Rorschach techniques in, 20
signs and symptoms in, 88–89
social class and, 89
somatoform disorders with, 153
substance abuse and, 67, 74
subtypes of, 96–97
suicide risk and, 254
thyrotropin-releasing hormone (TRH) stimulation test in, 29
treatment of, 98–102, 275
undifferentiated, 96, 97
very-high-dose therapy in, 287–288
violent behavior and, 260–261
viruses and, 94
visual average evoked response (AER) studies in, 31
Schizophreniform disorder, 27, 97
differential diagnosis in, 50
genetic factors in, 35
substance abuse patterns and, 68
thyrotropin-releasing hormone (TRH) stimulation test in, 29
treatment of, 102
Schizophreniform psychosis, 87, 247, 248
Schizotypal personality disorder, 188, 189, 191
clinical features of, 191, 198
differential diagnosis of, 191, 195
treatment of, 203
School problems, 8, 9
Secobarbital, 312
Sedative drug abuse, 59, 61, 64, 65, 71–72
Seeman, W., 18
Seizure disorders, 51, 55–57. *See also* Epilepsy
alcohol abuse and, 63, 71
barbiturate abuse and, 72
causes of, 55–56
depersonalization disorder with, 154
diagnosis of, 56–57
differential diagnosis with, 50
management of, 57
psychiatric complications of, 57
psychiatric interview on, 9
Self-esteem
in adolescence, 219
narcissistic personality disorder with, 192
suicide risk and, 255
violent behavior and, 262, 263
Self-help programs
bulimia and, 214
substance abuse and, 82
Seligman, M.E.P., 127
Selye, Hans, 177
Sensitivity training, 272

Sensorium, on mental status examination, 12
Sentence completion tests, 19, 21
Separation anxiety
adolescent disorders and, 231
anxiety disorders and, 144
psychiatric interview information on, 8–9
Serotonin
bipolar disorder and, 112
depressive disorders with, 127, 128, 292
electroconvulsive therapy (ECT) in, 322
mood disorders and, 27
stress and, 179
Sex differences, and suicide, 254
Sex offenders, treatment of, 170–171
Sex reassignment surgery, 164, 169–170
Sexual activity, and aging process, 234
Sexual development, on psychiatric interview, 9
Sexual dysfunction, 247. *See also* Psychosexual disorders
Shields, J., 93
Shopsin, B., 296
Sifneos, P., 178
Simple phobia, 135, 136–137
Simple schizophrenia, 96, 191
Slater, E., 152
Sleep patterns, 249
depression and, 119–120, 180
elderly and, 242
electroencephalographic (EEG) analysis of, 30–31, 124
Snyder, S.A., 283
Social class, and schizophrenia, 89, 92
Social history, in adolescent disorders, 222
Socialization disorders, 229
Social learning theory, 199
Social phobia, 134, 135, 136
DSM-III criteria for, 136
treatment of, 314
Sociocultural assessment in geriatric disorders, 239–240
Somatic delusions, on mental status examination, 11
Somatic therapy, in depressive disorders, 128
Somatization disorder, 151
Somatoform disorders, 151–153, 175
atypical, 151, 152
case examples of, 157–158
clinical features of, 151
cognitive style and, 156
differential diagnosis of, 152–153, 192
DSM-III on, 151
early work in, 155

etiology of, 155–156
psychiatric disorders associated with, 153
specific syndromes in, 151–152
treatment of, 156–157, 271
Sours, J.A., 207, 210
Speech, mental status examination of, 10
Splitting, 200
Standardized Luria-Nebraska Battery (SLNB), 23–24
Stanford-Binet intelligence test, 16, 17
Stefansson, J.G., 152
Stein, M., 177, 180
Steinberg, H., 279
Steroid drugs, 110, 111, 125, 247
Strauss, J.S., 90
Stress
anxiety disorders and, 144
autoregulatory techniques with, 182–183
biologic rhythms and, 180
bipolar disorder and, 113
brain and body reactions to, 179–180
dissociative states and, 156
illness and, 177–183
multiple personality and, 154
psychological defenses and, 177–179
treatment of disorders with, 180–183
Stuttering, 277
Sublimation, 201
Substance use disorders, 59–86. *See also* Alcohol abuse and alcoholism; Drug abuse; *specific substances*
addiction and, 60
adolescent, 229
aftercare in, 82
antisocial personality disorder and, 193
anxiety disorders and, 140, 142, 147
case examples of, 83–84
clarification of problems by patient, 81–82
classes of substances in, 59, 60–61
concept of dependence and, 60
confrontation in, 78–79
cross-dependence in, 60
denial in, 78–79
depressive disorders with, 125–126
diagnosis of, 77–83
differential diagnosis of, 50, 73–74
engaging patient in treatment in, 79–80
etiology of, 74–75
family illness and, 82–83
hospitalization in, 80–81

Substance use disorders (*continued*)
  medical descriptive model in, 60–76
  mixed patterns in, 69
  organic mental disorders with, 45, 48
  patient reaction to, 78
  physician in treatment of, 75
  recovery in, 82
  referral or consultation in, 79
  rehabilitative model of treatment in, 77–83
  selection of treatment setting in, 80
  suicide risk and, 255
  tolerance in, 60
  treatment of, 69–73, 74, 75–76, 311
  withdrawal syndromes in, 60
Succinimides, 56
Suicide risk, 253–258
  adolescent disorders and, 227, 248
  age and, 248
  antisocial personality disorder and, 193
  bipolar disorder and, 112
  case examples of, 257–258
  clinical conditions predisposing to, 254–255
  crisis intervention in, 256, 274
  demographic factors in, 248
  depression and, 120, 121, 122, 128, 129
  drug overdose and, 298
  epidemiology of, 253–254
  evaluation of, 255–256
  hospitalization for, 257
  management of, 256–257
  mental status examination and, 12
  rate and incidence of, 253
  schizophrenia and, 90
  somatization disorder with, 151
  substance abuse treatment and, 72
Sullivan, Harry Stack, 91
Sulpiride, 291
Sundberg, N.D., 16
Surgery, psychiatric effects of, 249
Systematic desensitization, 275
  anxiety disorders with, 147, 314
  psychosexual disorders with, 171
Systemic lupus erythematosus, 153, 249

Talbott, J.A., 153
Tardive dyskinesia, 286, 288–289
Temazepam, 242, 309
Temporal lobe epilepsy, 50, 55, 56, 154, 248
Tension headache, 175, 185, 276
Testosterone, 168
Tests. *See also* Psychological tests
  substance abuse diagnosis with, 77–78

Thematic Apperception Test (TAT), 19, 21, 24
  interpretation of, 21
  validity of, 21
Therapy. *See* Psychotherapy; Treatment
Thiamine deficiency, 53, 64, 70, 248
Thioridazine, 149–150, 284
  dementia treatment with, 54
  side effects of, 290
Thioxanthene derivatives, 155, 283
Thought broadcasting, 11
Thought insertion, 11
Thoughts, on mental status examination, 10–11
Thought withdrawal, 11
Thyroid gland disorders, 50, 125, 180
Thyroid-stimulating hormone (TSH), 29–30, 33, 40, 124
Thyrotoxicosis, 175
Thyrotropin-releasing hormone (TRH) stimulation test, 28–30
  clinical uses of, 28–29, 30, 40, 124
  procedure in, 29–30, 33
Tobacco dependence, 61, 69
Token economies, 202, 275
Tolerance, in substance abuse, 60
Tranquilizers. *See* Antipsychotic drugs
Transference, 267–268
Transference neurosis, 203
Transference psychosis, 203
Transsexualism
  DSM-III criteria in, 164
  sex reassignment surgery in, 164, 169–170
  treatment of, 169–170
Transvestism, 164, 277
Tranylcypromine, 241, 306, 314
Trazodone, 293, 307
Treatment, 251–323. *See also specific treatment modalities*
  psychiatric interview and recommendations for, 14
  psychological tests and, 15
TRH. *See* Thyrotropin-releasing hormone (THR) stimulation test
Tricyclic antidepressant drugs, 292–299
  acute anticholinergic syndrome with, 298
  anxiety disorders with, 146, 314, 315–317
  depression and, 37
  dosage level studies in, 32
  drug interactions with, 295–296
  geriatric disorders with, 240–241
  maintenance treatment with, 294–295
  mode of action of, 292–293, 316–317

  overdose with, 298–299
  plasma level measurements for, 32–33, 318
  predictors of response to, 293–294
  psychological factors affecting illness and, 182
  side effects of, 295–297
Trifluoperazine, 237
Trimipramine, 307
Twilight states, 56
Twin studies
  anxiety disorders in, 143
  bipolar disorder in, 112
  drug plasma levels in, 318
  homosexuality and, 168
  psychobiologic evaluation with, 34, 35, 38
  schizophrenia in, 93
Tyler, L.A., 16
Tylenol (acetaminophen), 65
Type A personality, 176, 181
Tyrer, P., 306

Ulcerative colitis, 175, 180, 184, 247
Uncomplicated bereavement, 124
Unconscious
  definition of, 267
  psychological therapies and, 267
  somatoform disorders and, 155
Undifferentiated schizophrenia, 96, 97
Undoing (defense mechanism), 200
Unipolar affective disorder
  adolescent, 229
  bipolar disorder differentiated from, 110
  definition of, 105
  genetic factors in, 34
  lithium in, 301–302
  maintenance treatment of, 294
  personality patterns in, 121
  use of term, 105, 123
Universal statements in interviews, 4
Uric acid, and stress, 177–178

Validity of psychological tests, 15–16, 19
Valium. *See* Diazepam (Valium)
Verbal ability, on intelligence tests, 17
Violent behavior, 259–265
  alcohol abuse and, 261
  case examples of, 264–265
  classification of, 260–262
  dangerousness concept and, 264
  drug abuse and, 261–262
  epilepsy and, 261
  epidemiology of, 259
  etiology of, 262–263
  family members and, 259
  general patterns of, 259
  management of, 263–264
  neurologic disorders and, 261

psychiatric conditions leading to, 260–261
social and professional responsibilities with, 264
toxic and organic conditions and, 261–262
Viruses
  dementia and, 53
  schizophrenia and, 94
Visual average evoked response (AER) studies, 31
Vitamin deficiencies, 53, 248

Wechsler, D., 17
Wechsler Adult Intelligence Scale (WAIS), 16–17, 20
  definition of intelligence in, 17
  interpretation of, 17–18
  mental retardation on, 24
  organic disorders and, 22, 23
  performance subtests in, 17
  scatter concept in, 17
  verbal subtests in, 17
Wechsler-Bellevue Scale, 16
Wechsler Intelligence Scale for Children (WISC), 16, 17
Weiner, H., 180, 181
Weissman, M.M., 122, 126
Wells, C.E., 51
Wender, P.H., 35
Wernicke-Korsakoff disorder, 64
Wernicke's encephalopathy, 70, 248
Wide Range Achievement Tests, 24

Wilson's disease, 52, 247
Winokur, G., 122, 127
Withdrawal, 60. *See also* Alcoholism and alcohol abuse; Drug abuse
  anxiety disorders with, 140
  organic mental disorders with, 45, 48
Women, and geriatric disorders, 234–235
Wooley, C.F., 141

Yalom, I.D., 272
Yoga, 183

Zimelidine, 293, 307
Zimmerman, I.L., 17